DERMOSCOPY
in Darker Skin

DERMOSCOPY in Darker Skin

Editors-in-Chief

Manas Chatterjee MD DNB (DVL)
Senior Adviser, Professor and Head
Department of Dermatology
INHS Asvini
Mumbai, Maharashtra, India

Shekhar Neema MD (Dermatology)
Assistant Professor
Department of Dermatology
Command Hospital
Kolkata, West Bengal, India

Subrata Malakar MD (Dermatology)
Director
Rita Skin Foundation
Kolkata, West Bengal, India

Assistant Editors

Biju Vasudevan MD (Dermatology)
Associate Professor
Department of Dermatology
Base Hospital
Barrackpore, West Bengal, India

Disha Dabbas MD (Dermatology)
Department of Dermatology
Military Hospital
Meerut, Uttar Pradesh, India

Foreword
Thomas Ruzicka

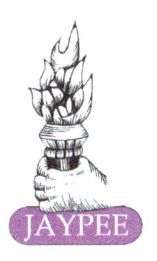

JAYPEE *The Health Sciences Publisher*
New Delhi | London | Panama

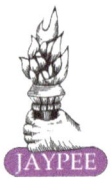

Jaypee Brothers Medical Publishers (P) Ltd

Headquarters

Jaypee Brothers Medical Publishers (P) Ltd
4838/24, Ansari Road, Daryaganj
New Delhi 110 002, India
Phone: +91-11-43574357
Fax: +91-11-43574314
Email: jaypee@jaypeebrothers.com

Overseas Offices

J.P. Medical Ltd
83 Victoria Street, London
SW1H 0HW (UK)
Phone: +44 20 3170 8910
Fax: +44 (0)20 3008 6180
Email: info@jpmedpub.com

Jaypee-Highlights Medical Publishers Inc
City of Knowledge, Bld. 235, 2nd Floor, Clayton
Panama City, Panama
Phone: +1 507-301-0496
Fax: +1 507-301-0499
Email: cservice@jphmedical.com

Jaypee Brothers Medical Publishers (P) Ltd
17/1-B Babar Road, Block-B, Shaymali
Mohammadpur, Dhaka-1207
Bangladesh
Mobile: +08801912003485
Email: jaypeedhaka@gmail.com

Jaypee Brothers Medical Publishers (P) Ltd
Bhotahity, Kathmandu
Nepal
Phone: +977-9741283608
Email: kathmandu@jaypeebrothers.com

Website: www.jaypeebrothers.com
Website: www.jaypeedigital.com

© 2017, Jaypee Brothers Medical Publishers

The views and opinions expressed in this book are solely those of the original contributor(s)/author(s) and do not necessarily represent those of editor(s) of the book.

All rights reserved. No part of this publication may be reproduced, stored or transmitted in any form or by any means, electronic, mechanical, photocopying, recording or otherwise, without the prior permission in writing of the publishers.

All brand names and product names used in this book are trade names, service marks, trademarks or registered trademarks of their respective owners. The publisher is not associated with any product or vendor mentioned in this book.

Medical knowledge and practice change constantly. This book is designed to provide accurate, authoritative information about the subject matter in question. However, readers are advised to check the most current information available on procedures included and check information from the manufacturer of each product to be administered, to verify the recommended dose, formula, method and duration of administration, adverse effects and contraindications. It is the responsibility of the practitioner to take all appropriate safety precautions. Neither the publisher nor the author(s)/editor(s) assume any liability for any injury and/or damage to persons or property arising from or related to use of material in this book.

This book is sold on the understanding that the publisher is not engaged in providing professional medical services. If such advice or services are required, the services of a competent medical professional should be sought.

Every effort has been made where necessary to contact holders of copyright to obtain permission to reproduce copyright material. If any have been inadvertently overlooked, the publisher will be pleased to make the necessary arrangements at the first opportunity.

Inquiries for bulk sales may be solicited at: jaypee@jaypeebrothers.com

Dermoscopy in Darker Skin

First Edition: **2017**

ISBN 978-93-86322-67-8

Dedicated to

My family, especially Dr Mrs Vibhu Chatterjee, my wife and Dr Miss Puja Chatterjee, my daughter as well as my parents, without whose support nothing in my life is ever possible
Manas Chatterjee

*My parents—Late Shri Krishnadasji Neema and Mrs Pushpa Neema,
for their unconditional love and support
My teachers—for being my inspiration
My wife Sweta and my children Advait and Avantika—my source of joy*
Shekhar Neema

*My late parents, to my late wife Dr Rita Shah Malakar and my son Surit Malakar
who constantly encourages me, for doing innovative things*
Subrata Malakar

Contributors

Balachandran S Ankad MD
Professor and Head
Department of Dermatology
SN Medical College
Bagalkot, Karnataka, India

Barnali Chowdhury MD
Consultant Dermatologist
Rita Skin Foundation
Kolkata, West Bengal, India

Biju Vasudevan MD (Dermatology)
Associate Professor
Department of Dermatology
Base Hospital
Barrackpore, West Bengal, India

BS Chandrashekar MD (Dermatology) DNB
Chief Dermatologist
Cutis Academy of Cutaneous Sciences
Bengaluru, Karnataka, India

Biswanath Behera MD
Senior Resident
Department of Dermatology
Jawaharlal Institute of Postgraduate
Medical Education and Research
Puducherry, India

Disha Dabbas MD (Dermatology)
Department of Dermatology
Military Hospital
Meerut, Uttar Pradesh, India

Laxmisha Chandrashekar MD
Additional Professor
Department of Dermatology
Jawaharlal Institute of Postgraduate
Medical Education and Research
Puducherry, India

Manas Chatterjee MD (Dermatology) DNB
Senior Adviser, Professor and Head
Department of Dermatology
INHS Asvini
Mumbai, Maharashtra, India

Nilendu Sarma MD FAAD
Associate Professor and Head
Department of Dermatology
Dr BC Roy Post Graduate Institute of Pediatric Sciences
Kolkata, West Bengal, India

Nirmal B MD
Assistant Professor
Department of Dermatology
Christian Medical College
Vellore, Tamil Nadu, India

Niti Khunger MD DDV DNB
Professor and Consultant Dermatologist
VM Medical College and Safdarjang Hospital
New Delhi, India

Protibha Pradhan DNB
Consultant Dermatologist
Rita Skin Foundation
Kolkata, West Bengal, India

Purva Mehta DNB
Consultant Dermatologist
Rita Skin Foundation
Kolkata, West Bengal, India

Rahul Arora MBBS MD DNB
Consultant Dermatologist
Arora Nursing Home
Shalimar Bagh, New Delhi, India

Samipa S Mukherjee DDV DDVL FRGUHS (Ped Dermatology)
Dermato-trichologist and Pediatric Dermatologist
Cutis Academy of Cutaneous Sciences
Bengaluru, Karnataka, India

Shekhar Neema MD (Dermatology)
Assistant Professor
Department of Dermatology
Command Hospital
Kolkata, West Bengal, India

Shubhangi Mahajan MD
Speciality Medical Officer
Department of Dermatology
Seth GS Medical College and KEM Hospital
Mumbai, Maharashtra, India

Subrata Malakar MD (Dermatology)
Director
Rita Skin Foundation
Kolkata, West Bengal, India

Sukesh MS MD
Consultant Dermato-trichologist and
Hair Transplant Surgeon
Bengaluru, Karnataka, India

Surit Malakar MBBS
Rita Skin Foundation
Kolkata, West Bengal, India

Uday Khopkar MD
Professor and Head
Department of Dermatology
Seth GS Medical College and KEM Hospital
Mumbai, Maharashtra, India

Foreword

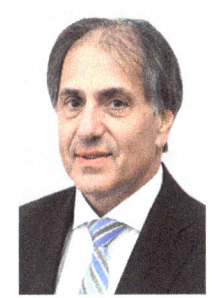

The textbook *Dermoscopy in Darker Skin* by Dr Manas Chatterjee, Dr Shekhar Neema and Dr Subrata Malakar is an illustrated guide to the practical use of this diagnostic tool in the types of skin prevalent predominantly in the Indian subcontinent. Its utility lies in its simplicity of format in which chapters are structured based on the images of the various conditions and their descriptions rather than text, to make this book a handy tool in the clinic of the busy dermatologists, in this part of the world where the large number of patients makes it impossible for a detailed reading during clinic/hospital hours.

The book emphasizes on areas of dermoscopic practice, which are more relevant to the Indian skin such as dermoscopy in pigmentary disorders, melasma and nonmelasma facial pigmentation of the face, granulomatous and other infectious disorders and vitiligo. The arrangement of the various chapters ensures that the clinician is quickly able to find the images that are relevant to the patient in front of him, increasing the immediate value of the book in his clinic.

It is indeed heartening to note that this book is a watershed in the literature on this speciality in India and surrounding countries and would be of value wherever in the world specialists are called upon to manage conditions in similar skin types. It is after long that a comprehensive set of images with descriptions and supporting text have been prepared in this readily readable and understandable form for its ready application in day-to-day practice. I am sure, this book will find its niche in the increasing amount of literature that is available to the practitioner looking after these patients and make a difference in the way he or she looks at dermoscopy as a diagnostic tool in his workplace scenario. The increased utility of this tool would, I am sure, improve patient-care delivery in large parts of the world.

Thomas Ruzicka
Professor and Head
Department of Dermatology and Allergy
Ludwig Maximilian University
Munich, Germany

Preface

This text on dermoscopy is an attempt to address those conditions in the type of skin found in the Indian subcontinent as well as in several other parts of the world, rather than in disorders which are not of day-to-day relevance in the types of patients we deal with. To this extent, we have attempted to illustrate those conditions that the reader who deals with patients of similar nature would have to assess and take a decision on diagnosis and therapy in his outpatient department/clinic every day. The format of the book has been kept as practical and user-friendly as possible with maximum emphasis on annotated images which would help the reader identify the specific diagnostic points in the dermoscopic images, which are from the personal collections of the editors and authors. Text has been kept to the barest minimum and only that which is relevant to the description of the dermoscopy images so that the book is kept of appropriate size and volume of material filtered to that which can be read even as the dermatologist is examining the patient so that the correct diagnosis and treatment can be administered in the same sitting as reviewing the contents of this treatise. The chapters also have been designed such that those of immediate relevance have been preferred to the esoteric for our routine clinical practice.

It is expected that the beginners as well as those in the regular practice of this fascinating diagnostic modality, which has the potential of being not only a supplement but also a supplant to dermatopathology in certain circumstances going ahead, are able to benefit from the typical as well as images of dermoscopic variants that adorn the pages of this book. We hope that with this illustrative text as we prefer to call it, dermoscopy is able to find its place in the routine diagnostic armamentarium in the hands of dermatology residents and consultants in several countries where we look at this amazing and simple instrument to be of utility beyond the confirmation and exclusion of melanoma.

We are thankful to Shri Jitendar P Vij (Group Chairman), Mr Ankit Vij (Group President) and the editorial team of M/s Jaypee Brothers Medical Publishers (P) Ltd, New Delhi, India, especially Mr Sabyasachi Hazra (Kolkata Branch), for printing and helping us with editing of this book.

Manas Chatterjee
Shekhar Neema
Subrata Malakar

Contents

Section 1 Basics of Dermoscopy
Subrata Malakar

Chapter 1. Introduction to Dermoscopy 3
Biju Vasudevan, Shekhar Neema
- How Does a Dermoscope Work? *3*
- Principles of Dermoscopy *4*
- Basis of Dermoscopic Study *4*
- Uses and Advantages of Dermoscopy *5*
- Limitations of the Dermoscope *5*

Chapter 2. Types of Dermoscope 7
Shekhar Neema, Manas Chatterjee
- Polarizing vs Nonpolarizing Dermoscope *7*
- Handheld Dermoscope or Video Dermoscope *7*
- Dermlite Dermoscopes *7*
- Heine Dermoscopes *8*
- Other Handheld and Video Dermoscopes *8*
- Which One to Buy? *8*
- How to Click Best Dermoscopic Images: Tips and Tricks *9*
- How to Archive Dermoscopic Images *9*

Chapter 3. Basic Patterns on Dermoscopy 12
Purva Mehta, Subrata Malakar, Barnali Chowdhury, Protibha Pradhan
- **Vascular Patterns 12**
- Vascular Patterns *12*
- **Melanocytic Patterns 20**
- Colors *20*
- Pigmented Network *20*
- Parallel Patterns or Acral Patterns *20*
- Dots and Globules *20*
- Cobblestone Morphology *21*
- Starburst Pattern *21*
- Homogenous Blue Pigmentation *21*
- Warning Signals of Melanoma *21*

Section 2 Disorders of Pigmentation
Manas Chatterjee

Chapter 4. Melasma 25
Shekhar Neema, Manas Chatterjee
- Melasma *25*

Chapter 5. Nonmelasma Facial Melanoses 27
Shekhar Neema, Manas Chatterjee
- Lichen Planus Pigmentosus *27*
- Pigmented Contact Dermatitis or Riehl-like Melanosis *28*

Erythema Dyschromicum Perstans or Ashy Dermatoses 29
Maturational Dyschromia or Maturational Hyperpigmentation 29
Acanthosis Nigricans 30
Pigmentary Demarcation Line 30

Chapter 6. Other Disorders of Hyperpigmentation — 31
Shekhar Neema
Primary Cutaneous Amyloidosis 31
Acanthosis Nigricans 32
Dowling-Degos Disease 32
Acropigmentation of Kitamura 33
Fixed Drug Eruption 33

Chapter 7. Vitiligo and Other Disorders of Hypopigmentation — 35
Shekhar Neema, Niti Khunger
Vitiligo 35
Differentiating Vitiligo from Idiopathic Guttate Hypomelanoses 36

Chapter 8. Differentiation of Nevus Depigmentosus, Ash Leaf Macules and Nevus Anemicus — 39
Surit Malakar, Samipa Mukherjee
Normal Pigmentary Pattern on Skin 39

Section 3 Papulosquamous Disorders
Shekhar Neema

Chapter 9. Papulosquamous Disorders — 45
Shekhar Neema
Psoriasis 45
Lichen Planus 49
Pityriasis Rosea and Pityriasis Rubra Pilaris 51

Section 4 Infectious Disorders
Manas Chatterjee

Chapter 10. Infectious Disorders — 55
Shekhar Neema, Manas Chatterjee
Scabies 55
Pediculosis 55
Viral Infection 56
Fungal Infections 56

Section 5 Autoimmune and Granulomatous Disorders
Subrata Malakar

Chapter 11. Autoimmune Diseases — 63
Rahul Arora, Shekhar Neema
Discoid Lupus Erythematosus 63
Lichen Sclerosus Et Atrophicus 64
Morphea 65
Systemic Sclerosis 65

Chapter 12. Dermoscopy of Granulomatous Disorders — 67
Uday Khopkar, Shubhangi Mahajan
Lupus Vulgaris 67
Tuberculosis Verrucosa Cutis 67
Post-kala-azar Dermal Leishmaniasis 68
Borderline Lepromatous Hansen's Disease 68

Section 6 Skin Tumors
Subrata Malakar

Chapter 13. Benign and Premalignant Tumors of Skin — 75
Subrata Malakar
Dermatofibroma *75*
Angiokeratoma *76*
Bowen's Disease *77*
Keratoacanthoma *77*
Seborrheic Keratosis *78*
Sebaceous Hyperplasia *79*

Chapter 14. Dermoscopy of Malignant Cutaneous Tumors — 81
Lakshmisha Chandrashekhar, Biswanath Behera
Dermoscopy of Basal Cell Carcinoma *81*
Dermoscopy of Squamous Cell Carcinoma and Keratoacanthoma *82*
Dermoscopy of Malignant Melanoma *82*
Dermoscopy of Bowen's Disease *84*
Dermoscopy of Actinic Keratosis *84*

Section 7 Onychoscopy
Nirmal B

Chapter 15. Onychoscopy — 89
Nirmal B
Relevant Anatomy of Nail Unit *89*
Indications of Onychoscopy in Dermatology *89*
Subungual Hematoma *90*
Pseudomonas Superinfection *90*
Onychomycosis *90*
Psoriasis *90*
Nail Melanonychia *90*
Nailfold Capillaroscopy *90*

Section 8 Trichoscopy
BS Chandrashekhar

Chapter 16. Trichoscopy — 97
BS Chandrashekhar, Samipa S Mukherjee
Normal Scalp 97
Hair *97*
Interfollicular Space *97*
Pigmentary Pattern *97*
Vascular Pattern *98*
Scales *99*
Trichoscopy of Nonscarring Alopecias 100
Patterned Hair Loss *100*
Alopecia Areata *100*
Alopecia Areata Incognito *102*
Telogen Effluvium: Acute and Chronic *104*
Trichotillomania *104*
Nutritional Deficiency *105*
Congenital Atrichia with Papular Eruption *106*
Congenital Triangular Alopecia *106*

Trichoscopy of Scarring Alopecias 108
Lichen Planopilaris 108
Frontal Fibrosing Alopecia 108
Discoid Lupus Erythematosus 108
Tractional Alopecia 111
Folliculitis Decalvans 112
Pseudopelade of Brocq 112
Trichoscopy of Scaly Scalp Conditions 113
Seborrhea Capitis or Pityriasis Sicca 113
Scalp Psoriasis 114
Seborrheic Dermatitis 114
Pityriasis Amiantacea 114
Scale Mimickers: Hair Color Residue and Nits 114
Tinea Capitis 117
Classification 117

Section 9   Miscellaneous
Shekhar Neema

Chapter 17.   Disorder of Vessels 121
Shekhar Neema
Vascular Anomalies (Malformations and Hemangioma) 121
Pyogenic Granuloma 122
Lymphangioma Circumscriptum 124
Vasculitis, Venous Disorders and Pigmented Purpuric Dermatoses 124

Chapter 18.   Dermoscopy in Nevoid Disorders 127
Nilendu Sarma, Balachandran Ankad
Nevus Depigmentosus 127
Congenital Melanocytic Nevus 128
Nevus Spilus 129
Becker's Nevus 130
Nevus Sebaceous 131
Epidermal Nevi 132
Shagreen Patch 132

Chapter 19.   Dermoscopy of Miscellaneous Disorders 134
Sukesh MS
Phrynoderma 134
Keratosis Pilaris 134
Trichostasis Spinulosa 137
Follicular Lichen Planus 138
Follicular Eczema 139
Sebaceous Hyperplasia 141
Rosacea 141
Human Papillomavirus Infections 142
Porokeratosis 142
Arsenic Keratosis 143
Terra Firma-Forme Dermatosis 143

Index 147

SECTION 1: Basics of Dermoscopy

Subrata Malakar

Section Outline

- Introduction to Dermoscopy
- Types of Dermoscope
- Basic Patterns on Dermoscopy
  - Vascular Patterns
  - Melanocytic Patterns

CHAPTER 1

Introduction to Dermoscopy

Biju Vasudevan, Shekhar Neema

INTRODUCTION

Dermoscope or dermoscope is a handheld device which has a magnification lens and light source. It improves diagnostic accuracy of skin lesion as it allows subsurface structures to be visualized. Utilization of dermoscope in examination of skin lesion has opened a new dimension in dermatologic examination, as various details other than size, shape, color and structure can be visualized with this instrument.

HOW DOES A DERMOSCOPE WORK?

How is dermoscope different from simple magnifying glass and light source?
Why does dermoscope allow visualization of subsurface structure which magnifying glass with light source does not?

- Answer to these questions lie in optical principles of dermoscopy.
- Refractive index of stratum corneum is higher than air. Majority of incident light on skin, thus, gets reflected off the surface of the skin, thereby overwhelming the retina and any light reflected from subsurface structure cannot be visualized. Some amount of refraction also adds to the problem.
- The dermoscope circumvents this problem by allowing light which is reflected from subsurface structure to reach the eye so that these deeper structures can be visualized. Dermoscope consists of a magnifying lens and light source giving it inbuilt illumination. The light source can be halogen lamp or light-emitting diode (LED). The yellow light of the halogen lamp and high-intensity white light of LED, both aid in better visualization (Figs 1A and B).

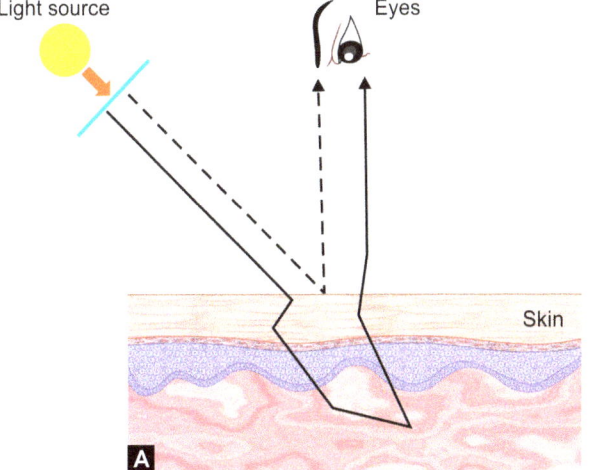 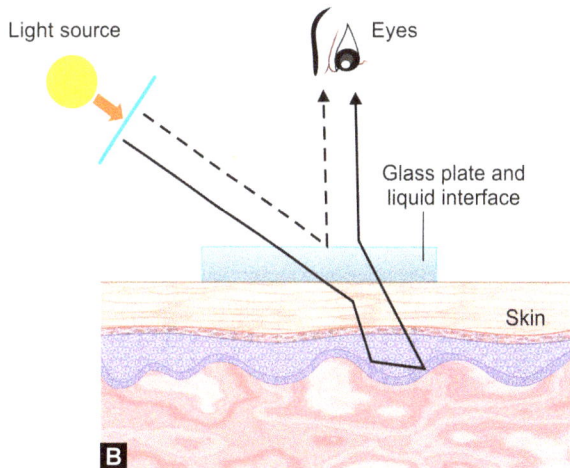

Figs 1A and B: (A) Without use of dermoscope: Most of incident light which falls on skin gets reflected from surface (dotted line) and light which reflects from deeper part does not reach the eye, thus deeper structures are not visible; (B) With use of dermoscope: More incident light reaching deeper part of skin gets reflected and makes deeper structure visible

PRINCIPLES OF DERMOSCOPY

Dermoscopy, also called epiluminescence microscopy, episcopy, skin surface microscopy or incident light microscopy is a noninvasive imaging technique which provides a good horizontal view of the skin subsurface. It improves the diagnostic accuracy as well as the confidence of the clinicians assessing the skin lesions. The angle at which the light falls is usually 20º. The presence of melanin and hemoglobin in various layers helps this differential viewing.

Dermoscopy allows visualization of colors, structures and patterns in the subsurface of skin lesions which are not visible to naked eye. This provides additional diagnostic information which in turn helps users to correctly identify the skin lesions.

There are two types of dermoscopy:
1. Nonpolarized
2. Polarized.

Nonpolarized Dermoscopy

To examine skin lesion, a liquid interface (ideally with refractive index equal to that of skin) is required to convert skin-air interface to skin-liquid-glass interface. This skin-liquid interface is more translucent, reduces light reflection and, leads to better visualization of the superficial epidermis and dermis.

Different immersion liquids like mineral oil, alcohol, water or ultrasound gel can be used as an interface. Seventy percent alcohol appears to be best immersion liquid as it produces less air bubbles and decreases chance of cross contamination, though it evaporates fast. Air bubbles can reduce the image quality. Ultrasound jelly is particularly useful for onychoscopy, as gel fills up the curved area. It is also useful in area around the eye region as it has less tendency to flow into the eyes. Liquid paraffin is an inexpensive, safe and easily available option. Immersion oils are to be avoided as they contain chlorinated paraffin and dibutyl phthalate which can be teratogenic, fetotoxic and carcinogenic.

The glass plate of dermoscope comes in contact with linkage fluid applied on the lesion. The contact plates are usually made of multicoated silicone glass and have inscribed graduated scales for measuring the lesion. Smaller plates with small contact areas are better for difficult to access areas like web spaces, flexures and nail folds in capillaroscopy. These plates can be sterilized using 2% glutaraldehyde, methylated spirit, by boiling or autoclaving.

Polarized Dermoscopy

Introduction of polarized dermoscopy changed the way dermoscopy is performed. It does not require liquid interface system or direct contact with the skin. It uses two polarizers with orthogonal axes to achieve cross polarization. In this noncontact technique, there is no contact of lens with the lesion and the crosspolarized lens absorbs the entire scattered light, thereby, allowing only light in a single plane to pass through. The crosspolarizing filters accept light more preferentially from deeper layers of skin allowing visualization of the skin structures that were not so easily visible with the nonpolarized dermoscopy. It also allows faster screening of the skin lesions. The noncontact technique prevents nosocomial infections, while this advantage is offset by disadvantage of reduced illumination and decreased resolution.

Hybrid Dermoscopy

Hybrid dermoscopes, where polarized and nonpolarized modes can be switched with a click are now available (DermLite DL3N-3rd generation). Both the dermoscopic techniques offer complementary information along with knowledge and these differences can further help in differentiating benign from malignant skin lesions. The polarized dermoscopy is more sensitive when it comes to detection of skin cancer while nonpolarized dermoscopy can improve the specificity in diagnosis, especially in conditions such as seborrheic keratosis.

The following differences exist between the polarized and nonpolarized dermoscopy (Table 1).

BASICS OF DERMOSCOPIC STUDY

- Dermoscopy helps in studying various conditions by looking at patterns, colors and structures. For example the five basic structures or elements which are used to describe pigment abnormalities are lines, pseudopods, circles, clods and dots.
- A pattern is formed actually by the multiple repetitions of various basic elements over sufficient proportions of a lesion that can be recognized on scanning rapidly.

Table 1: Differences between the polarized and nonpolarized dermoscopy

	Nonpolarized	Polarized
Colors enhanced	Blue-white	Pink-red
Obvious structures	Milia-like cysts, comedo-like openings, regression structures	Vascular structures, white-scar-like areas, shiny white structures, blue nevi

- An area which is large enough to constitute a pattern, but having no basic element which dominates is called "structureless".
- Four parameters which should be assessed in dermoscopy of inflammatory and infectious conditions include: (1) morphological vascular patterns; (2) arrangement of vascular structures; (3) colors; and (4) follicular abnormalities. Specific features of each condition should also be considered while evaluating them.
- In malignancies, however, rather than patterns, small distinctive features may be more important.
- Colors have great diagnostic value in dermoscopy. Melanin and hemoglobin, the two most important pigments appear differently at different depths in the skin layers. Very superficial melanin may look black, but deeper down in the epidermis it may appear brown. In the dermis, it may appear as either gray or blue. So the level of the lesion can be gauged by the color, which especially helps in diagnosing invasive malignancies.
- The "ugly duckling" sign which signifies lesions that are distinctly different from everything else in the neighborhood, should always raise eyebrows.

USES AND ADVANTAGES OF DERMOSCOPY

- Dermoscopy is useful for visualization of subsurface structures not visible to naked eye.
- Dermoscopy is useful for diagnosis of melanoma. It increases diagnostic accuracy, decreases unnecessary biopsy and increase confidence of treating physician in making a diagnosis of melanoma.
- First observed by Rona MacKie in 1971, pattern analysis and seven-point technique along with the modified ABCD technique has led to a great revolution in the use of dermoscopy as a very important diagnostic tool for this condition. It has vastly increased the sensitivity and specificity of diagnosing melanoma in the hands of the experienced users. It is now recognized as a good screening test for melanoma, leading to decreased morbidity and mortality caused by this dreaded condition.[1]
- It is useful for diagnosis of nonmelanoma skin cancer- like squamous cell carcinoma, basal cell carcinoma and Bowen's disease.[2]
- Dermoscopy is increasingly being utilized in general dermatology. It is now being utilized for diagnosis of inflammatory and infectious disorders.[3] It is being used for diagnosis of psoriasis, lichen planus, dermatitis and pityriasis rosea.[4] Scabies, pediculosis and tungiasis are also being diagnosed with its help.[5] It can also be used for diagnosis of benign neoplasm-like clear cell acanthoma, seborrheic keratosis, dermatofibroma, vascular lesions- like hemangioma, capillary malformations and urticarial vasculitis.
- It can be used to differentiate scalp psoriasis from seborrheic dermatoses.
- It is used for trichoscopy and onychoscopy for rapid diagnosis of hair and nail diseases. It can be useful in differentiating the common hair disorders like alopecia areata, androgenetic alopecia, female pattern hair loss and telogen effluvium from one another. It can also be used to calculate follicular density of donor area before hair transplantation. It can be used to diagnose lichen planopilaris as well as structural hair defects like monilethrix.
- It can also be used for nailfold capillaroscopy in diagnosis of connective tissue diseases.
- It tries to bridge the gap between clinical findings and invasive investigations especially in case of suspicious lesions so that a better decision regarding whether a lesion needs to be excised or can be left alone, can be taken.
- It has reduced the need for skin biopsies in some instances.
- It is a handy portable diagnostic instrument.
- The facility for storage of images and results of findings being immediately available is an added advantage. Some dermoscopes have inbuilt photography systems with either attachable cameras or inbuilt cameras with supporting software which helps in capture, storage, retrieval and sometimes even interpretation of images. Few dermoscopes can also capture videos of findings.
- By reducing the number of excisions, it will help in reducing cost of treatment.

LIMITATIONS OF THE DERMOSCOPE

- Cost
- Requires training
- Role still not defined in various inflammatory, pigmentary and infectious disorders.
- Standardization of findings of various conditions needs to be done
- Diagnosis of very early melanomas is still circumspect. Digital dermoscopy may overcome this. Sequential digital dermoscopy imaging may allow storage of images and their comparison over prolonged period.

CONCLUSION

Dermoscopy is rapidly advancing field in diagnosis of skin diseases. Its utility for inflammatory, infectious and pigmentary dermatoses makes it an important tool in hand of Indian dermatologist, where melanoma is not so common. With increase in available literature and development of specific signs, dermoscopic characterization of diseases are becoming more specific and dermoscope has become an important diagnostic armamenterium for dermatologist. For those who are studying the subject of dermatology, knowledge about dermoscopic signs of various diseases has become inevitable.

REFERENCES

1. Bafounta ML, Beauchet A, Aegerter P, Saiag P. Is dermoscopy (epiluminescence microscopy) useful for the diagnosis of melanoma? Results of a meta-analysis using techniques adapted to the evaluation of diagnostic tests. Arch Dermatol. 2001;137(10):1343-50.
2. Fargnoli MC, Kostaki D, Piccioni A, Micantonio T, Peris K. Dermoscopy in the diagnosis and management of non-melanoma skin cancers. Eur J Dermatol. 2012;22(4):456-63.
3. Errichetti E, Stinco G. The practical usefulness of dermoscopy in general dermatology. G Ital Dermatol Venereol. 2015;150(5):533-46.
4. Lallas A, Kyrgidis A, Tzellos TG, Apalla Z, Karakyriou E, Karatolias A, et al. Accuracy of dermoscopic criteria for the diagnosis of psoriasis, dermatitis, lichen planus and pityriasis rosea. Br J Dermatol. 2012;166(6):1198-205.
5. Dupuy A, Dehen L, Bourrat E, Lacroix C, Benderdouche M, Dubertret L, et al. Accuracy of standard dermoscopy for diagnosing scabies. J Am Acad Dermatol. 2007;56(1):53-62.

CHAPTER 2

Types of Dermoscope

Shekhar Neema, Manas Chatterjee

INTRODUCTION

Dermoscopy is an expanding field of noninvasive diagnostic dermatology. Its easy availability, portability and ability to increase confidence of physicians in diagnosis of lesions has led to increased interest in buying this handy equipment. In this chapter, we will try to discuss as to which device will suit your need.

With availability of so many devices in market, rapid improvement in technology and improved resolution, it has become increasingly difficult to choose which device to buy from so many available devices. In our opinion, for physicians who practice in multiple offices two most important considerations are portability and economic considerations. Device that he intends to buy should be portable, which not only means that it should be easy to carry but it should also have a system by which images can also be stored for future reference. Resolution of images should be good enough that images can be used for teledermatology, teleconsultation as well as publication.

POLARIZING VS NONPOLARIZING DERMOSCOPE

As has already been discussed in the last chapter (Chapter 1), depending on the source of light a dermoscope can be divided into polarizing and nonpolarizing dermoscope. While most of the newer dermoscopes, which are now available, are either polarizing dermoscope or hybrid dermoscope (polarizing plus nonpolarizing), there were fewer older dermoscopes which were available only in nonpolarizing mode. Polarizing dermoscope is beneficial in many ways as it does not require liquid interface, does not require contact with skin and therefore vessel morphology is better visualized, and chances of transmission of infection is less. Surface scales are better visualized in nonpolarizing light, nonpolarizing dermoscopes are cheaper and they are sufficient for certain indications like trichoscopy in nonscarring alopecia (Figs 1A and B).

HANDHELD DERMOSCOPE OR VIDEO DERMOSCOPE

Handheld dermoscopes are easier to carry, cheaper and are easier to maintain. However, handheld dermoscopes have their limitations that they have limited magnification, only limited area can be visualized at a time and person who is not an expert cannot rapidly screen large area in less time.

Video dermoscopes require computer or any other screen for output to visualize the structures. They have higher magnification so lesions can be visualized in better details (like vascular morphology). Video dermoscopes are very good for teaching purpose where exact structure can be shown to student. Since images can be saved directly to computer with patient data, it does not require separate camera and computer to acquire and store image. Video dermoscopes, however, are more expensive and difficult to carry if one has to travel for consultation.

DERMLITE DERMOSCOPES

DermLite dermoscopes are one of the most commonly used hand held dermoscopes by dermatologists world over. These dermoscopes have light weight, bright light source and good optics resulting in good image quality and resolution. Field of vision of DermLite dermoscope is generally bigger. It also comes with an added advantage of accessories where a dermoscope can be attached to most commonly used phones and tablets (iPhone, iPad, Samsung Galaxy), and

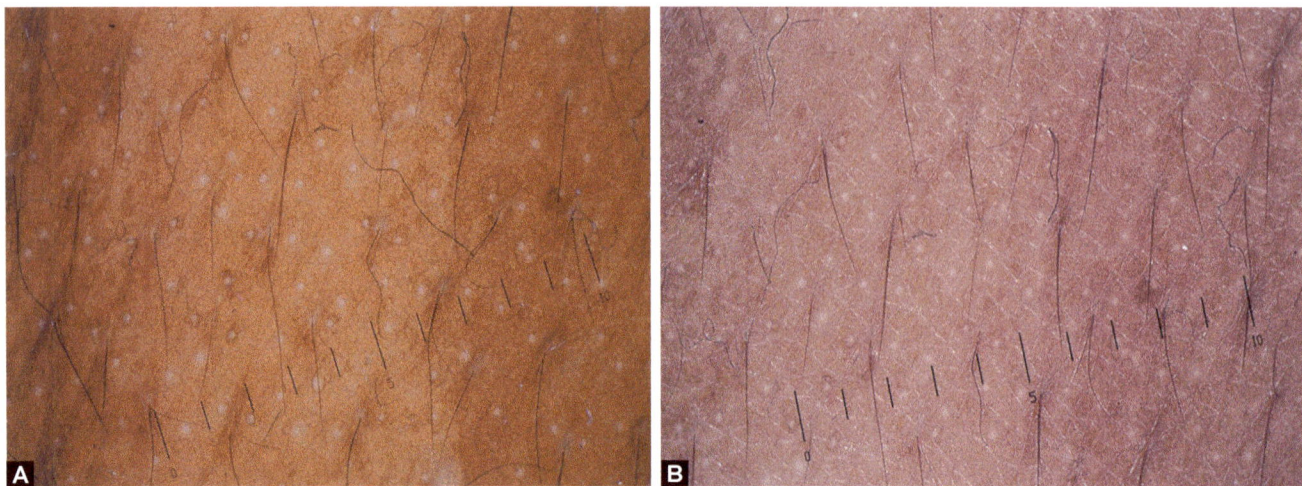

Figs 1A and B: (A) Captured in polarizing light; (B) Captured in nonpolarizing light. Surface scales are prominent in nonpolarizing light

the phone can be used to click and store images. It has many advantages. With availability of advance camera in phone, high-quality publishable images can be captured from phone camera, it increases the chance of capturing dermoscopic image manifold as one tends to carry phone everywhere, it is very easy to archive phone images as phone detects location and date of the image clicked. With all the advantages of DermLite products, the only disadvantage is financial constraint of using it especially for a beginner.

There are many DermLite dermoscopes available, starting from DermLite DL100 to latest being DermLite DL4. These products can be procured from Timpac health care pvt ltd, Dermlite.com or Amazon.in (Figs 2 and 3).

HEINE DERMOSCOPE

Heine Delta 20 is a versatile hand-held dermoscope. It has a bright light-emitting diode (LED) light source, good optics and rechargeable battery. This dermoscope results in good resolution images and many images published in this book have been clicked by Heine Delta 20. It is a sturdy dermoscope and is good for multiple users as in academic settings. It has its own drawback for image capturing as it requires a digital single-lens reflex (DSLR) camera and an adapter for DSLR, which is expensive besides being bulky (Figs 4A and B). While dermoscope itself is handy and can be carried anywhere, it is impractical to carry entire image capturing facilities if consultant is travelling to more than one place.

OTHER HANDHELD AND VIDEO DERMOSCOPES

Firfly has digital polarizing dermoscope (DE 300), it wirelessly streams images and videos directly to the computer in which software is installed. It is easy to use, image capturing is easier and affordable for beginner though resolution of image is not great (Fig. 5A).

Dinolite also has a universal serial bus (USB) based polarizing dermoscope which can capture image directly in computer (Fig. 5B).

Dermaindia has a dermoscope called Ultracam Triple Light Source, which has three light sources: (1) normal light, (2) ultraviolet light and (3) polarized light. It can be connected to a computer and images can be captured in the computer (Fig. 5C).

WHICH ONE TO BUY?

After all the discussions on availability of various dermoscopes, the question remains is, *if you want to start using dermoscope in your practice, which one should you buy?*

It depends on certain factors like how much is your mobility for practice, how do you want to archive the images, how many people are going to use single dermoscope in your set up and of course how much you are willing to spend and, most importantly, are you willing to learn the art and science of dermoscopy and make it part of your routine practice.

- If you are a beginner and do not want to invest, yet want to see how lesions look under dermoscope. USB-based dermoscope is a good choice.
- For a person, who works in a setting where multiple doctors work and more than one doctor is going to use your scope, Heine Delta 20 is a good choice as it is a sturdy dermoscope.
- A consultant who works in multiple offices and needs a portable device which can capture image in mobile phone or tablets, DermLite dermoscopes are the devices to go for (see Figs 3A to C).

Chapter 2 Types of Dermoscope

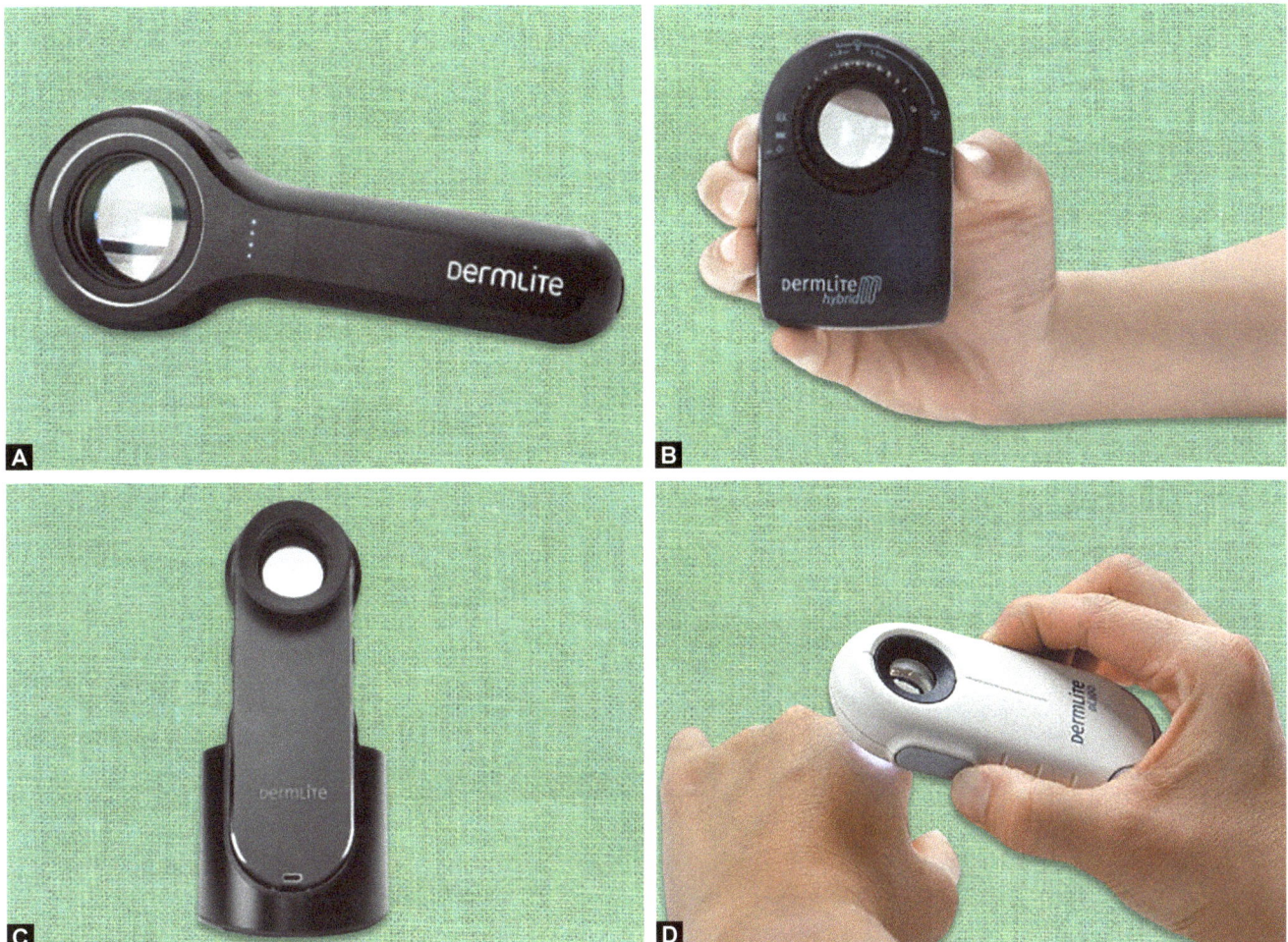

Figs 2A to D: DermLite dermoscopes: (A) DermLite DL4; (B) DermLite II hybrid M; (C) DermLite DL3N; (D) DermLite DL 100

- Video dermoscope is definitely useful if you are working only from one office as it has an advantage that you can show images to patients especially trichoscopic images, which is important to gain confidence of patient in therapy.

HOW TO CLICK BEST DERMOSCOPIC IMAGES: TIPS AND TRICKS

- Keep dermoscope fully charged. Poor light leads to poor images. When using Heine dermoscope in heavily pigmented skin, it is important to increase exposure time by decreasing shutter speed to get brighter images (1/4–1/10).
- Use gel interface for onychoscopy, it results in better images and less glare from curved angles.
- Use of minimum pressure on lesion is important especially when vessel architecture is important for diagnosis (basal cell carcinoma, psoriasis). One trick is to stabilize the dermoscope with use of hand at the same level as contact plate, thereby decreasing pressure of dermoscope on lesion. Use of ultrasound gel on lesion also reduces pressure (Figs 6A and B).

HOW TO ARCHIVE DERMOSCOPIC IMAGES

- It is best to click clinical and dermoscopic images from the same camera. Using different camera for clinical and dermoscopic images leads to confusion in archiving especially if archiving is delayed.
- Applications like DermLite or DermLite X can be used for archiving dermoscopic images when using DermLite dermoscopes with iPhone or iPad. These applications make the process of archiving and retrieving dermoscopic images much simpler.

Section 1 Basics of Dermoscopy

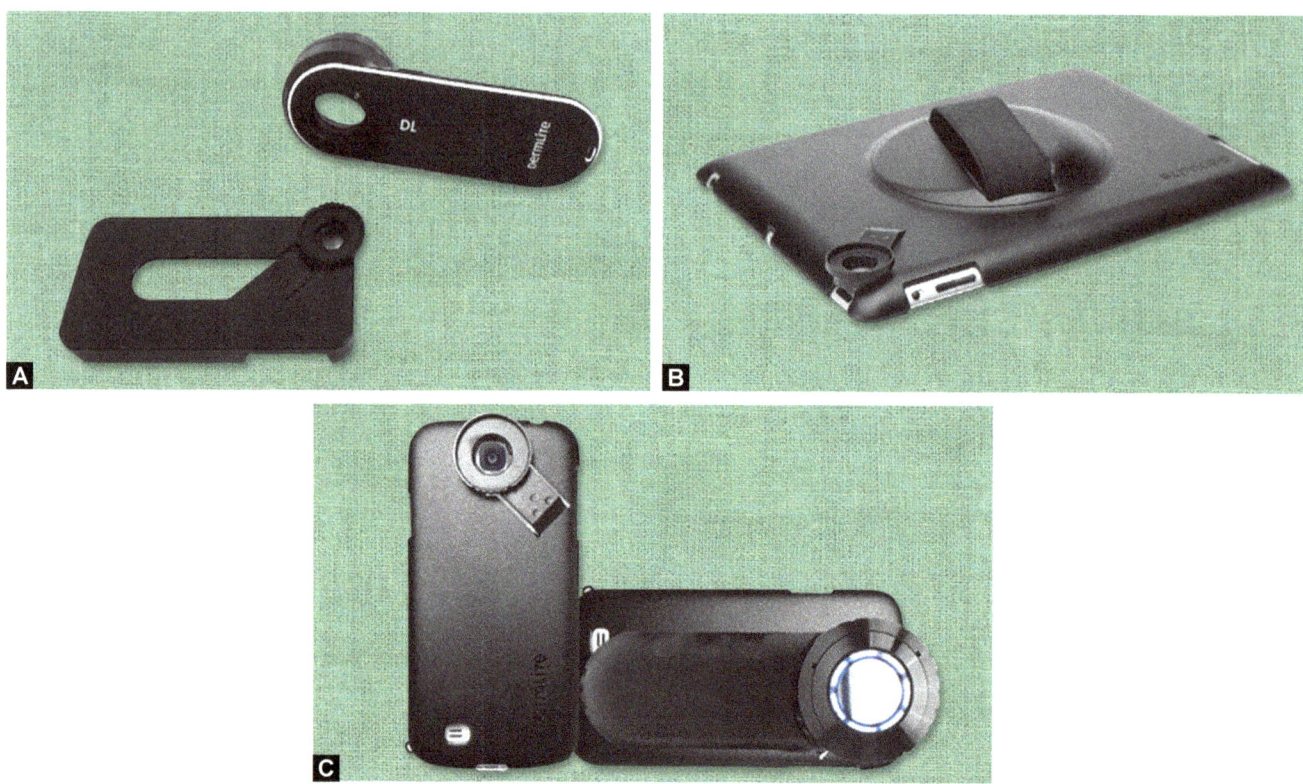

Figs 3A to C: (A) Connection kit for iPhone; (B) Connection kit for iPad; (C) Connection kit for Samsung Galaxy series phone to connect DermLite devices

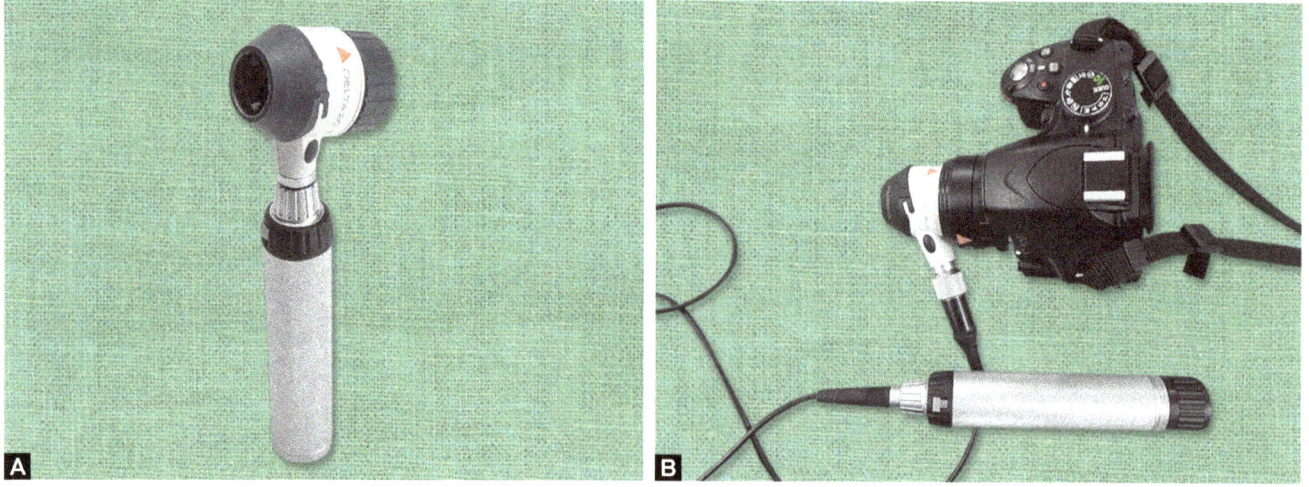

Figs 4A and B: (A) Heine delta 20 dermoscope; (B) Adapter to connect Heine delta 20 dermoscope to DSLR camera

Chapter 2 Types of Dermoscope 11

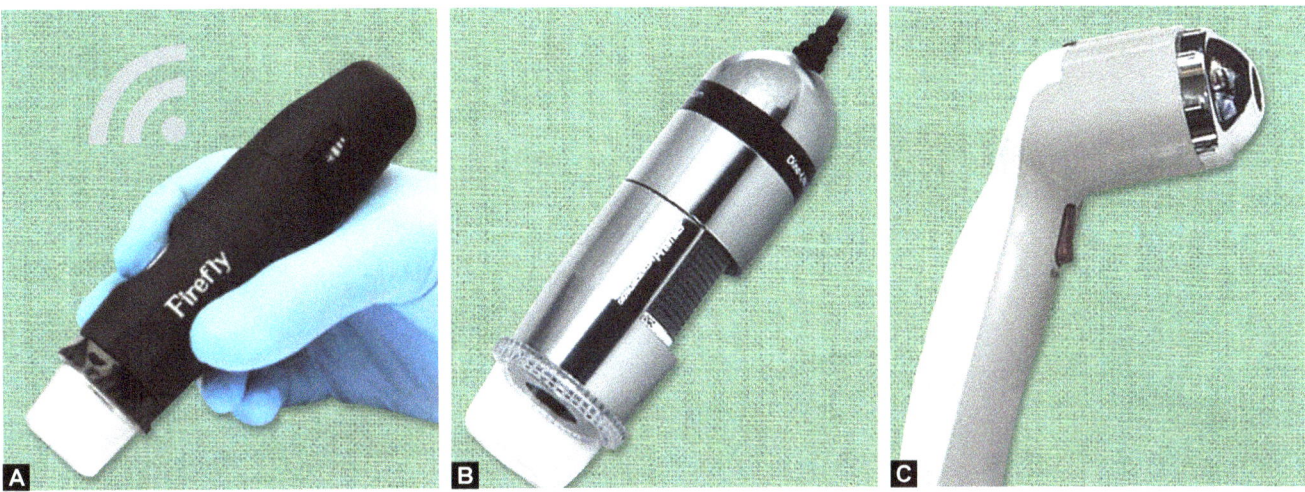

Figs 5A to C: (A) Firefly DE350 wireless dermoscope; (B) Dinolite dermoscope; (C) Ultracam TLS Dermaindia video dermoscope with ultraviolet light source

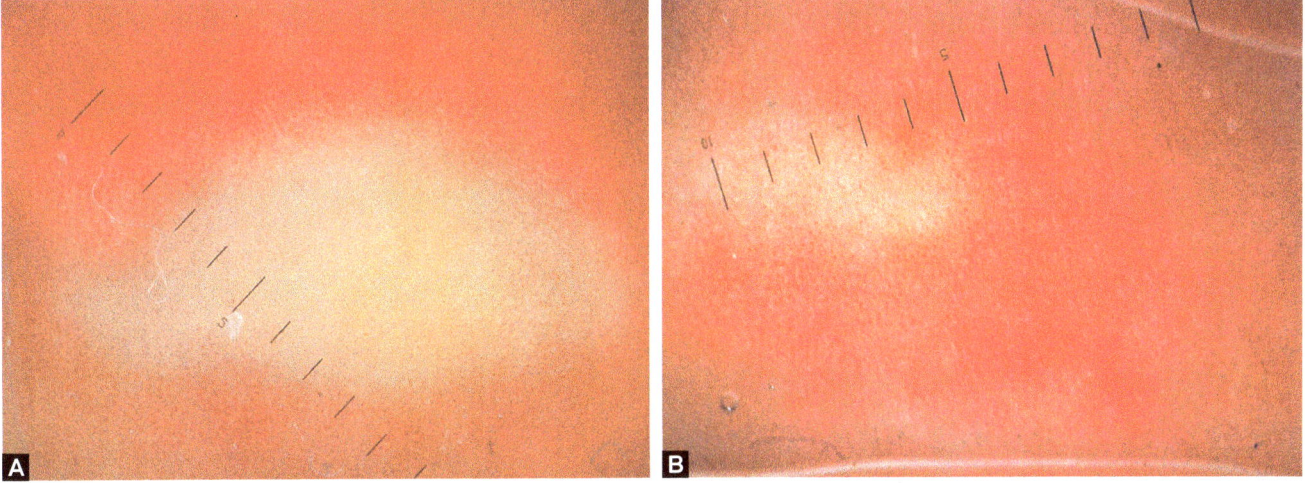

Figs 6A and B: (A) Captured with Heine delta 20 without any interface media; (B) Captured with ultrasound gel as interface media. These images are of psoriasis lesion, where use of pressure during dry dermoscopy has resulted in blanching of lesions

CONCLUSION

Dermoscope is rightly called dermatologist stethoscope, it provides insight into the dermatopathology and increases the physician's confidence in diagnosis of skin lesion. Increasing use of dermoscopic images and signs in clinical dermatology makes it imperative that all clinicians should be aware of basics of dermoscopy and should utilize its potential in diagnosis of skin diseases in routine practice.

CHAPTER 3

Basic Patterns on Dermoscopy

Purva Mehta, Subrata Malakar, Barnali Chowdhury, Protibha Pradhan

VASCULAR PATTERNS

Purva Mehta, Subrata Malakar

INTRODUCTION

The introduction of dermoscopy in the field of dermatology is an asset to clinical diagnosis. It not only reveals the intricacies of the subsurface structures, but also highlights the underlying vascular pattern. Identification of vascular pattern on dermoscopy is crucial as it is diagnostic of a multitude of dermatological lesions.

VASCULAR PATTERNS

The location of the blood vessels can be determined by their color (Box 1).

Connective tissue in the lower dermis causes dispersion of light, which causes the deeper dermal vessels to appear pink in color (Figs 1 and 2).[1]

As dermoscopy provides a horizontal view of the lesion, the shape of the vessel indicates its course (Figs 3 and 4, and Boxes 2 to 4).[1]

Dotted vessels in psoriasis correspond to dilated capillaries present in the papillary dermis (Box 5). Dermoscopy also serves as a therapeutic index in psoriasis as clinical improvement will be marked by reduction in the density of dotted vessels (Figs 5 and 6).[2]

Comma vessels are an important differentiating feature for melanoma as their presence rules out the diagnosis of melanoma.[3,4] Also, comma vessels are far more numerous in Spitz nevi as compared to dysplastic nevi (Figs 9 and 10, and Box 7).[1]

Hairpin vessels will be arranged in a peripheral manner in keratoacanthoma whereas in seborrheic keratosis they will be coursing evenly and consistently throughout the lesion.[1] Moreover, these vessels will be monomorphic and

Box 1: Determining the location of the blood vessels by their color

- Red in color and prominent: Vessel lies close to the surface of the lesion, in the superficial dermis
- Pink in color and not very prominent: Vessel lies in the deeper dermis

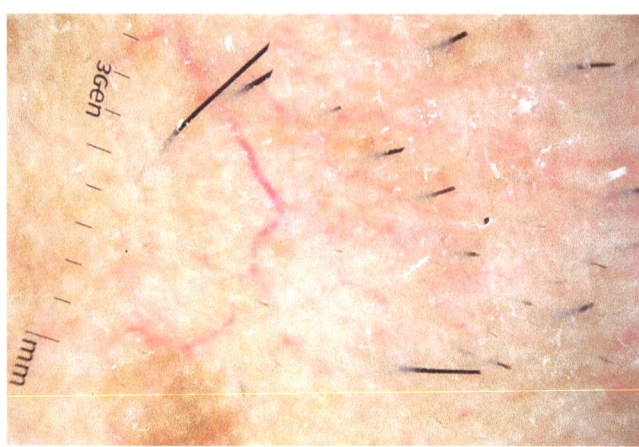

Fig. 1: Superficial vessels: Bright red and in focus

Chapter 3 Basic Patterns on Dermoscopy

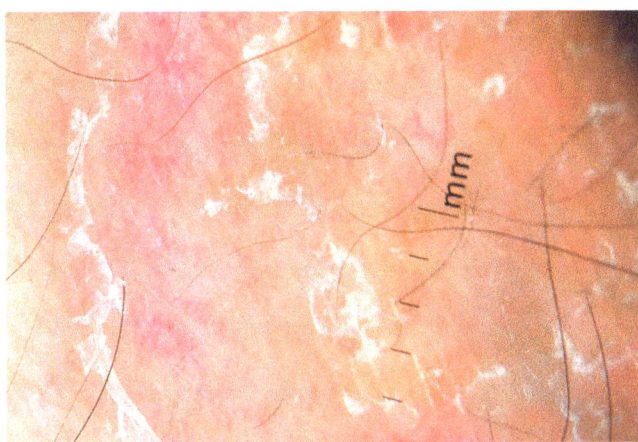

Fig. 2: Deep vessels: Pink and out of focus

Box 3: Diagnostic logarithm to evaluate vascular structures with a dermoscope

- Morphology of the vessels
- Structural arrangement of the vessels
- Presence or absence of other features

Box 4: Vascular morphological patterns

- Dotted vessels
- Crown vessels
- Comma vessels
- Hairpin vessels
- Arborizing vessels
- Telangiectatic vessels
- Glomerular vessels
- Corkscrew vessels
- Linear irregular vessels
- Polymorphous vessels
- Lacunae

Box 5: Dotted vessels

- Circular in shape resembling a pinhead with a small diameter
- Seen in psoriasis, viral warts, lichen planus, Spitz nevus and melanoma

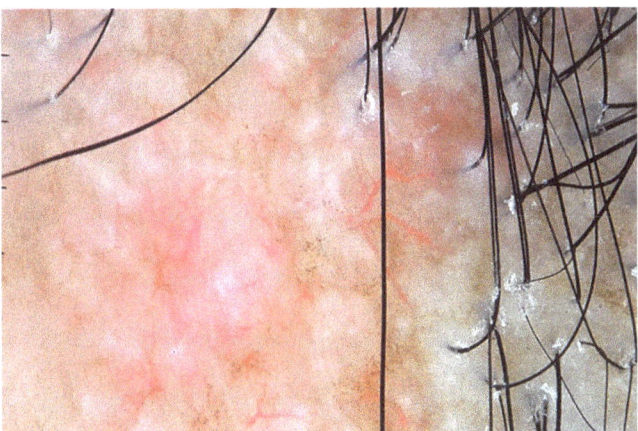

Fig. 3: Vessels parallel to skin surface: Linear

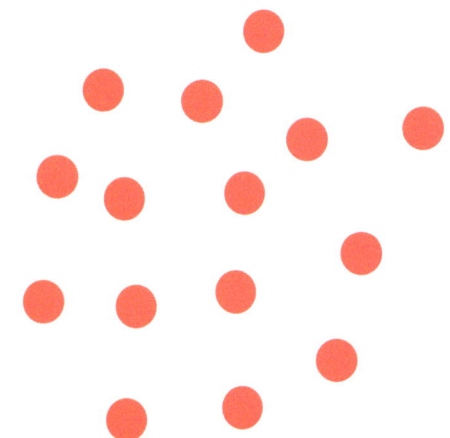

Fig. 5: Schematic diagram of dotted vessels

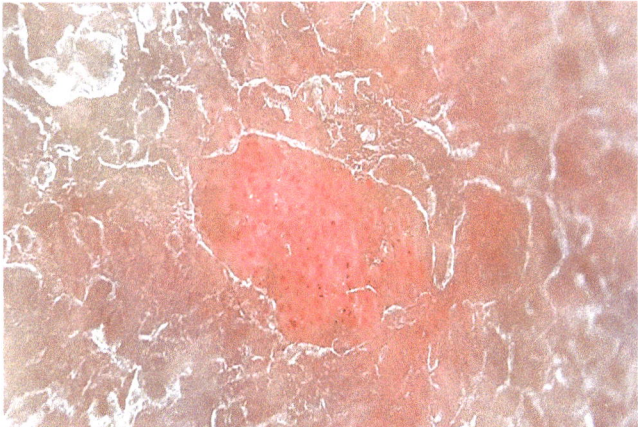

Fig. 4: Vessels perpendicular to skin surface: Dots or loops

Box 2: Shape of the vessel indicating its course

- Vessels that run parallel to the skin surface: Linear in nature
- Vessels that run perpendicular to the skin surface: Dots or loops

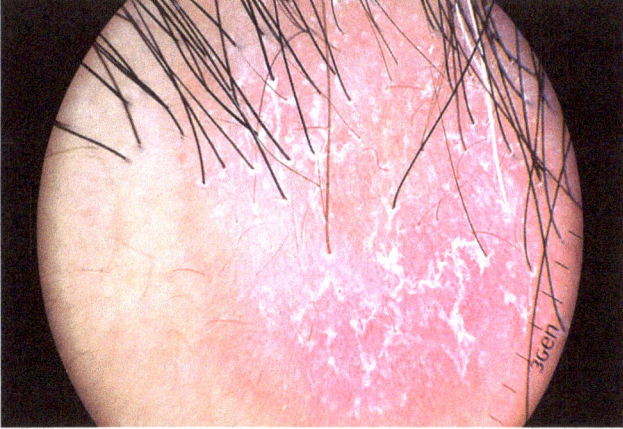

Fig. 6: Dotted vessels on dermoscopy

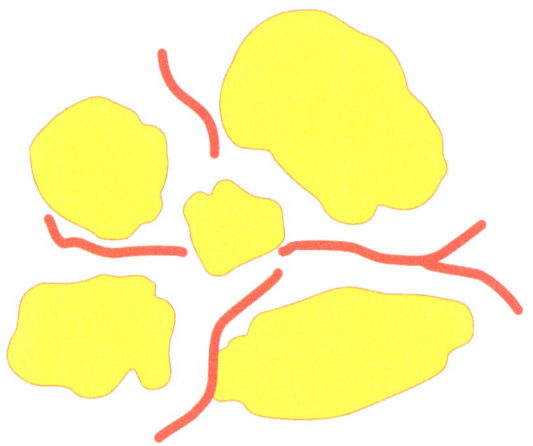

Fig. 7: Schematic diagram of crown vessels

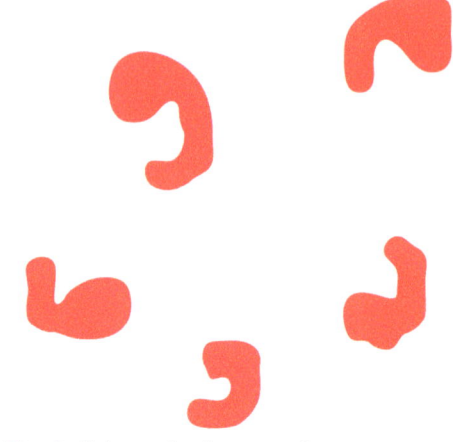

Fig. 9: Schematic diagram of comma vessels

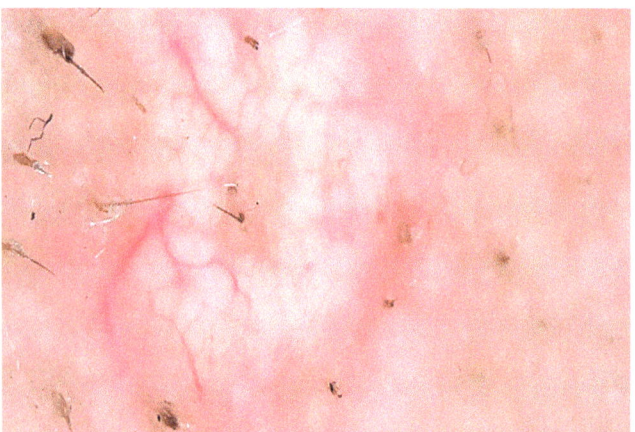

Fig. 8: Crown vessels on dermoscopy in sebaceous hyperplasia

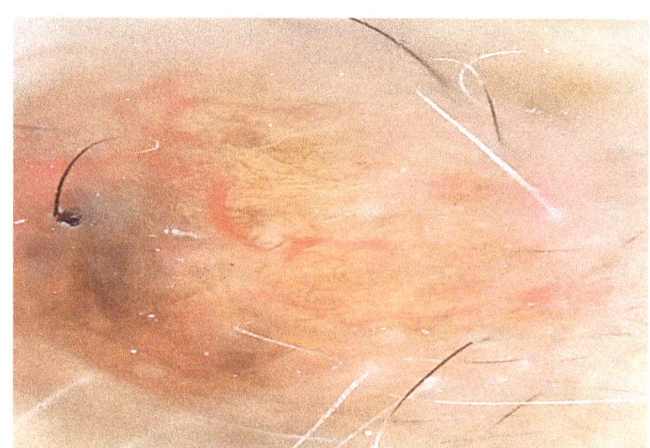

Fig. 10: Dermoscopic image of comma vessels

Box 6: Crown vessels

- Branching vessels peripherally arranged not coursing through the center of the lesion
- Seen in molluscum contagiosum and sebaceous hyperplasia

Box 8: Hairpin vessels

- Vessels with a U-shaped bend resembling a hairpin
- Seen in seborrheic keratosis, keratoacanthoma, Spitz nevi and melanoma

Box 7: Comma vessels

- Vessels that are curved with one end being thicker than the other
- Seen in compound nevi, intradermal nevi, Spitz nevi and dysplastic nevi

homogenous in lesions of seborrheic keratosis (Box 8, and Figs 11 and 12).[5]

The dermoscopic lacunae correspond to dilated vascular spaces in the papillary dermis histologically. The color of the lacunae is clinically significant, as dark brown to black lacunae signify thrombosis within the hemangioma, while

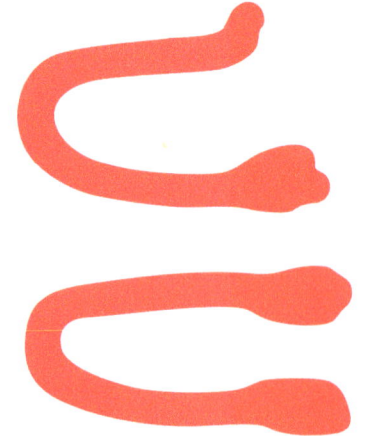

Fig. 11: Schematic diagram of hairpin vessels

Chapter 3   Basic Patterns on Dermoscopy   15

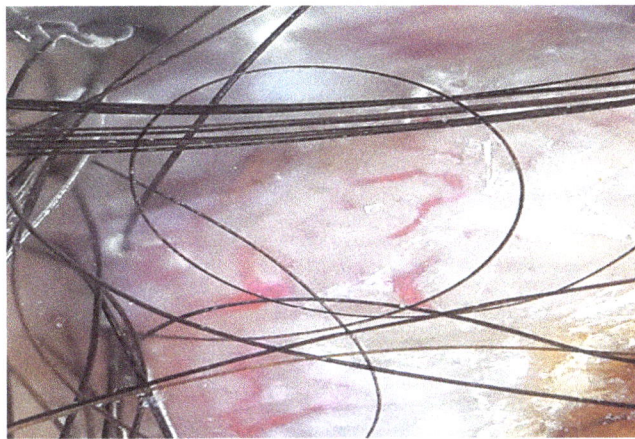

Fig. 12: Hairpin vessels on dermoscopy

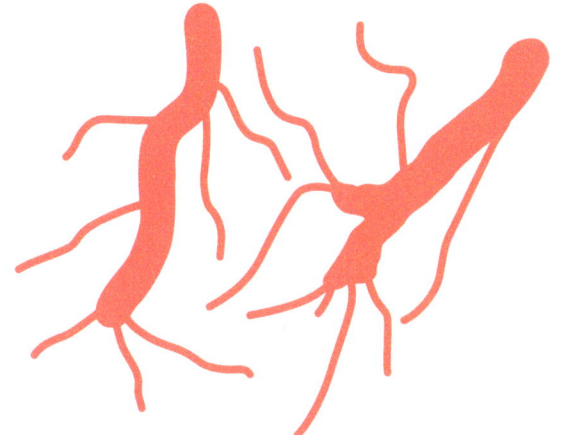

Fig. 13: Schematic diagram of arborizing vessels

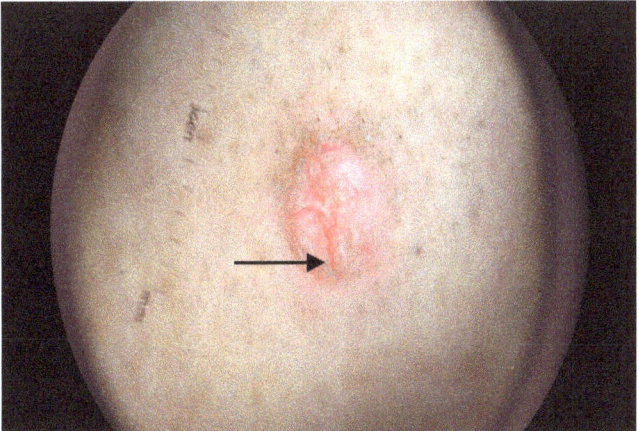

Fig. 14: Arborizing vessels (arrow) in basal cell carcinoma

Box 9: Arborizing vessels

- Large bore vessels branching into smaller terminal vessels
- Seen in adnexal tumors and basal cell carcinoma

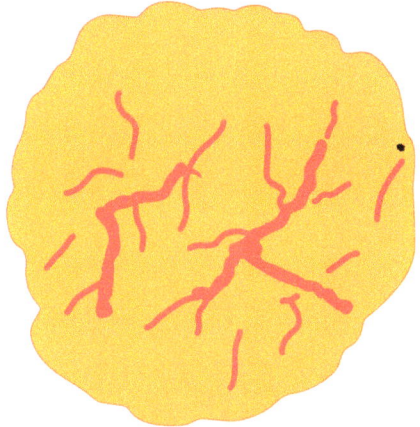

Fig. 15: Schematic diagram of telangiectatic vessels

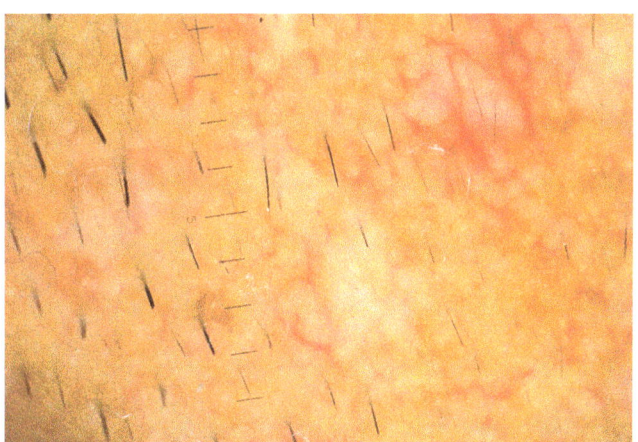

Fig. 16: Dermoscopic picture of telangiectatic vessels in steroid damaged facies

Box 10: Telangiectatic vessels

- Vessels that branch into other vessels albeit with a uniform diameter
- Seen in dermatofibroma and steroid damaged facies

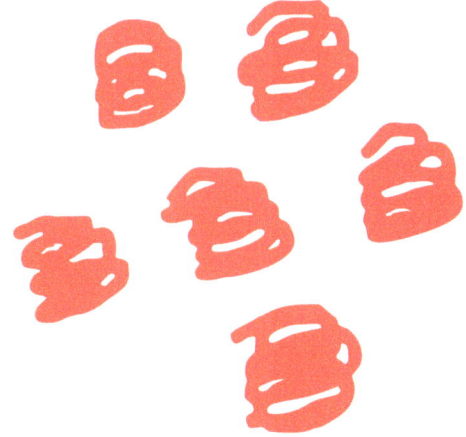

Fig. 17: Schematic diagram of glomerular vessels

Section 1 Basics of Dermoscopy

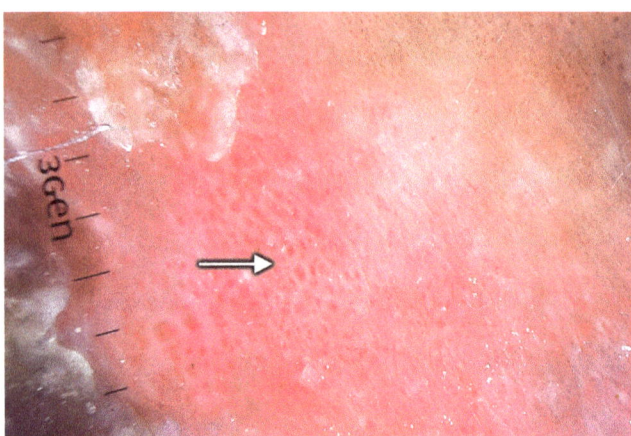

Fig. 18: Dermoscopic picture of glomerular vessels in Bowen's disease

Box 11: Glomerular vessels

- Vessels curling up on each other in a tortuous fashion
- Seen in Bowen's disease and stasis dermatitis

Box 12: Corkscrew vessels

- Spiral vessels in an irregular pattern
- Seen in melanoma

Box 13: Linear irregular vessels

- Vessels following a straight course but in an irregular fashion
- Seen in melanoma

Box 14: Polymorphous vessels

- Vessels with varied morphologies existing in the same lesion
- Seen in malignancies like melanoma and carcinomas

Box 15: Lacunae

- Oval vascular structures with a reddish blue hue
- Seen in hemangiomas and angiokeratomas

white scar-like areas will signify a regressing hemangioma.[6] On the other hand, the lacunae in angiokeratomas are dark and are accompanied by a whitish veil (Figs 19 and 20).[7]

Once the morphology of the vessels has been established, identifying the structural arrangement of the vessels helps in differentiating between similar morphological vascular patterns (Boxes 16 and 17).

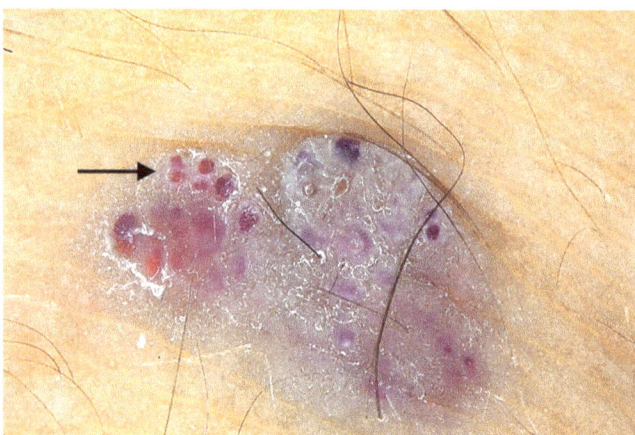

Fig. 20: Well-demarcated, round to oval, red to blue lacunae (arrow) in angiokeratoma

Box 16: Structural arrangement of vessels

- Radial
- Branching
- Regular
- Irregular
- Clustered
- String of pearls

Features to differentiate basal cell carcinoma and sebaceous hyperplasia on dermoscopy are presence of sebaceous lobules and the opening of the sebaceous gland which will be visible as a crater, seen in sebaceous hyperplasia (Figs 21 and 22).[8,9]

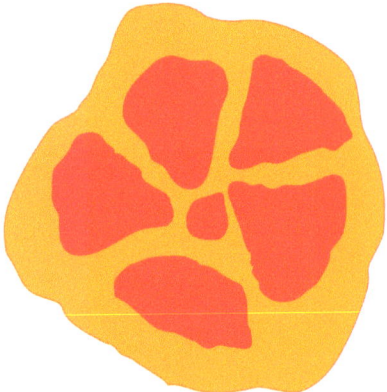

Fig. 19: Schematic diagram of lacuna

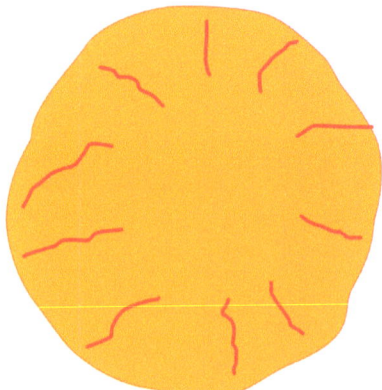

Fig. 21: Schematic diagram of radial distribution

Chapter 3   Basic Patterns on Dermoscopy

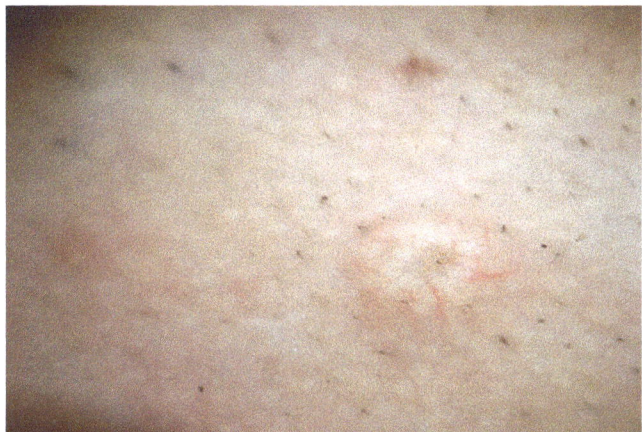

Fig. 22: Dermoscopic picture of radial distribution

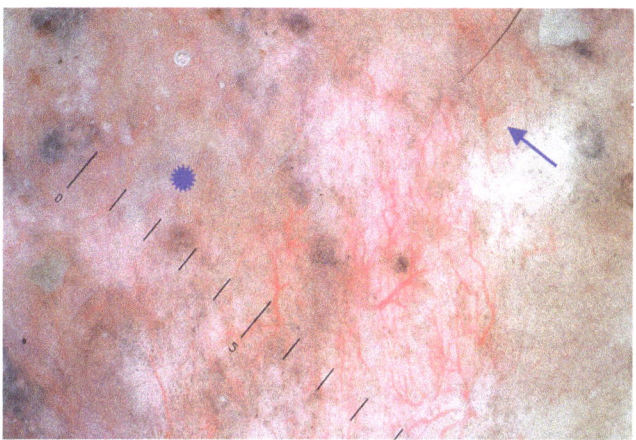

Fig. 24: Dermoscopic picture of branching distribution in basal cell carcinoma

Box 17: Radial distribution of vessels

- Vessels arranged in the periphery of the lesion radially
- Seen in sebaceous hyperplasia and molluscum contagiosum

Box 18: Branching distribution

- Large diameter vessels branching into finer ones
- Seen in basal cell carcinoma and adnexal tumors

Additional features to distinguish between basal cell carcinoma and adnexal tumor would be that the vessels in basal cell carcinoma would be branching irregularly and they would be bright red in color and prominent, thus signifying their superficial location in the dermis (Figs 23 and 24, and Box 18).[3,10]

The regular distribution of the dotted vessels in Spitz nevus helps to differentiate it from dysplastic nevus on dermoscopy as the vessels will be scattered in Spitz naevi (Figs 25 and 26, and Box 19).[1]

Dotted, irregularly arranged vessels packed in milky red globules should arouse a dermoscopic suspicion of melanoma (Box 20).[4,11]

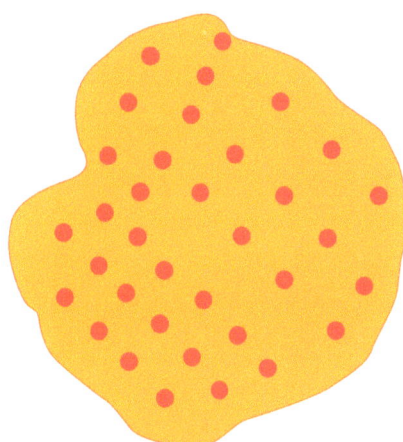

Fig. 25: Schematic diagram of regular pattern

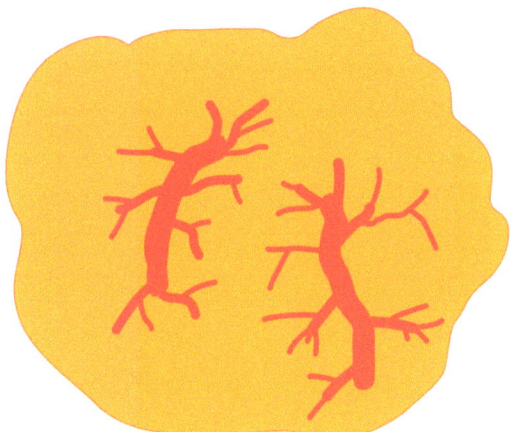

Fig. 23: Schematic diagram of branching distribution

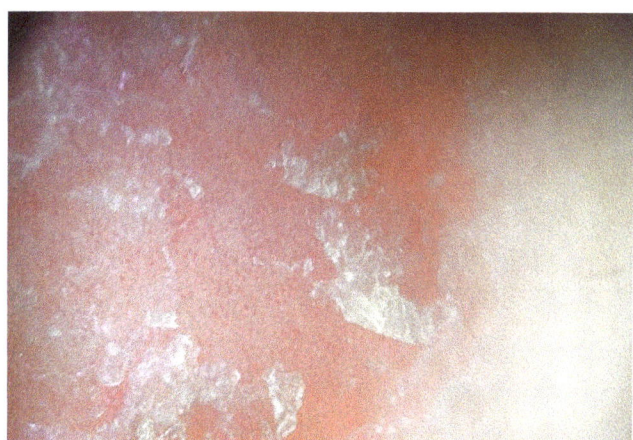

Fig. 26: Dermoscopic image of regular pattern

Box 19: Regular distribution

* Vessels are evenly arranged at regular intervals
* Seen in Spitz nevus and psoriasis

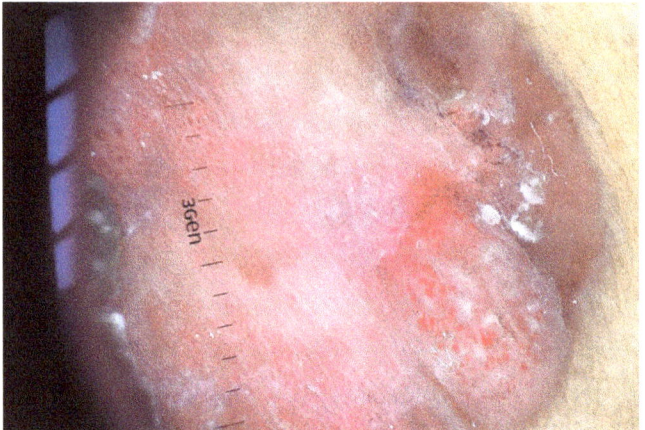

Fig. 29: Dermoscopic picture of clustered distribution in Bowen's disease

Box 21: Clustered arrangement

* Vessels grouped together within a lesion
* Seen in Bowen's disease

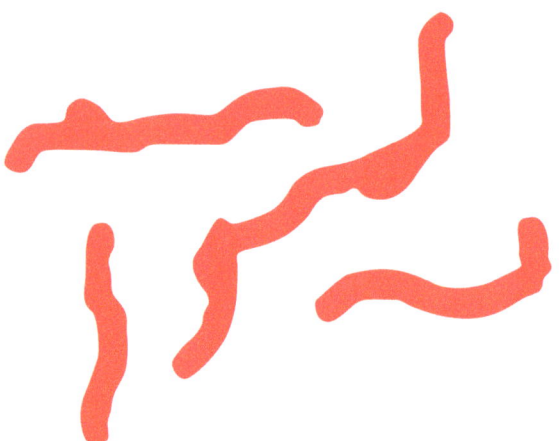

Fig. 27: Schematic diagram of irregular distribution

Box 20: Irregular distribution

* Vessels with varied morphologies haphazardly distributed
* Seen in melanoma, basal cell carcinoma and squamous cell carcinoma

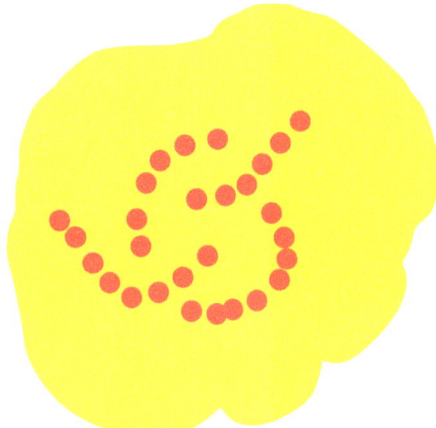

Fig. 30: Schematic diagram of string of pearls distribution

Box 22: String of pearls arrangement

* Linear arrangement of dotted vessels simulating a string of pearls
* Seen in clear cell acanthoma

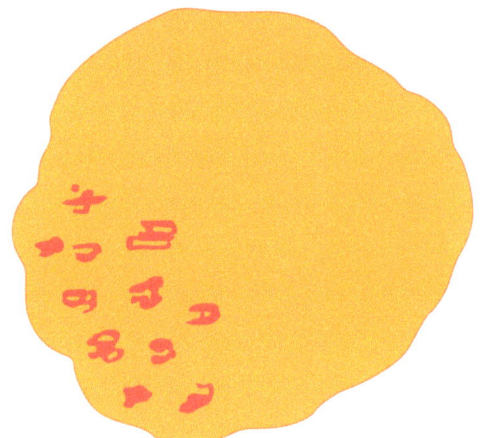

Fig. 28: Schematic diagram of clustered distribution

CONCLUSION

Vascular patterns on dermoscopy are of utmost significance. Identification of these patterns is essential for an accurate diagnosis.

REFERENCES

1. Zalaudek I, Kreusch J, Giacomel J, Ferrara G, Catricala C, Argenziano G. How to diagnose nonpigmented skin tumors: A review of vascular structures seen with dermoscopy: part I. Melanocytic skin tumors. J Am Acad Dermatol. 2010;63:361-74.
2. Micali G, Lacarrubba F, Musumeci ML, Massimino D, Nasca MR. Cutaneous vascular patterns in psoriasis. Int J Dermatol. 2010;49:249-56.
3. Argenziano G, Zalaudek I, Corona R, Sera F, Cicale L, Petrillo G, et al. Vascular structures in skin tumors: a dermoscopy study. Arch Dermatol. 2004;140:1485-9.
4. Menzies SW, Kreusch J, Byth K, Pizzichetta MA, Marghoob A, Braun R, et al. Dermoscopic evaluation of amelanotic and hypomelanotic melanoma. Arch Dermatol. 2008;144:1120-7.
5. Braun RP, Rabinovitz HS, Krischer J, Kreusch J, Oliviero M, Naldi L, et al. Dermoscopy of pigmented seborrheic keratosis: a morphological study. Arch Dermatol. 2002;138:1556-60.
6. Wolf IH. Dermoscopic diagnosis of vascular lesions. Clin Dermatol. 2002;20:273-5.
7. Zaballos P, Daufi C, Puig S, Argenziano G, Moreno-Ramirez D, Cabo H, et al. Dermoscopy of solitary angiokeratomas: a morphological study. Arch Dermatol. 2007;143:318-25.
8. Zaballos P, Ara M, Puig S, Malvehy J. Dermoscopy of sebaceous hyperplasia. Arch Dermatol. 2005;141:808.
9. Bryden AM, Dawe RS, Fleming C. Dermatoscopic features of benign sebaceous proliferation. Clin Exp Dermatol. 2004;29:676-7.
10. Menzies SW, Westerhoff K, Rabinovitz H, Kopt AW, McCarthy WH, Katz B. Surface microscopy of pigmented basal cell carcinoma. Arch Dermatol. 2000;136:1012-6.
11. Carli P, Massi D, de Giorgi V, Giannotti B. Clinically and dermoscopically featureless melanoma: when prevention fails. J Am Acad Dermatol. 2002;46:957-9.

MELANOCYTIC PATTERNS

Barnali Chowdhury, Protibha Pradhan, Subrata Malakar

INTRODUCTION

Dermoscopic pattern analysis is the first step in differentiating a melanocytic lesion from a nonmelanocytic lesion and malignant lesion. The application of this noninvasive instrument can help a physician avoid unnecessary excision of lesions. Melanin is the most important chromophore in the skin, which is responsible for generation of different colors and patterns on dermoscopy depending upon its depth of location and concentration.[1-4]

COLORS

The following are the colors reflected on dermoscopy:
- Black color is reflected when melanin lies in stratum corneum of the epidermis (Fig. 31)
- Dark- or light-brown color, if it lies in the other epidermal strata, including the dermoepidermal junction (DEJ)
- Blue-gray: Melanin in the papillary dermis
- Steel-blue: In the reticular dermis.

PIGMENTED NETWORK

It consists of pigmented lines and pigment-free holes giving a honeycomb appearance.[5] The network holes are produced by melanin in the suprapapillary epidermis, while the pigmented lines are due to melanin in the rete ridges.[1,5] The chromatique of a pigmented network varies from light or dark brown to black, to gray and it can be even or uneven. The other patterns are given as follows:
- *Negative network*: Bony white network-like structures seen in pink naevi, Spitz naevi, melanoma and dermatofibroma. However, it is not a primary criteria to diagnose melanocytic lesions.
- *Pseudo-network*: These are uniform round white or yellowish structures seen in head and neck region as the skin is thin with not so developed rete ridges. Gray pseudo-network is associated with benign lesion, e.g. lichen planus-like keratosis and malignant lesions like melanoma.[1-5]
- *Atypical pigment network*: There can be variability in the thickness of the pigment network which reflects fusion of rete ridges in dysplastic lesions (Figs 32 to 34).

PARALLEL PATTERNS OR ACRAL PATTERNS

These are furrows or fissures and ridges seen on palms and soles (dermatoglyphics) (Fig. 35).[6]

DOTS AND GLOBULES

Dots are round dermoscopic structures under 0.1 mm in diameter of different colors.[1,7] Dots are caused by free melanin or melanin present in melanocytes, melanophages or keratinocytes.[2] Globules are round sometimes angular structures over 0.1 mm in diameter, which are caused by

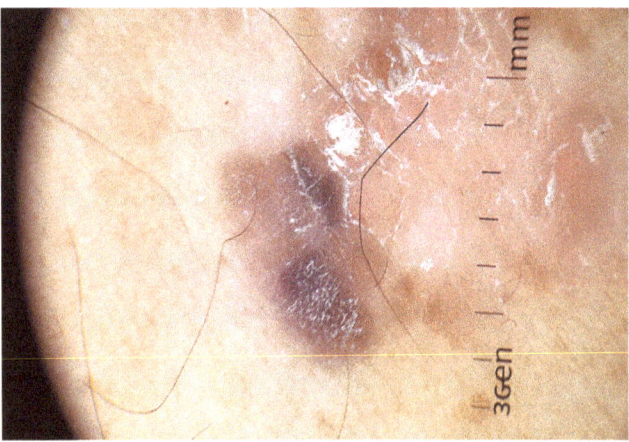

Fig. 31: Dermoscopic picture showing brown-black pigment

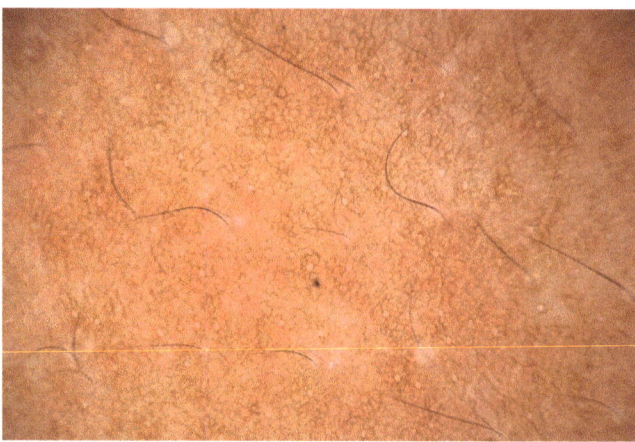

Fig. 32: Reticular pigment pattern: Seen in extremities
Courtesy: Shekhar Neema, Command Hospital, Kolkata

Chapter 3 Basic Patterns on Dermoscopy

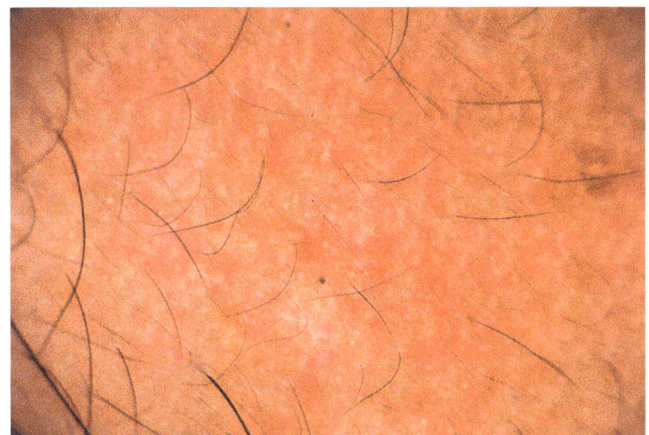

Fig. 33: Pseudoreticular pattern: Seen in head and neck
Courtesy: Shekhar Neema, Command Hospital, Kolkata

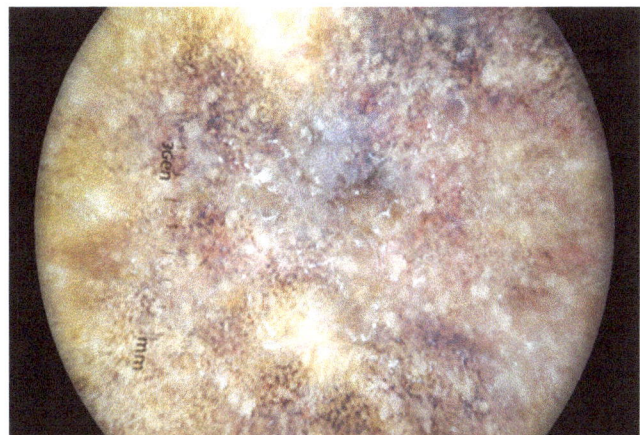

Fig. 36: Dots and globules

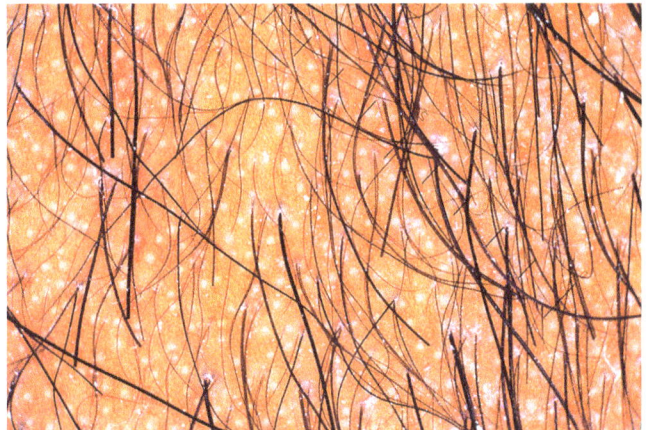

Fig. 34: Honeycomb pattern: Seen in scalp in pigmented skin
Courtesy: Shekhar Neema, Command Hospital, Kolkata

Fig. 35: Acral pattern

free melanin, melanocytes or melanophages clusters in the deep epidermal strata, at DEJ, in the papillary dermis and rarely in the reticular dermis (Fig. 36).[1,8] Types of dots and globules are given as follows:

- *Black*: Atypical melanocytes in epidermis
- *Regular brown dots and globules*: Nests of melanocytes at the DEJ
- *Irregular brown dots and globules*: Nests of atypical melanocytes at DEJ
- *Grayish dots*: Free melanin or melanophages in papillary dermis
- *Reddish globules*: Melanoma (neovascularization).

COBBLESTONE MORPHOLOGY

It reflects large dermal nests of melanocytes seen in dermal naevi.[6]

STARBURST PATTERN

There is a central homogenous pigmentation with circumferential pigmented streaks, typically seen in Spitz nevus (Fig. 37).[6]

HOMOGENOUS BLUE PIGMENTATION

These are structureless blue color in the absence of dots and globules and pigment network usually seen in blue nevus.[9]

WARNING SIGNALS OF MELANOMA

Melanoma accounts for few skin malignancies among Indian population. Literature reports a very low age-specific incidence rates of less than 0.5 per 1,000,000.[10] Hence, there is a low index of suspicion among clinicians, which may lead to delayed diagnosis and treatment. A consensus net meeting on dermoscopy has formulated the following checkpoints for diagnosing melanoma.[10]

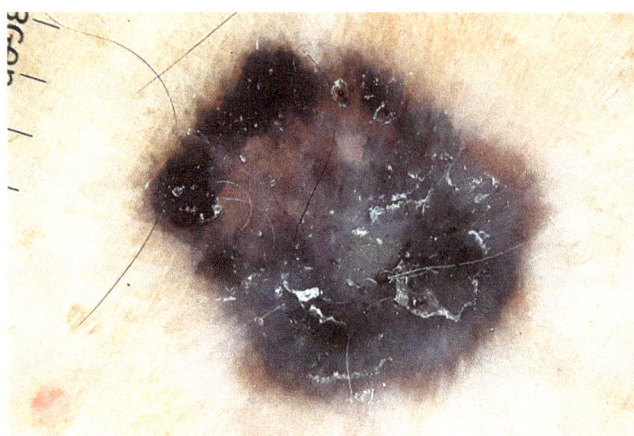

Fig. 37: Starburst pattern in Spitz naevi

Three-point checklist is given as follows:
1. Asymmetry of color and structure (in one or two perpendicular axes).
2. Atypical pigment network (irregular holes and thick lines).
3. Blue white structures.

REFERENCES

1. Stolz W, Braun-Falco O, Bilek P, Landthaler M, Burgdorf WHC. Color Atlas of Dermatoscopy, 2nd edition. Berlin: Blackwell Wissenschafts-Verlag; 2002.
2. Marghoob AA, Braun RP, Kopf AW. Atlas of Dermoscopy. London: Taylor & Francis Group; 2005.
3. Johr RH, Soyer HP, Argenziano G, Hofman-Wellenhof R, Scalvenzi M. Dermoscopy: The Essentials, 1st edition. London: Mosby; 2004.
4. Soyer HP, Hofmann-Wellenhof R, Argenziano G, Johr RH. Color Atlas of Melanocytic Lesions of the Skin. Berlin Heidelberg: Springer-Verlag; 2007.
5. Malvehy J, Puig S. Principles of Dermoscopy. Barcelona: CEGE; 2002.
6. Neila J, Soyer HP. Key points in dermoscopy for diagnosis of melanomas, including difficult to diagnose melanomas, on the trunk and extremities. J Dermatol. 2011;38:3-9.
7. Carli P, De Giorgi V, Soyer HP, Stante M, Mannone F, Giannotti B. Dermatoscopy in the diagnosis of pigmented skin lesions: a new semiology for the dermatologist. J Eur Acad Dermatol Venereol. 2000;14:353-69.
8. Bowling J, Argenziano G, Azenha A, Bandic J, Bergman R, Blum A, et al. Dermoscopy key points: recommendations from the International Dermoscopy Society. Dermatology. 2007;214(1):3-5.
9. de Giorgi V, Massi D, Salvini C, Trez E, Mannone F, Carli P. Dermoscopic features of combined melanocytic nevi. J Cutan Pathol. 2004; 31(9):600-4.
10. Argenziano G, Soyer HP, Chimenti S, Talamini R, Corona R, Sera F, et al. Dermoscopy of pigmented skin lesions: results of a consensus meeting via the Internet. J Am Acad Dermatol. 2003;48(5):679-93.

SECTION 2
Disorders of Pigmentation

Manas Chatterjee

Section Outline

- Melasma
- Nonmelasma Facial Melanoses
- Other Disorders of Hyperpigmentation
- Vitiligo and Other Disorders of Hypopigmentation
- Differentiation of Nevus Depigmentosus, Ash Leaf Macules and Nevus Anemicus

CHAPTER 4

Melasma

Shekhar Neema, Manas Chatterjee

INTRODUCTION

Melasma is an acquired hypermelanosis of uncertain etiology that occurs exclusively in sun-exposed areas, mostly on face and rarely on neck and forearms.[1] It is more common in women and in Asians. Exact pathogenesis is unknown, however, genetic predisposition and ultraviolet light exposure seems to play an important role.[2]

MELASMA

Diagnosis of melasma remains clinical and aided by Wood's lamp examination. Melasma needs to be differentiated from other causes of facial hypermelanoses like pigmented contact dermatitis, lichen planus pigmentosus and erythema dyschromicum perstans. Histopathology is not performed routinely for diagnosis of facial hypermelanoses because of reluctance on part of the patient and physician, alike, as there is a risk of development of unsightly scar or postinflammatory dyschromia.

Dermoscopy of normal facial skin shows opening of sweat glands and hair follicles on the background of diffuse pigmentation creating a pseudo-network pattern. Melanin is the main chromophore in pigmented skin lesions, and anatomical location of melanin determines color perceived on dermoscopy. Melanin present in stratum corneum appears as black, dermoepidermal junction appears as brown and dermis appears as blue to gray.[3] Dermoscopy of pigmented lesions of face can be used for diagnosis as well as prognosis of the clinical condition. Color of the pigment on dermoscopy can determine depth of pigment and has obvious therapeutic implications as dermal pigment is difficult to treat by conventional therapy. Dermoscopic pattern in melasma has been described as reticuloglobular pattern, perifollicular brown black globules, arcuate and honeycomb-like pattern (Figs 1 to 5).[4-6]

Dermoscopy is also useful for detection of adverse effects of therapy. It is useful for detection of exogenous ochronosis and steroid-induced telangiectasia and atrophy of skin. Dermoscopic features of exogenous ochronosis have been described as blue-gray, brown-gray, amorphous areas obliterating follicular openings; a "worm-like" pattern has also been described.[7-9]

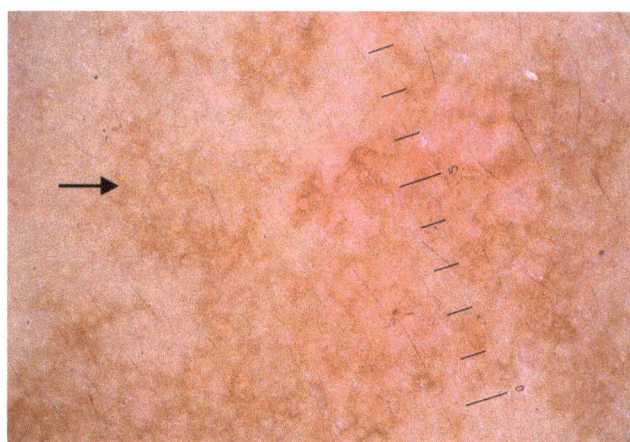

Fig. 1: Reticuloglobular pattern—reticular pigmented pattern accentuated with globules of pigment and network of pigment is broken with acrosyringium (black arrow)

Section 2 Disorders of Pigmentation

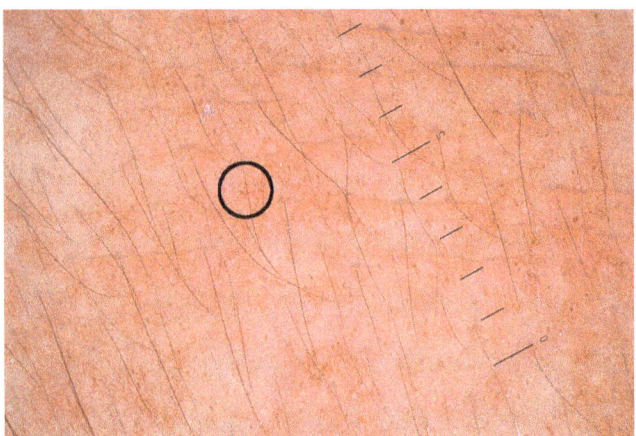

Fig. 2: Granular pigment on background of reticular pigment suggestive of dermal component of melasma

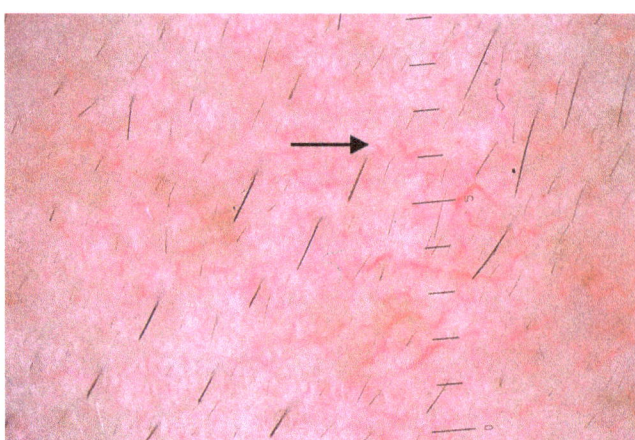

Fig. 5: Telangiectasia in partially treated case of melasma with triple combination suggestive of steroid damaged face. Dermoscopy can be used for rapid screening of patients prior to prescribing them triple combination therapy as many patients come after self-medication with topical steroid containing cream

Fig. 3: Unpatterned or nonspecific pattern

CONCLUSION

Dermoscopy is a useful tool for diagnosis and prognosis of melasma. It can be used as a screening tool in all cases of melasma before starting steroid-based triple combination therapy as first-line agent and during follow-up, as many patients come after self-medicating with topical steroid cream and early signs of steroid damage may not be detectable with naked eye examination alone.

REFERENCES

1. Bandyopadhyay D. Topical treatment of melasma. Indian J Dermatol. 2009;54:303-9.
2. Handel AC, Miot LD, Miot HA. Melasma: a clinical and epidemiological review. An Bras Dermatol. 2014;89:771-82.
3. Mahajan SA. Melasma. In: Khopkar U (Ed). Dermoscopy and Trichoscopy in Diseases of Brown Skin, 1st edition. New Delhi: Jaypee; 2012. pp. 50-9.
4. Li Y, Liu J, Sun QN. Characteristic Dermoscopic Features of Melasma. Zhongguo Yi Xue Ke Xue Yuan Xue Bao. 2015;37:226-9.
5. Tamler C, Fonseca RMR, Pereira FBC, Barcauí CB. Classificação do melasma pela dermatoscopia: estudo comparativo com lâmpada de Wood. Surg Cosmetic Dermatol. 2009;1(3):115-9.
6. Stolz W. Color Atlas of Dermoscopy, 2nd edition. Berlin: Blackwell Wissenschafts-Verlag G; 2002. pp. 121-31.
7. Charlín R, Barcaui CB, Kac BK, Soares DB, Rabello-Fonseca R, Azulay-Abulafia L. Hydroquinone-induced exogenous ochronosis: A report of four cases and usefulness of dermoscopy. Int J Dermatol. 2008;47:19-23.
8. Gil I, Segura S, Martínez-Escala E, Lloreta J, Puig S, Vélez M, et al. Dermoscopic and reflectance confocal microscopic features of exogenous ochronosis. Arch Dermatol. 2010;146:1021-5.
9. Khunger N, Kandhari R. Dermoscopic criteria for differentiating exogenous ochronosis from melasma. Indian J Dermatol Venereol Leprol. 2013;79:819-21.

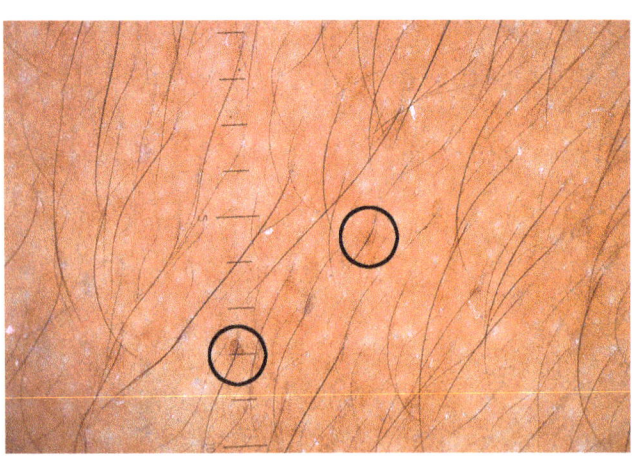

Fig. 4: Perifollicular accentuation of pigmentation on background of reticular pigmentation (black circle)

CHAPTER 5

Nonmelasma Facial Melanoses

Shekhar Neema, Manas Chatterjee

INTRODUCTION

Pigmentary disorders involving face are very common in outpatient dermatology practice. Dermoscopy can provide clues to diagnose various pigmentary disorder of face, since performing histopathology is not always possible. Various pigmentary disorders involving face like lichen planus pigmentosus (LPP), pigmented contact dermatitis, macular amyloidosis, maturational hyperpigmentation, postinflammatory hyperpigmentation and pigmentary demarcation lines (PDLs) will be discussed in this chapter.

LICHEN PLANUS PIGMENTOSUS

Lichen planus pigmentosus is a disease of unknown etiology, characterized by presence of dark brown colored macules in sun-exposed parts of the body. This disease is more common in women, in individual with darker skin and may be associated with pruritus. Pigmentation can be diffuse, reticular, blotchy, or perifollicular. Pigmentation involves face, neck and flexures.[1,2] Dermoscopy of LPP shows the following:

- Hem-like distribution of cluster of pigments
- Perifollicular pigment deposition
- Perieccrine pigment deposition
- Granules appear bluish to slate gray in color and appear larger as compared to pigmented contact dermatitis (Figs 1 to 4).

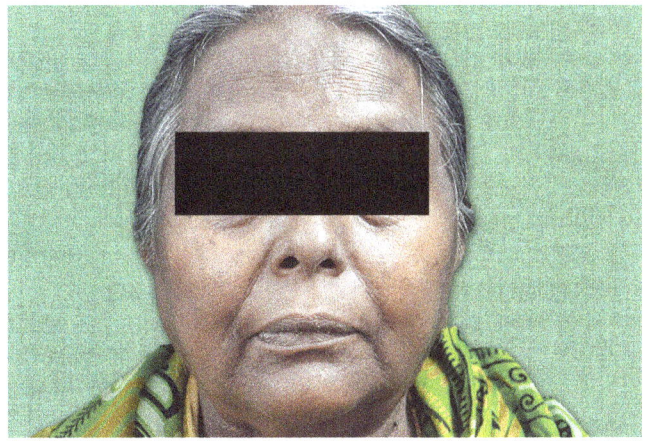

Fig. 1: Lichen planus pigmentosus: Presence of dark brown macules on sun-exposed parts of the body

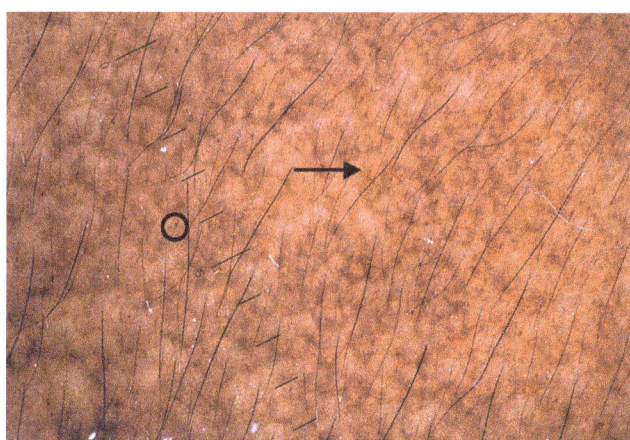

Fig. 2: Reticular network of pigmentation
Note: Hem-like pattern, reticulations are thicker as compared to pigmented contact dermatitis (black arrow). Granules are also thicker (black circle)

Section 2 Disorders of Pigmentation

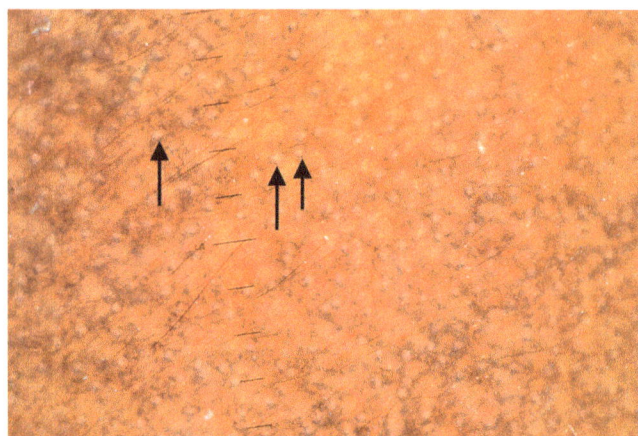

Fig. 3: Presence of pigment granules around eccrine openings (black arrow). Granules are slate gray in color suggesting deep dermal location of pigment

PIGMENTED CONTACT DERMATITIS OR RIEHL-LIKE MELANOSIS

Pigmented contact dermatitis is a noneczematous variant of contact dermatitis. It is characterized clinically by hyperpigmentation, which results from repeated contact with allergen. The most common cosmetic agents causing pigmented contact dermatitis in Indian patients are kumkum and hair dye. Face is the most common site involved.[3,4] Dermoscopy of pigmented contact dermatitis shows the following:

- Reticular pigment network
- Regular distribution of fine pigment granules
- As compared to LPP, in pigmented contact dermatitis granules are smaller, appear black in color and arranged regularly. This occurs possibly because of extensive basal cell damage and lymphocytic infiltrate at dermoepidermal junction in LPP (Figs 5 to 8).

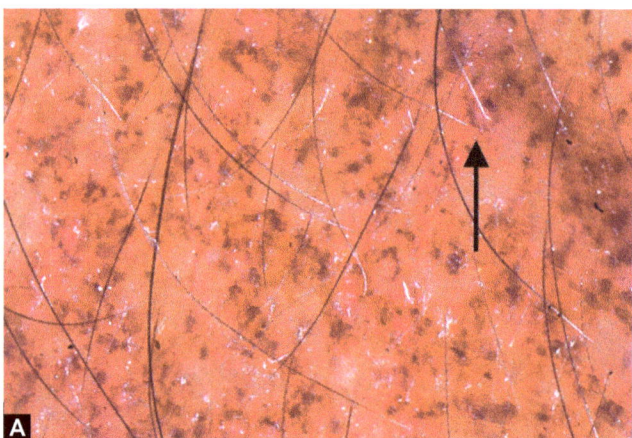

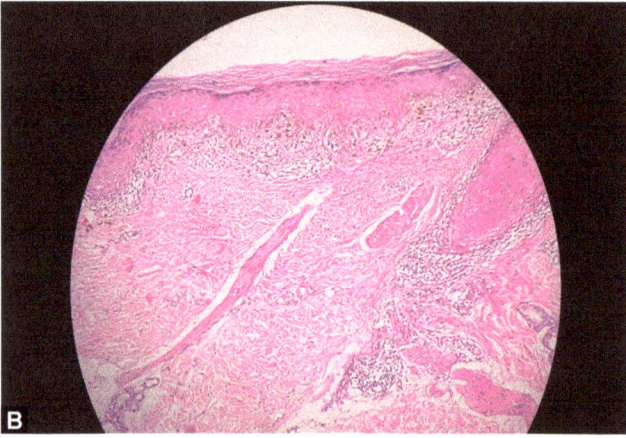

Figs 4A and B: (A) Perifollicular pigment granules in lichen planus pigmentosus (black arrow) in a digitally magnified image; (B) Histopathology (H&E 10X): Shows band-like lymphomononuclear infiltration at dermoepidermal junction and pigment incontinence in upper epidermis

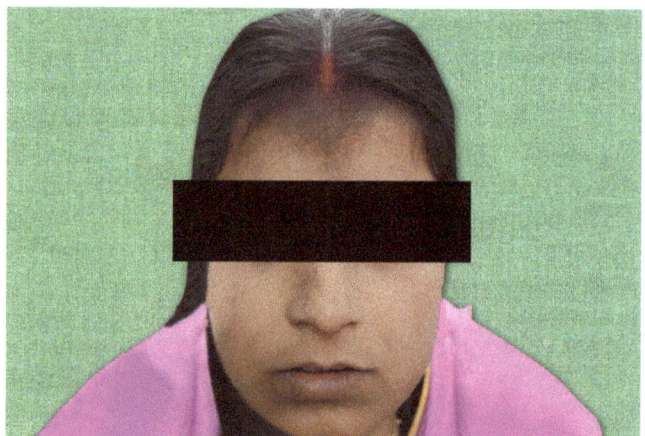

Fig. 5: Pigmented contact dermatitis: Presence of dark brown macules in area of kumkum application

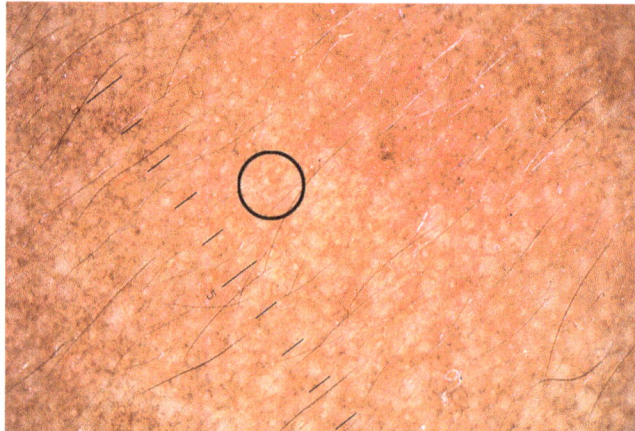

Fig. 6: Reticular network of pigmentation. Presence of fine granules superimposed on reticular network of pigmentation suggests pigmented contact dermatitis

Chapter 5 Nonmelasma Facial Melanoses

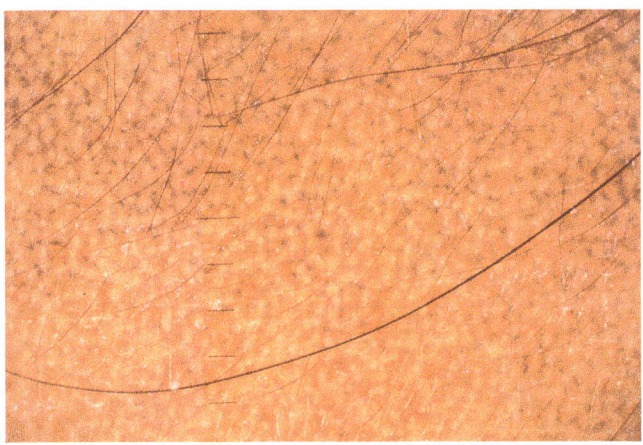

Fig. 7: Reticular network of pigmentation. Pigment granules are larger as compared to previous image and are more akin to lichen planus pigmentosus, however, arrangement of granules is regular giving it a net-like appearance

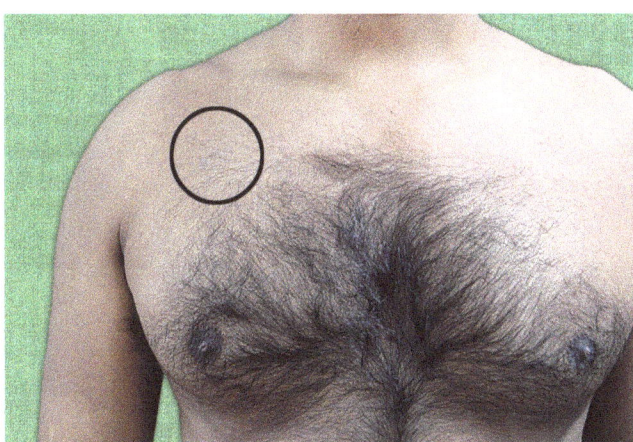

Fig. 9: Erythema dyschromicum perstans: Slate-gray macules on trunk and extremities (black circle)

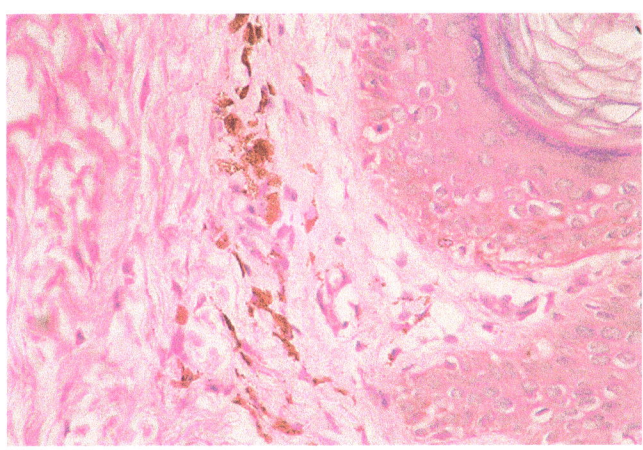

Fig. 8: Histopathology (H & E 40X): Shows pigment incontinence in upper dermis, mild basal vacuolation is seen. No lichenoid infiltrate is seen as opposed to lichen planus pigmentosus. Spongiosis is not prominent, hence it is known as noneczematous contact dermatitis

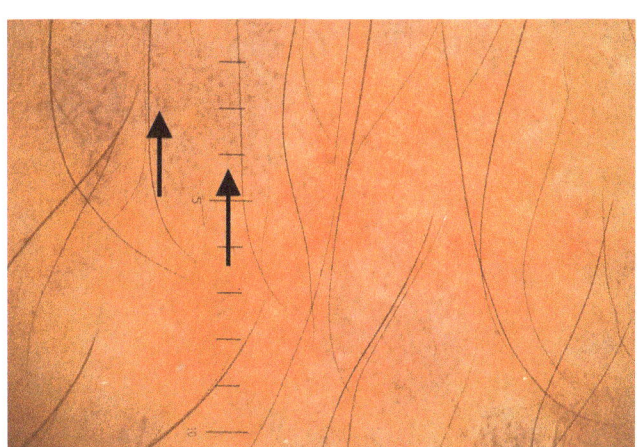

Fig. 10: Normal reticular network of pigment appears broader but becomes blunt and broken at places. Color of the pigment is slate gray (black arrow)

ERYTHEMA DYSCHROMICUM PERSTANS OR ASHY DERMATOSES

Erythema dyschromicum perstans (EDP) is a pigmentary disorder of unknown etiology and overlaps with LPP and Riehl melanoses, not only in morphology, but also in etiology to some extent creating a nosological confusion. It is characterized by presence of slate-gray macules with erythematous borders, present over face, trunk and extremities.[5] Dermoscopy shows exaggeration of normal pigmentary reticular pattern. Reticulations become broader, blunted and broken at places. Color of pigment is slate-gray on dermoscopy (Figs 9 and 10).

MATURATIONAL DYSCHROMIA OR MATURATIONAL HYPERPIGMENTATION

It is a common pigmentary disorder of face, which occurs in middle-aged individuals. Sun exposure may play a role in its etiology. It is characterized by presence of homogenous, symmetrical, hyperpigmented macules on lateral forehead and cheek bones. Dermoscopy shows presence of perifollicular pigment (Figs 11A and B).

Section 2 Disorders of Pigmentation

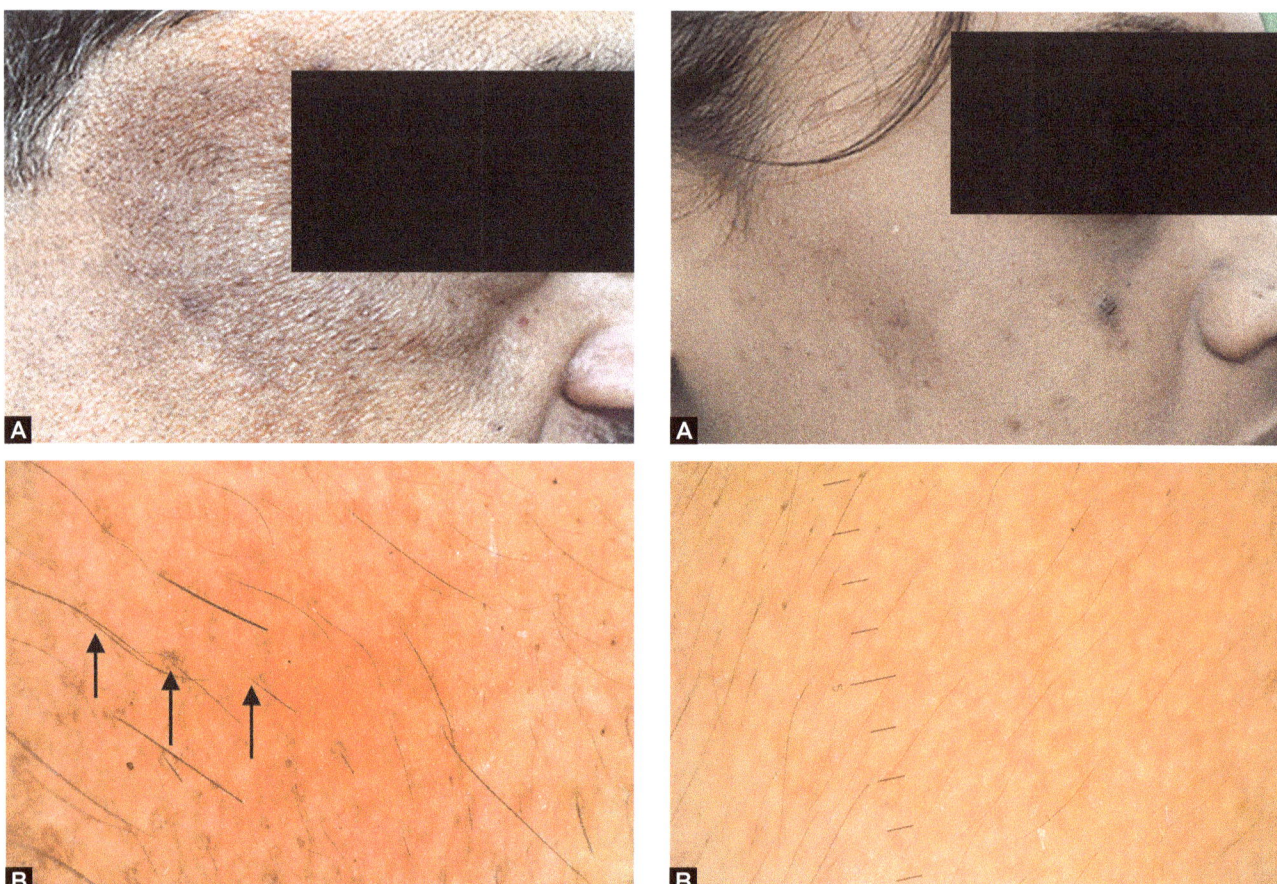

Figs 11 A and B: (A) Clinical photograph of maturational hyperpigmentation; (B) Dermoscopy shows perifollicular pigmentation

Figs 12 A and B: (A) Clinical photograph showing pigmentary demarcation line-face (PDL-F); (B) Dermoscopy showing exaggerated pseudoreticular pattern

ACANTHOSIS NIGRICANS

Acanthosis nigricans is characterized by presence of symmetric hyperpigmented plaque involving the malar region, tending to spare the zygomatic area. It tends to occur in individuals who are obese and diabetic. Examination of neck, axilla and groin shows similar involvement with presence of velvety hyperpigmented plaque.

PIGMENTARY DEMARCATION LINE

Pigmentary demarcation line-face (PDL-F) are V-shaped hyperpigmented patches, bilaterally symmetrical, present between malar prominence and temple.[6] Dermoscopy shows either normal pseudoreticular pattern or exaggeration of this pseudoreticular pattern. Because there is no specific pattern other than what is normally seen on the face, it is often termed as "patternless" (Figs 12A and B).

REFERENCES

1. Rieder E, Kaplan J, Kamino H, Sanchez M, Pomeranz MK. Lichen planus pigmentosus. Dermatol Online J. 2013;19:20713.
2. Kanwar AJ, Dogra S, Handa S, Parsad D, Radotra BD. A study of 124 Indian patients with lichen planus pigmentosus. Clin Exp Dermatol. 2003;28:481-5.
3. Nath AK, Thappa DM. Kumkum-induced dermatitis: An analysis of 46 cases. Clin Exp Dermatol. 2007;32:385-7.
4. Shenoi SD, Rao R. Pigmented contact dermatitis. Indian J Dermatol Venereol Leprol. 2007;73:285-7
5. Zaynoun S, Rubeiz N, Kibbi AG. Ashy dermatoses-a critical review of the literature and a proposed simplified clinical classification. Int J Dermatol. 2008;47:542-4.
6. Somani VK, Razvi F, Sita VV. Pigmentary demarcation lines over the face. Indian J Dermatol Venereol Leprol. 2004;70:336-41

CHAPTER 6

Other Disorders of Hyperpigmentation

Shekhar Neema

INTRODUCTION

Dermoscopy can be used for diagnosis of various other disorders of hyperpigmentation like acanthosis nigricans, primary cutaneous amyloidosis, fixed-drug eruption, acropigmentation of Kitamura and Dowling-Degos disease (DDD).

PRIMARY CUTANEOUS AMYLOIDOSIS

Primary cutaneous amyloidosis is a common pigmentary disorder and is composed of macular amyloidosis, lichen amyloidosis and biphasic amyloidosis. It can be diagnosed clinically; however, differential diagnosis includes lichen simplex chronicus, postinflammatory hyperpigmentation and prurigo nodularis. Dermoscopy can help in diagnosis in atypical cases. Dermoscopy reveals central hub which can either be brown or white in color and presence of fine streaks around that central hub in some cases, typically called as "hub and spoke" pattern (Figs 1 and 2).[1]

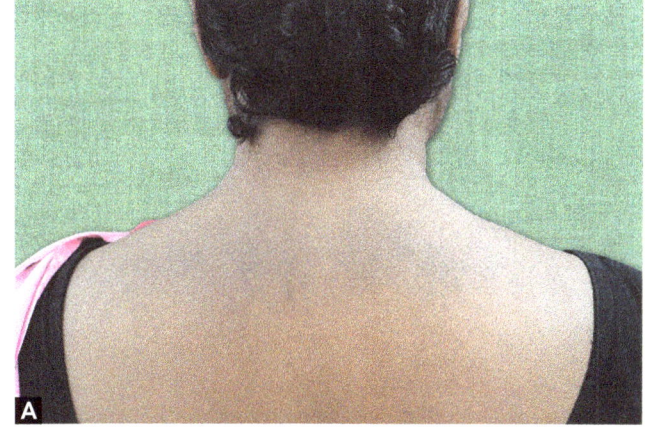

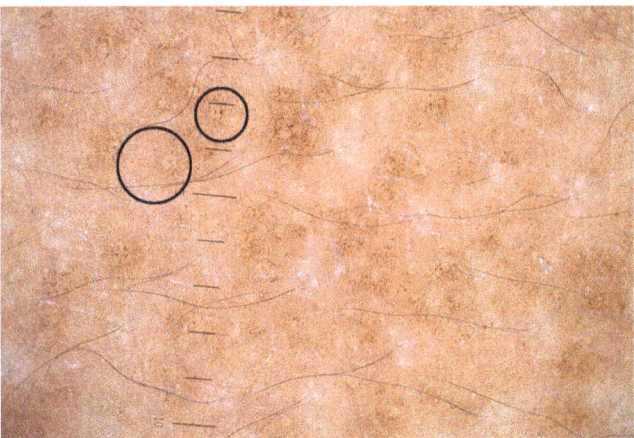

Fig. 1: Dermoscopy of macular amyloidosis: Central brown hub and radiating fine streaks (black circle)

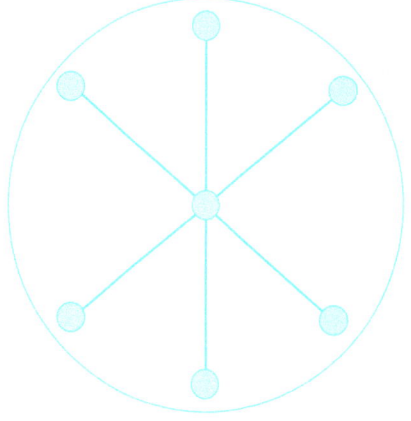

Figs 2A and B: (A) Clinical photograph: Macular amyloidosis; (B) Hub and spoke pattern: Schematic diagram

ACANTHOSIS NIGRICANS

It is characterized by velvety hyperpigmented plaque and involves mainly intertriginous area. It is commonly associated with obesity and diabetes mellitus, other causes being familial, acral, drug induced and malignancy associated. Dermoscopy of acanthosis nigricans has been described as linear crista cutis and sulcus cutis and hyperpigmented dots in crista cutis (Figs 3 to 5).[2]

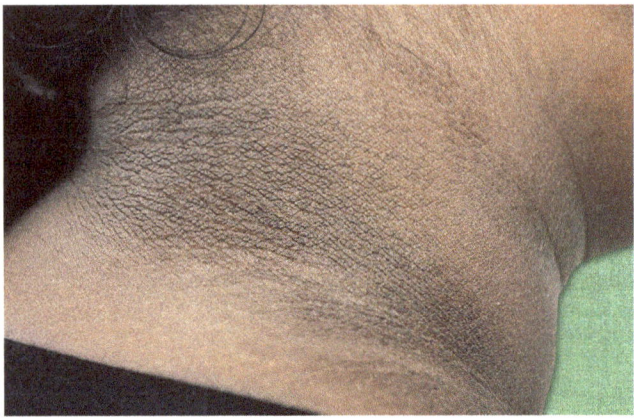

Fig. 3: Clinical photograph: Acanthosis nigricans

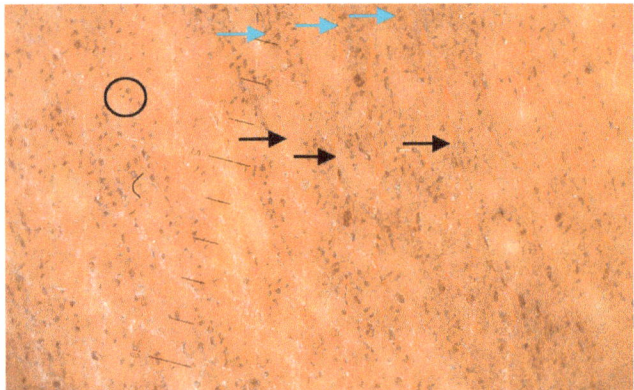

Fig. 4: Dermoscopy picture showing linear crista cutis (blue arrow) and sulcus cutis (black arrow), they appear like sulci and gyri in brain. Presence of hyperpigmented dots in crista cutis (black circle)

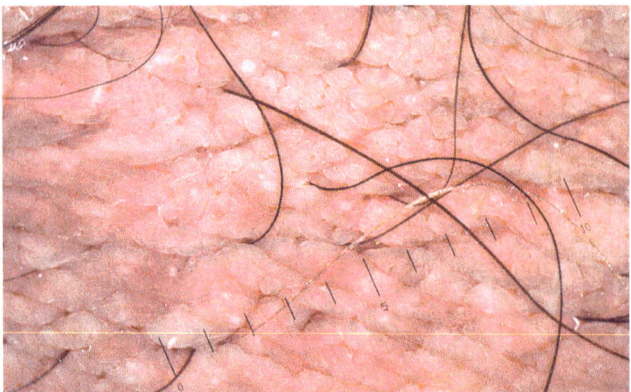

Fig. 5: Digitally magnified view showing linear crista cutis and sulcus cutis

DOWLING-DEGOS DISEASE

It is a genodermatosis characterized by gradually progressive hyperpigmented macules involving flexures, other features being follicular papules and pitted perioral scars. Hypopigmented macules can also be present in generalized variant of DDD. Dyschromatosis universalis hereditaria can overlap clinically with this variant with presence of hypopigmented and hyperpigmented macules. Dermoscopy of hyperpigmented macule shows accentuation of reticular pattern and palmar pits shows keratinous plugging (Figs 6 to 8).[3]

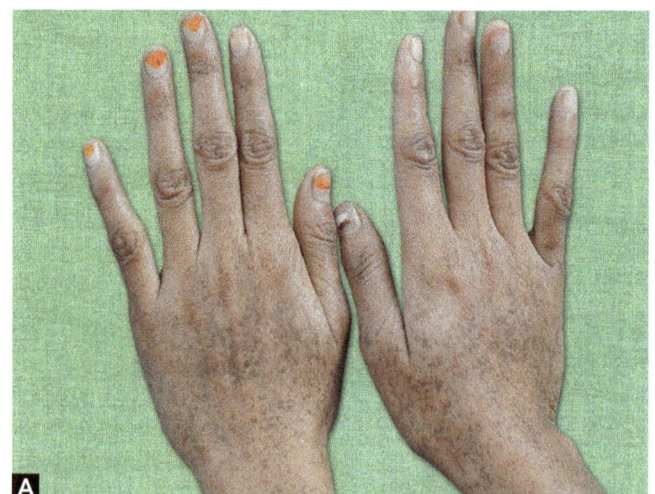

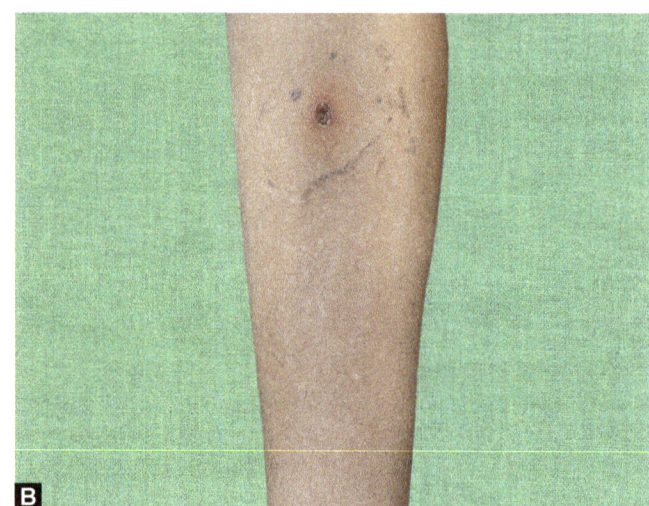

Figs 6A and B: (A) Reticulate hyperpigmentation on dorsum of hands; (B) Hypopigmented macules on leg

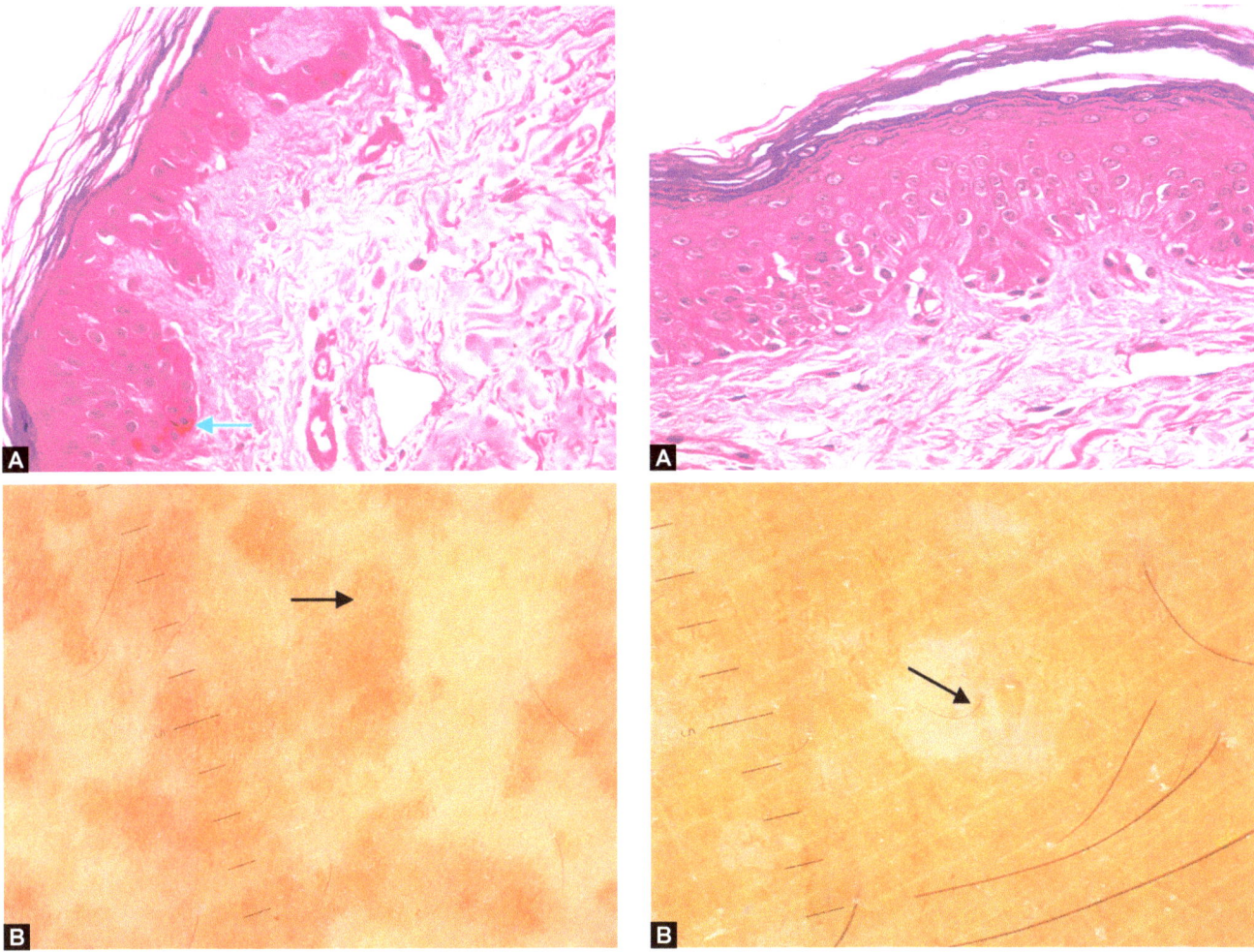

Figs 7A and B: (A) Histopathology of hyperpigmented macule (H&E stain 40X)—irregular elongation of rete ridges with presence of pigment at tip of rete ridges (blue arrow); (B) Dermoscopy of hyperpigmented macule (Heine Delta 20–20X, polarised light)—accentuation of reticular pattern and presence of thick branching reticular pattern (black arrow)

Figs 8A and B: (A) Histopathology of hypopigmented macule (H&E stain 40X)—absence of pigment in basal layer; (B) Dermoscopy of hypopigmented macule (Heine Delta 20–20X, polarised light)—circumscribed absence of pigmentation with retention of perifollicular pigment (arrow)

ACROPIGMENTATION OF KITAMURA

It is characterized by presence of hyperpigmented brownish macules on acral areas of body, absence of hypopigmented macule anywhere on body, presence of slight depression corresponding to areas of pigmentation and punctate depression on palms and soles. Dermoscopy of hyperpigmented macules shows presence of fine reticular pigment network.[4]

FIXED DRUG ERUPTION

Fixed drug eruption (FDE) is clinically characterized by solitary to multiple hyperpigmented macules. Dermoscopy shows multiple slate-gray pigmented granules of varying size, suggesting deep dermal location of pigment (Figs 9A and B).

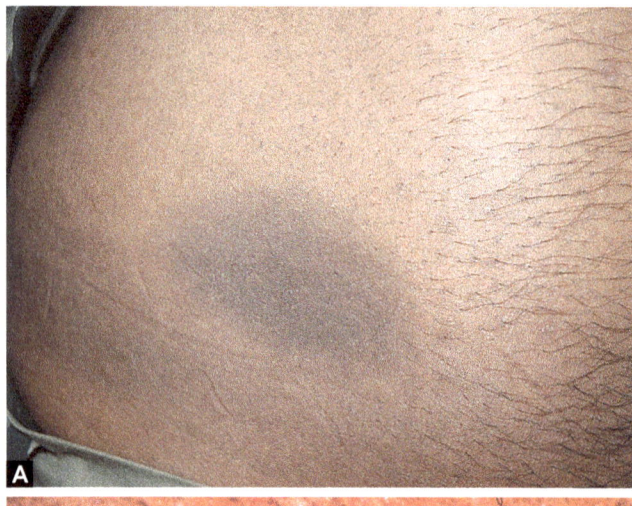

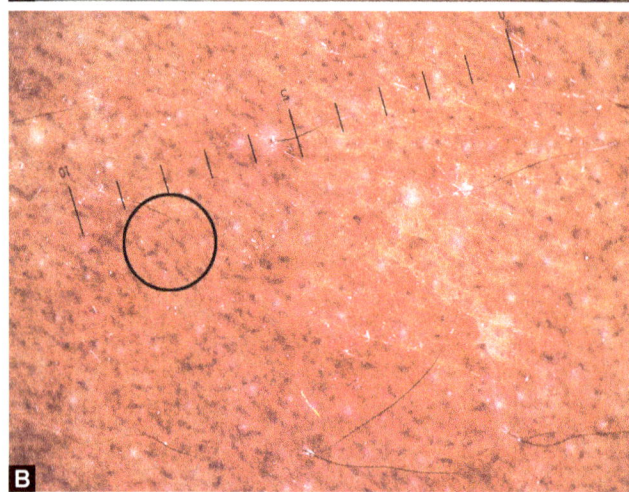

Figs 9A and B: (A) Clinical picture: Fixed drug eruption; (B) Multiple slate-gray colored pigmented granules of varying size can be seen

CONCLUSION

Dermoscopic criteria for diagnosis of disorders of hyperpigmentation will continue to evolve as it is going to be used more and more for their diagnosis in conjunction with histopathology.

REFERENCES

1. Chuang YY, Lee DD, Lin CS, Chang YJ, Tanaka M, Chang YT, Liu HN. Characteristic dermoscopic features of primary cutaneous amyloidosis: a study of 35 cases. Br J Dermatol. 2012;167(3):548-54.
2. Uchida S, Oiso N, Suzuki T, Kawada A. Dermoscopic features of hyperpigmented dots in crista cutis in two siblings in a Japanese family with inherited acanthosis nigricans. J Cosmetics Dermatol Sci Appl. 2012;2:252-3.
3. Nirmal B, Dongre AM, Khopkar US. Dermatoscopic features of hyper and hypopigmented lesions of Dowling-Degos disease. Indian J Dermatol. 2015;61(1):125.
4. Koguchi H, Ujiie H, Aoyagi S, Osawa R, Shimizu H. Characteristic findings of handprint and dermoscopy in reticulate acropigmentation of Kitamura. Clin Exp Dermatol. 2014;39(1):85-7.

CHAPTER 7

Vitiligo and Other Disorders of Hypopigmentation

Shekhar Neema, Niti Khunger

INTRODUCTION

Pigmentary disorders of skin are quite common in dermatology practice in the Indian population. Disorders of hypopigmentation can result from varied etiology like infectious, inflammatory, genetic, autoimmune or malignancy. These disorders especially vitiligo and leprosy are associated with social stigma in dark-skinned individuals. Dermoscopy can be a useful tool in differentiating various hypopigmentary disorders.

VITILIGO

Vitiligo is an acquired, depigmenting disorder of the skin characterized clinically by white macules and histopathologically by an absence of functional melanocytes in the affected area.[1] It has a severe psychosocial impact in the affected person, greatly affecting the quality of life. The relative prevalence is higher in India, being 0.46–8.8% as compared to the worldwide incidence of 0.1–2%. Vitiligo is usually classified into two broad types: (1) nonsegmental vitiligo (NSV) and segmental vitiligo (SV). The natural course of the disease varies greatly. NSV usually has a chronic, slowly progressive course and may show periods of sudden activity. Patients with SV usually have rapid progression following an abrupt onset, which later becomes quiescent and stable. Stability in vitiligo is important from the therapeutic and prognostic point of view. Since, there are no definite criteria to prove stability, dermoscopy may be used as a noninvasive procedure.

Leukotrichia (presence of white hairs) is generally present and Koebner's phenomenon suggests active disease. Trichrome, quadrichrome, pentachrome, blue vitiligo and inflammatory vitiligo are morphological variants of vitiligo.[1]

Various dermoscopy patterns which have been described in vitiligo are trichrome pattern, reticular pattern, perifollicular pigmentation, salt and pepper pigmentation, star-burst pattern, polka-dot pattern, comet-tail appearance, marginal hyperpigmentation, reversed pigmentary network and leukotrichia.[2] Different dermoscopy patterns have been described in association with various stages of vitiligo like evolving vitiligo, stable vitiligo, unstable vitiligo and repigmenting vitiligo.

Utility of Dermoscopy in Vitiligo

The utility of dermoscopy in vitiligo has been studied recently and appears to be a promising new technique to differentiate, evaluate and prognosticate the response to treatment. Following are few of the uses of dermoscopy in vitiligo:
- To differentiate vitiligo from other hypo- and depigmenting disorders
- To assess stability of vitiligo: Lesional and global
- To aid in selecting treatment modality: Medical or surgical
- To evaluate the response to treatment
- To assist in prognosis of the disease.

Stability in Vitiligo

Stability in vitiligo is the most important criteria before any surgical treatment can be performed. Indian Association of Dermatologists, Venereologists and Leprologists (IADVL) task force recommends period of 1 year of clinical stability of disease before any surgical procedure can be carried out.[3] However, this concept of stability has been challenged and a new concept of lesional stability has been introduced.[4] Dermoscopy can be useful in finding out lesional stability.

- Following dermoscopy patterns have been described with unstable disease, however, they require further validation with larger studies:[2,5]
    - Trichrome appearance
    - Comet-tail appearance
    - Star-burst appearance
    - Polka-dot appearance
- Marginal hyperpigmentation, perifollicular repigmentation and reticular pigmentation were associated with stability of disease.
- Salt and pepper pattern has been described with unstable disease in one study, while stable disease in another study. In our opinion, salt and pepper pattern indicates unstable disease.[2,5]

Use of Dermoscopy for Evolving Vitiligo

Evolving vitiligo has been studied by Thatte and Khopkar. They have described reduced pigmentary network, absent pigmentary network and reverse pigmentary network as common dermoscopic finding of evolving vitiligo. Diffuse white glow was seen in majority of patient with evolving vitiligo (Figs 1 to 6).[6]

DIFFERENTIATING VITILIGO FROM IDIOPATHIC GUTTATE HYPOMELANOSES

Idiopathic guttate hypomelanoses (IGH) is a disorder of unknown etiology, characterized by presence of 2–5 mm size porcelain white hypopigmented macules on extremities. It is generally seen in older individuals and in sun-exposed areas.[7] Dermoscopy can be helpful in distinguishing IGH from guttate vitiligo.[8] Dermoscopic pattern seen in IGH are as follows (Figs 7 to 9):

- Ameboid pattern
- Feathery pattern
- Petaloid pattern
- Nebuloid pattern

CONCLUSION

Dermoscopy is an important non-invasive tool to diagnose vitiligo, to know the stability of vitiligo and to differentiate it from other disorders of hypopigmentation.

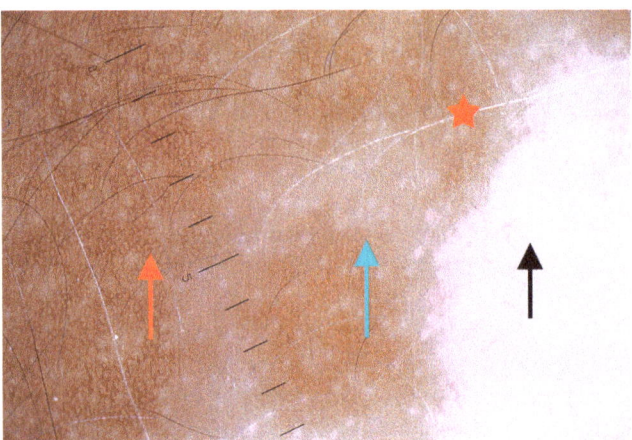

Fig. 1: Trichrome pattern on dermoscopy suggests unstable disease
Note: Normal skin (red arrow), hypopigmented zone (blue arrow) and depigmented zone (black arrow). Leukotrichia can also be seen (red star)

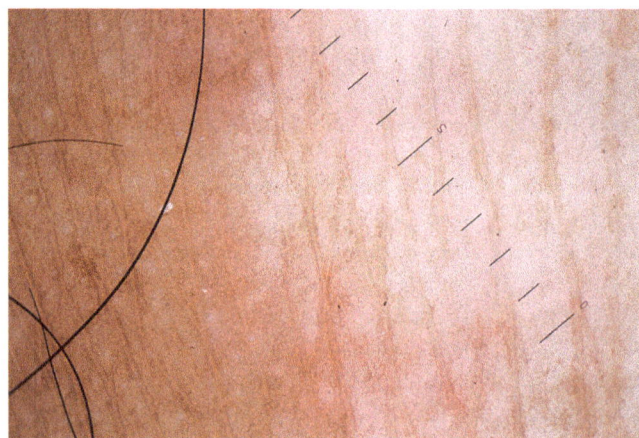

Fig. 2: Reduced pigmentary network in evolving vitiligo

Chapter 7 Vitiligo and Other Disorders of Hypopigmentation

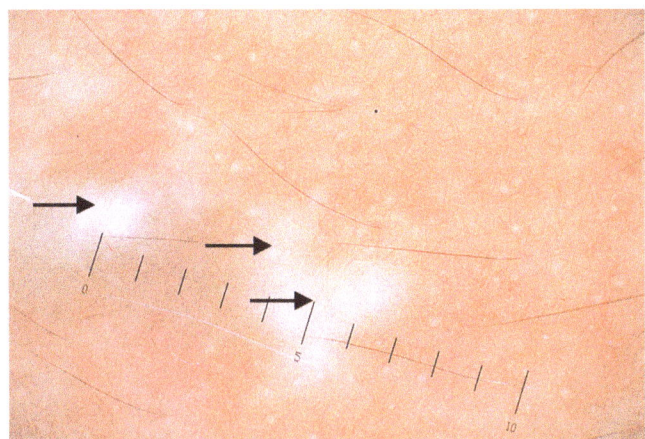

Fig. 3: Evolving vitiligo with reversal of pigmentary network (black arrow)

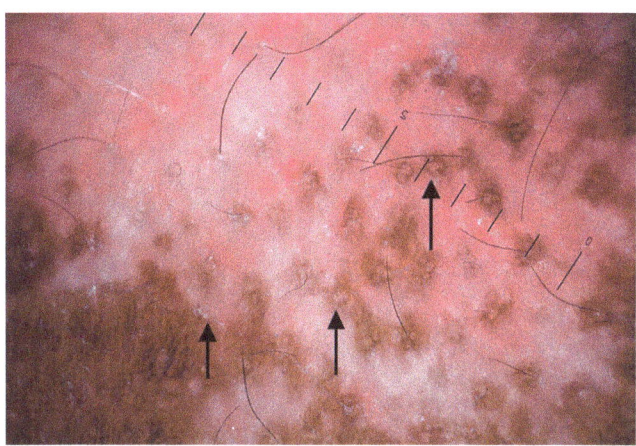

Fig. 6: Perifollicular pigmentation and marginal hyperpigmentation (black arrow) suggest stable disease and repigmenting vitiligo

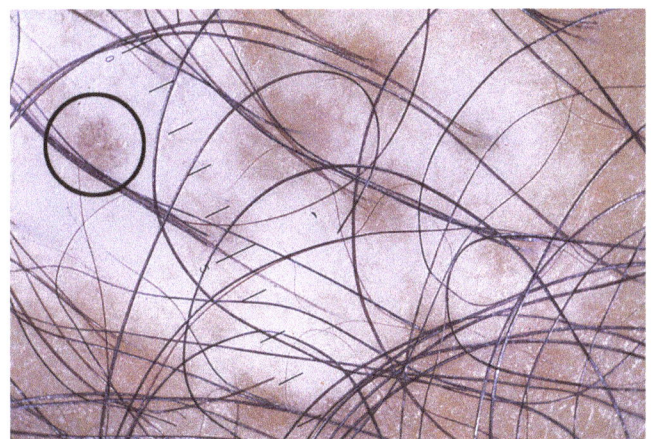

Fig. 4: Stable vitiligo: Reticular pattern of pigmentation is associated with stability and repigmentation

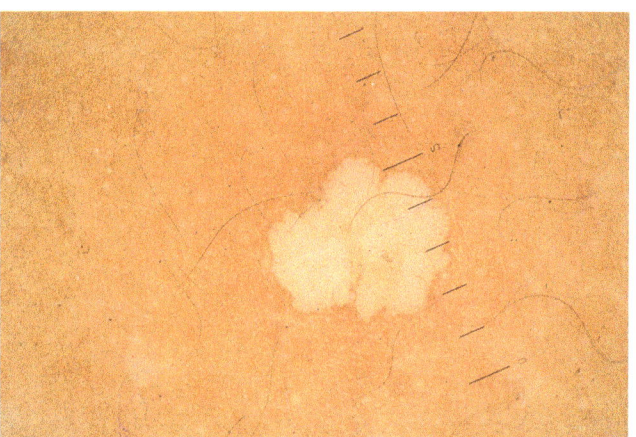

Fig. 7: Petaloid pattern seen in idiopathic guttate hypomelanoses (IGH). It has well-defined borders

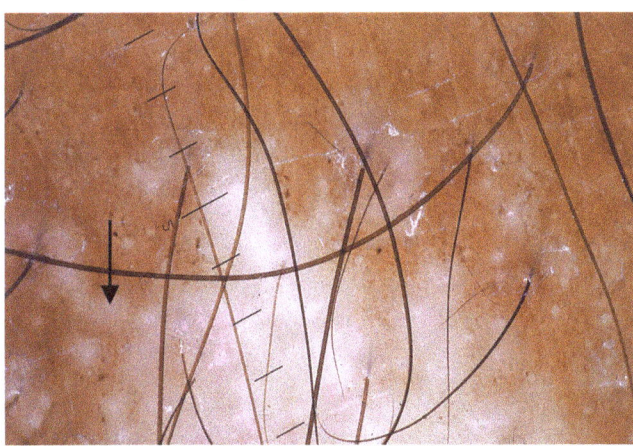

Fig. 5: Comet-tail appearance (black arrow): Indicates Koebner's phenomenon and active disease

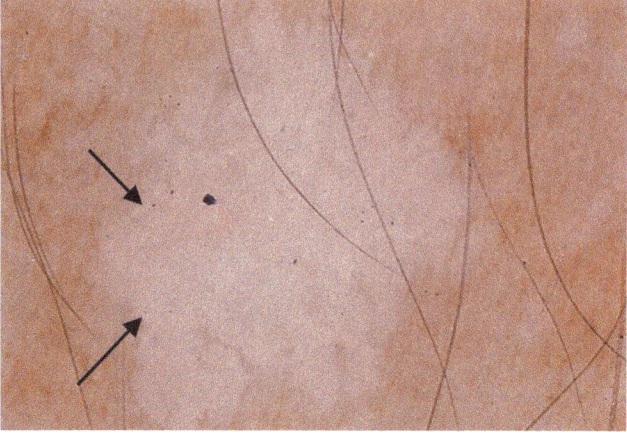

Fig. 8: Ameboid pattern seen in idiopathic guttate hypomelanoses (IGH). Borders resembling pseudopodia (black arrow)

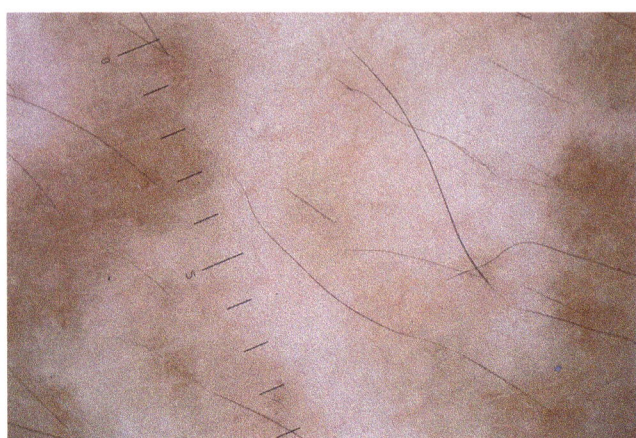

Fig. 9: In contrast to Figure 8, in active vitiligo borders are blurred

REFERENCES

1. Sehgal VN, Srivastava G. Vitiligo: Compendium of clinico-epidemiological features. Indian J Dermatol Venereol Leprol. 2007;73:149-56.
2. Wali V, Deepali M, Hogade AS, Hogade S. A panoramic study of dermascopic patterns in vitiligo. Int Med J. 2016;3(4):4.
3. Parsad D, Gupta S, IADVL Dermatosurgery Task Force. Standard guidelines of care for vitiligo surgery. Indian J Dermatol Venereol Leprol. 2008;74 Suppl:S37-45.
4. Majid I, Mysore V, Salim T, Lahiri K, Chatterji M, Khunger N, et al. Is lesional stability in vitiligo more important than disease stability for performing surgical interventions? Results from a multicentric study. J Cutan Aesthet Surg. 2016;9:13-9.
5. Chandrashekhar L. Dermoscopy: A tool to assess stability in vitiligo. Khopkar U (Ed). Dermoscopy and Trichoscopy in Diseases of Brown Skin: Atlas and Short Text. New Delhi: Jaypee; 2012. pp. 91-6.
6. Thatte SS, Khopkar US. The utility of dermoscopy in the diagnosis of evolving lesions of vitiligo. Indian J Dermatol Venereol Leprol. 2014;80:505-8.
7. Kim SK, Kim EH, Kang HY, Lee ES, Sohn S, Kim YC. Comprehensive understanding of idiopathic guttate hypomelanosis: Clinical and histopathological correlation. Int J Dermatol. 2010;49:162-6.
8. Ankad BS, Beergouder SL. Dermoscopic evaluation of idiopathic guttate hypomelanosis: A preliminary observation. Indian Dermatol Online J. 2015;6:164-7

CHAPTER 8

Differentiation of Nevus Depigmentosus, Ash Leaf Macules and Nevus Anemicus

Surit Malakar, Samipa Mukherjee

INTRODUCTION

Nevus depigmentosus (ND) is a localized hypopigmentation which most of the time is congenital and not uncommonly a diagnostic challenge. The parent generally notices the lesion at birth or few months subsequently after birth. The lesions have a strong psychological impact due to the cosmetic concerns and also due to resemblance with vitiligo.

Simple diagnostic techniques like diascopy help in arriving at a conclusion. With the advent of newer noninvasive diagnostic tools like dermoscopy, it helps in easy diagnosis, documentation and alleviates the anxiety of parents.

Common differentials include the following:
- Ash leaf macule
- Nevus anemicus
- Vitiligo.

NORMAL PIGMENTARY PATTERN ON SKIN

The normal pigmentary pattern on skin is represented by a reticulate pigmentary pattern which corresponds to the rete ridges histologically (Figs 1A and B).

Nevus Anemicus

It is defined as patchy hypopigmentation due to a localized hypersensitivity to catecholamines with resultant vasoconstriction (Figs 2A and B).

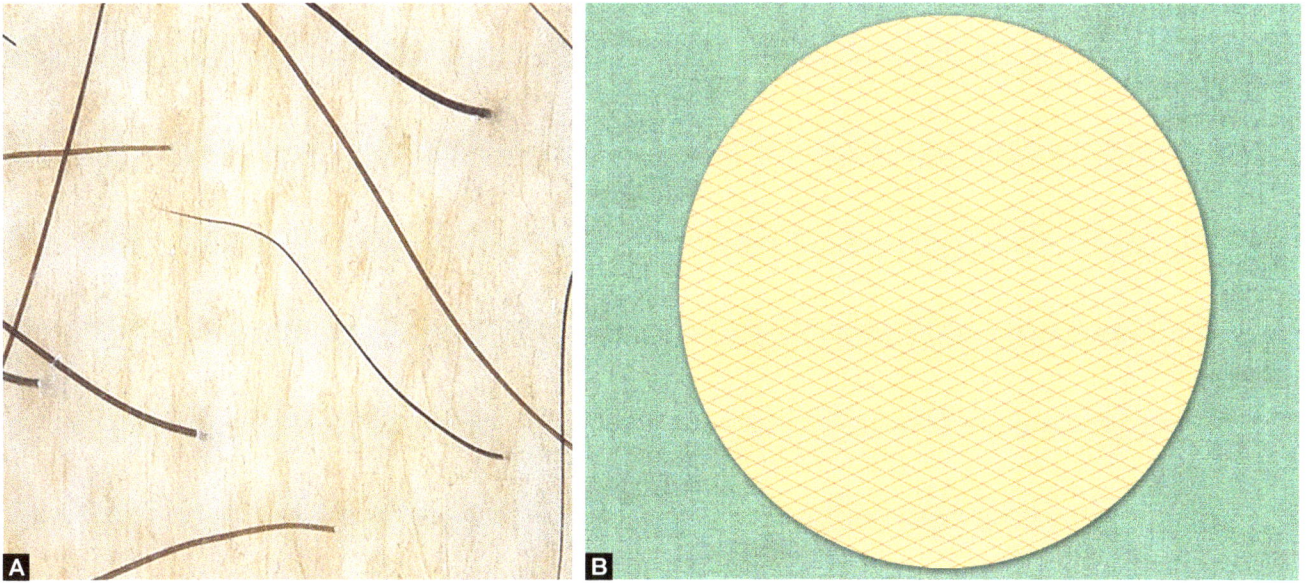

Figs 1A and B: (A) Reticular pigmentary pattern on skin; (B) Schematic diagram of reticular pigmentary pattern

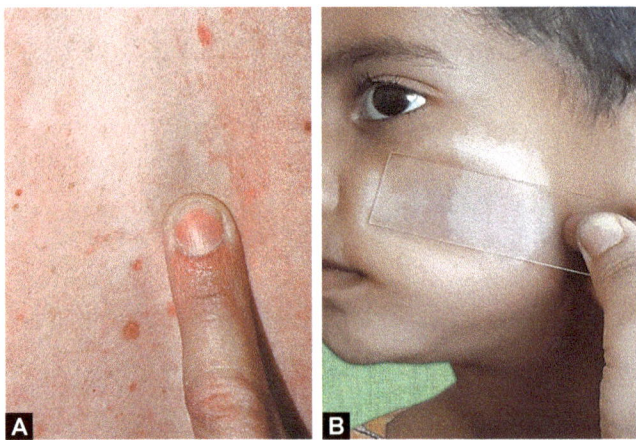

Figs 2A and B: (A) Nevus anemicus; (B) Nevus depigmentosus

Vitiligo

Vitiligo is an autoimmune disease of unknown etiology characterized by destruction and absence of melanocytes. Clinically, it presents as well-defined hypo- to depigmented patches on the skin.

Dermoscopically, vitiligo lesions show complete absence of reticulate pigmentary network as opposed to the normal skin (Fig. 3).

Fig. 3: Vitiligo: Dermoscopy shows absence of reticular pigmentary network

Ash Leaf Macule

This lesion has acquired its name from the resemblance of its morphology to an ash leaf which is invariably lanceolate in shape. Less than two ash leaf macule (ALM) can be seen in normal individuals without tuberous sclerosis complex (TSC). However, three or more ALM is a major diagnostic criteria for TSC. In more than 90% of cases, ALM is the first to appear at birth or during infancy (when other clinical features of TSC may not be evident) and likely to go unnoticed or remain under diagnosed or may be misdiagnosed for a benign lesion without any association to the untrained eye. Hence, ALM can produce a diagnostic challenge (if the child presents very early after birth or there are less than three lesions).

Differentiation of ALM from nevus depigmentosus (ND) becomes difficult clinically as both can present as irregular hypopigmented macules and can be segmental.

On dermoscopy, ash leaf macules are characterized by areas of faint reticular pigmentation and zones of total loss of any pigmentary pattern (Fig. 4).

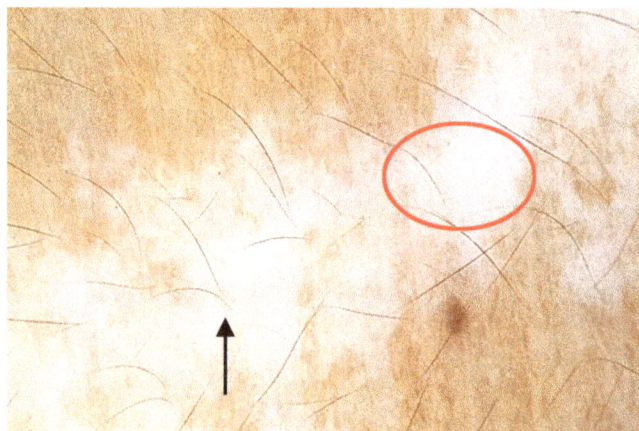

Fig. 4: Ash leaf macules: Dermoscopy shows faint reticular pigmentation (black arrow) and zones of total loss of any pigmentary pattern (red circle)

Nevus Depigmentosus

This is a lesion often present at birth. Hypopigmentation is due to the defect in transfer of melanosomes from melanocytes to keratinocytes rather than total loss of pigment. This pathology manifests itself dermoscopically as the presence of faint reticular pigment pattern as opposed to total loss of pigment (due to absent melanocytes) as in vitiligo. Melanocytes usually are normal in number and size.

Nevus depigmentosus on dermoscopy reveals uniform faint melanocytic network which correlates with the transfer defect of melanosomes. In comparison to this, dermoscopy of ALM reveals faint pigmentary network interspersed with amelanotic areas (Fig. 5).

Fig. 5: Nevus depigmentosus: Dermoscopy shows uniform faint melanocytic network

CONCLUSION

To summarize, differentiation of nevus anemicus from ND is done by dermoscopy and firmly stroking lesional area. Vitiligo shows absence of melanocytic network.

Nevus depigmentosus reveals uniform faint melanocytic network whereas faint melanocytic network interspersed with total loss of the network characterizes ALM dermoscopically.

SECTION 3
Papulosquamous Disorders

Shekhar Neema

Section Outline

- Papulosquamous Disorders

CHAPTER 9

Papulosquamous Disorders

Shekhar Neema

INTRODUCTION

Dermoscopy is an important tool for diagnosis of pigmented lesions of skin. Use of dermoscopy in inflammatory disorder has been described recently and is also known as inflammoscopy.[1] Dermoscopy in papulosquamous disorder is increasingly being utilized as an adjunct to histopathology.

Papulosquamous group of disorders are heterogenous disorders and consists of psoriasis, parapsoriasis, lichen planus, lichen striatus, lichen nitidus, pityriasis rosea, pityriasis rubra pilaris, seborrheic dermatitis, etc.[2] Dermoscopy of papulosquamous disorders has two main components: (1) presence of scales and (2) vascular pattern. Apart from psoriasis, lichen planus and pityriasis rosea, dermoscopy in most of other papulosquamous disorder is not so well defined.

PSORIASIS

Clinical diagnosis of psoriasis is not difficult. However, atypical presentations like inverse psoriasis, presence of few plaques and guttate psoriasis can be difficult to diagnose. Presence of regularly distributed dotted vessels over light red background and white scales are characteristics of psoriasis on dermoscopy.[3] Presence of homogenous vascular pattern, red dots and light red background gives a diagnostic probability of 99% for psoriasis if all three features are present.[4] This dermoscopic pattern is constant in almost all variants of psoriasis. Dermoscopic features of psoriasis are reasonably specific to allow rapid diagnosis in cases where clinical diagnosis is doubtful.

Dermoscopy can differentiate between plaque psoriasis, pityriasis rosea, lichen planus and dermatitis.[5] Psoriasis shows dotted vessels in regular arrangement and presence of white scales. Dermatitis shows patchy distribution of vessels with presence of yellow scales. Pityriasis rosea has yellowish background color associated with dotted

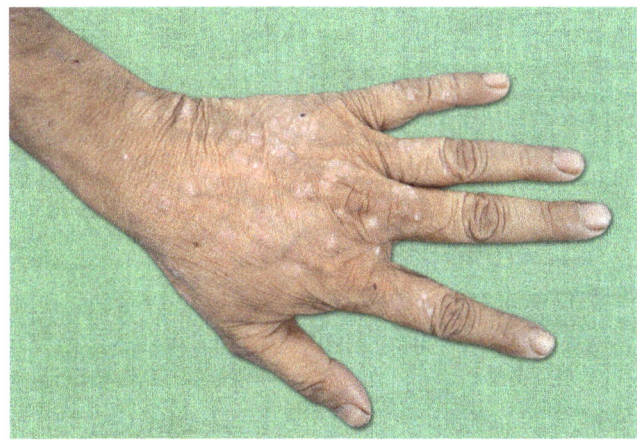

Fig. 1: Clinical photograph: Chronic plaque psoriasis

vessels and scales are peripheral. Lichen planus shows characteristic Wickham striae and peripheral arrangement of scales (Figs 1 to 6).

Section 3 Papulosquamous Disorders

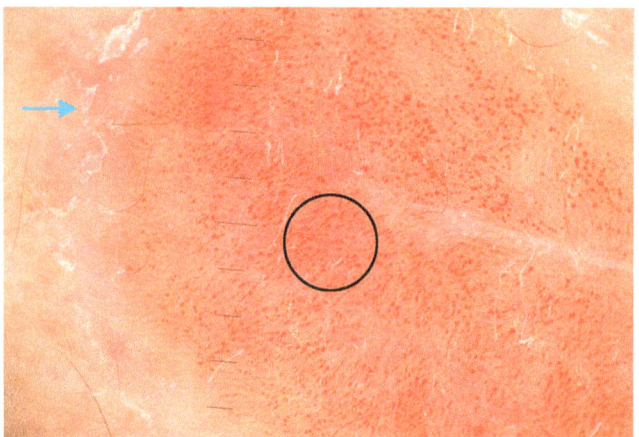

Fig. 2: Dermoscopy of chronic plaque psoriasis shows regular arrangement of dotted vessels (black circle) over homogenous red background and white scales (blue arrow)

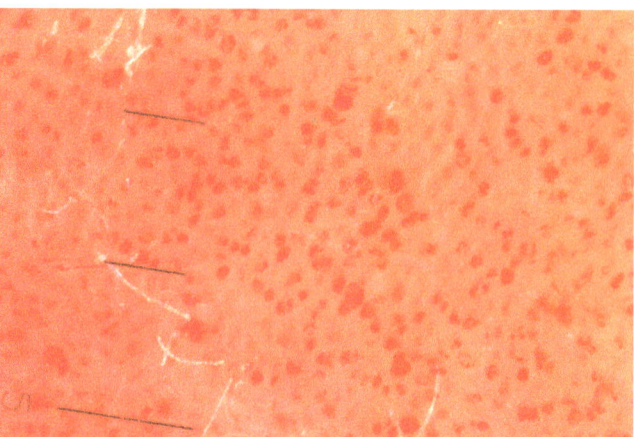

Fig. 3: Digitally magnified dermoscopic image of chronic plaque psoriasis shows regular arrangement of bushy dilated capillaries on light red background

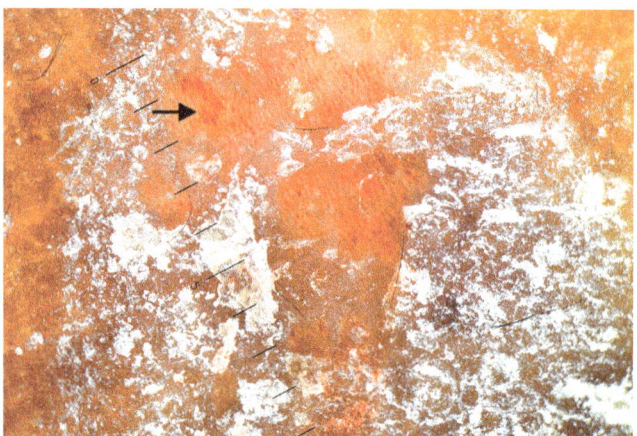

Fig. 4: Scraping of psoriatic lesion shows pinpoint bleeding, known as dermoscopic Auspitz sign (black arrow)

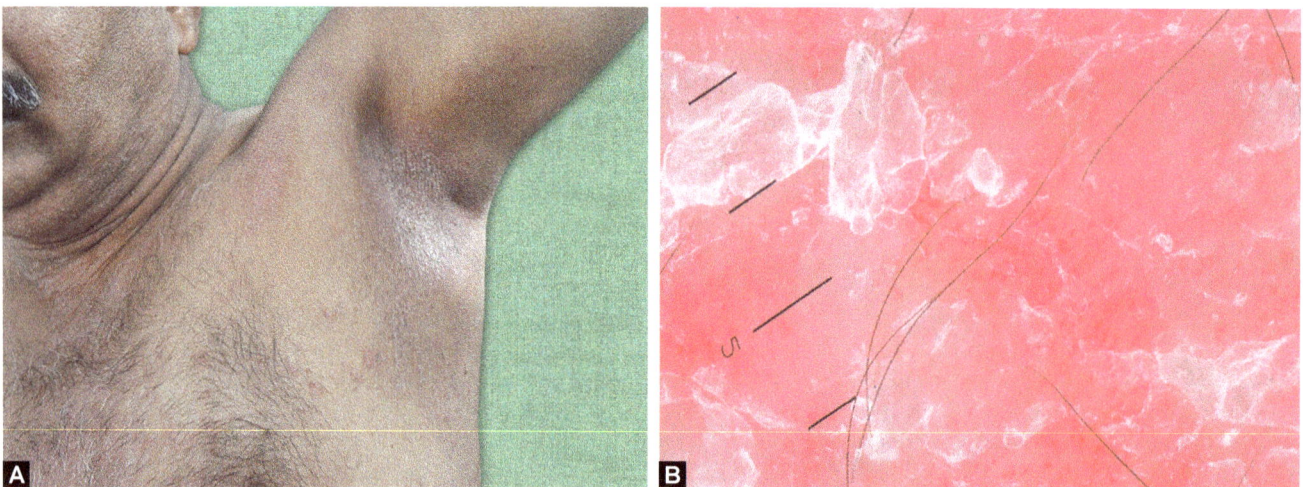

Figs 5A and B: Inverse psoriasis: Shows characteristic white scales, homogenous light red background and regular arrangement of dilated capillaries

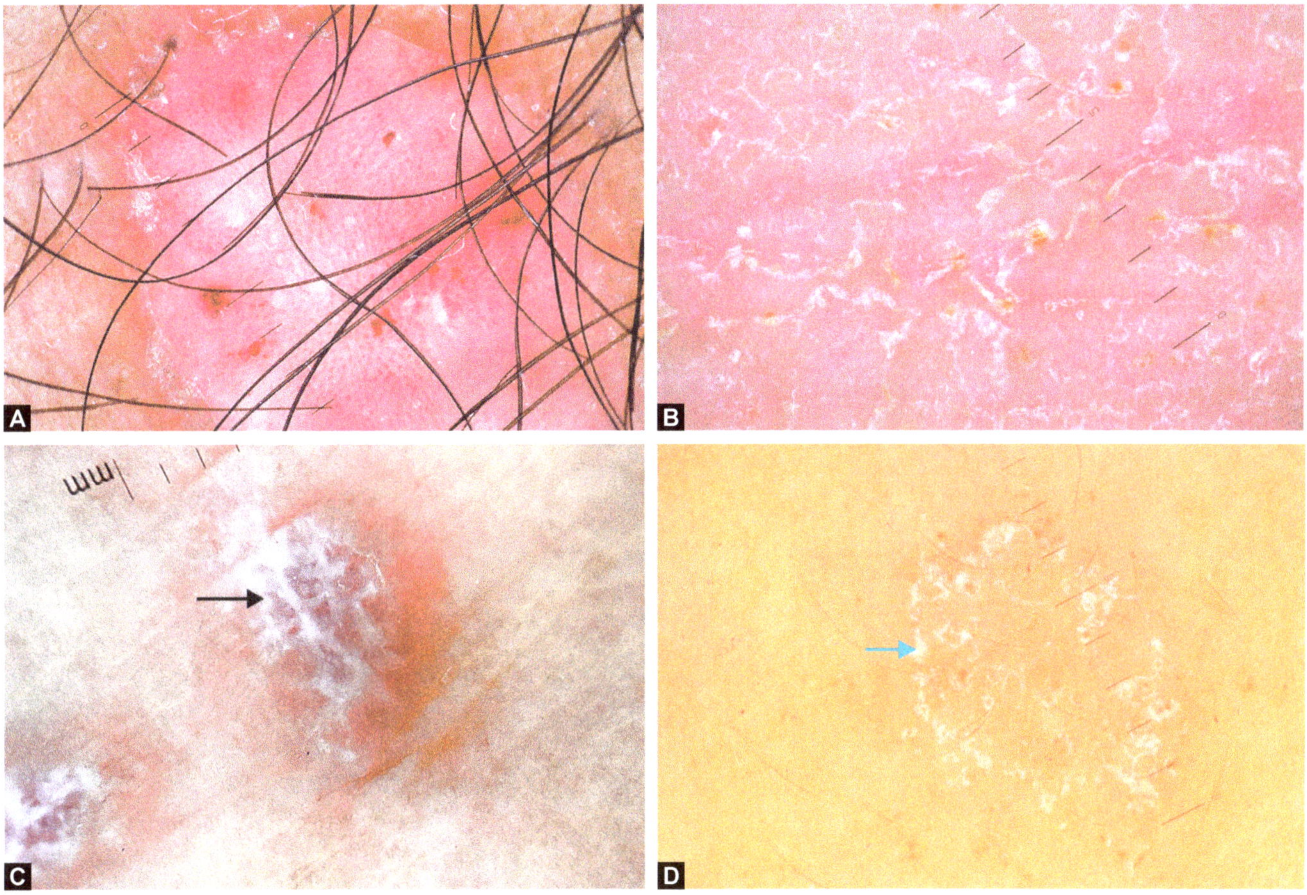

Figs 6A to D: Comparison amongst dermatitis, lichen planus, psoriasis and pityriasis rosea. (A) Presence of regular arrangement of dotted vessels on light red background and white scales seen in psoriasis; (B) Presence of yellow crusts and patchy distribution of dotted vessels is characteristic feature of dermatitis; (C) Presence of crossing white lines (Wickham's striae) is seen in lichen planus (black arrow); (D) Peripheral white collarete of scale seen in pityriasis rosea (blue arrow)

Scalp Psoriasis

Scalp psoriasis shows presence of regularly arranged dotted vessels and white scales similar to psoriasis on other parts of the body. However, presence of white scales are more common dermoscopic finding in scalp psoriasis and removal of overlying scale shows characteristic vascular pattern (Figs 7 and 8).[6]

Dermoscopy can also be used to differentiate seborrheic dermatitis of scalp from scalp psoriasis. Scales are seen in both diseases. Scalp psoriasis shows red dot and globules, glomerular vessels and annular vessels, while seborrheic dermatitis shows atypical vessels and arborizing vessels (Fig. 9).[7] Vascular morphology is visible in higher magnification (50X).

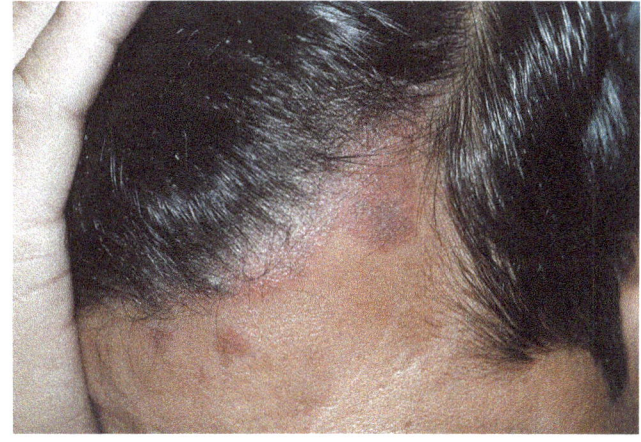

Fig. 7: Clinical photograph: Scalp psoriasis

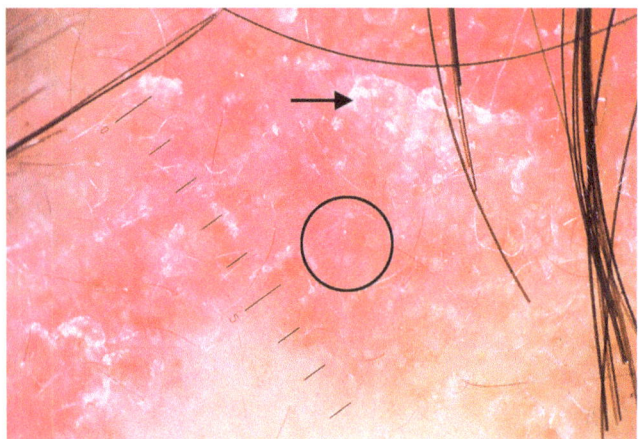

Fig. 8: Scalp psoriasis: Dermoscopy shows white scales (black arrow) and regular arrangement of dilated capillaries (black circle)

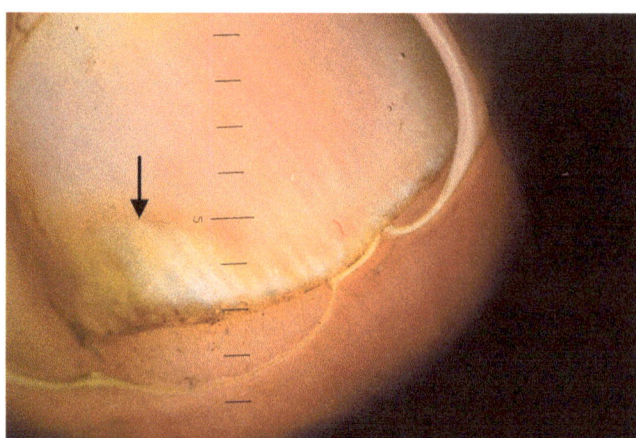

Fig. 10: Nail psoriasis: Dermoscopy shows onycholysis (yellowish white area surrounded by homogenous orange stain) (black arrow)

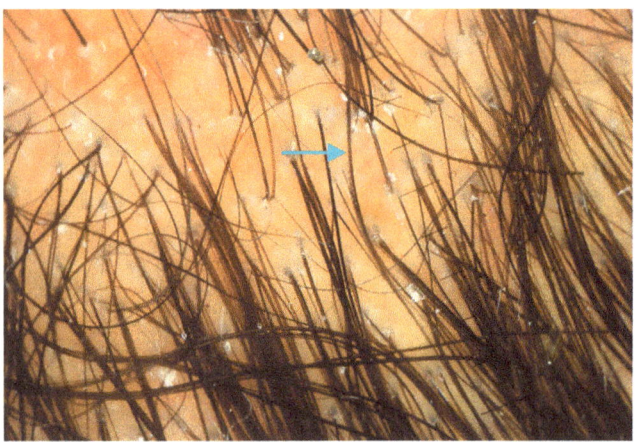

Fig. 9: Seborrheic dermatitis: Dermoscopy shows white scales and arborizing vessels (blue arrow)

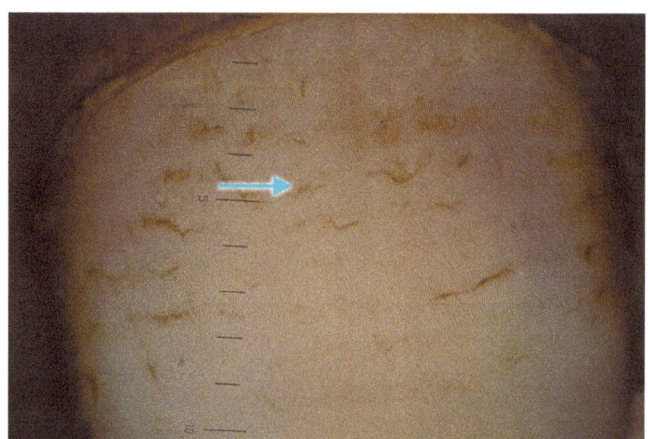

Fig. 11: Nail psoriasis: Dermoscopy shows presence of irregular pits (blue arrow)

Nail Psoriasis

Dermoscopy of nails or onychoscopy can be used to differentiate nail psoriasis from onychomycosis and detection of subtle nail involvement in psoriasis. Nail findings in psoriasis on dermoscopy are pitting, splinter hemorrhage, onycholysis, salmon patch, oil spots, presence of subungual hyperkeratosis and regular arrangements of dotted vessels in hyponychium (Figs 10 and 11).[8,9]

Palmoplantar Psoriasis

Dermoscopy of palmoplantar psoriasis is similar to other variant of psoriasis, however, vascular morphology is not well visualized because of thick scales in palmoplantar region. Dermoscopy can be used to differentiate palmoplantar psoriasis from hand eczema (Figs 12A and B).

Chapter 9 Papulosquamous Disorders

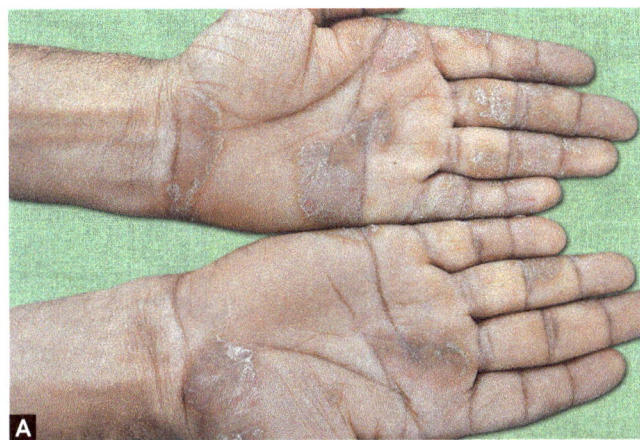

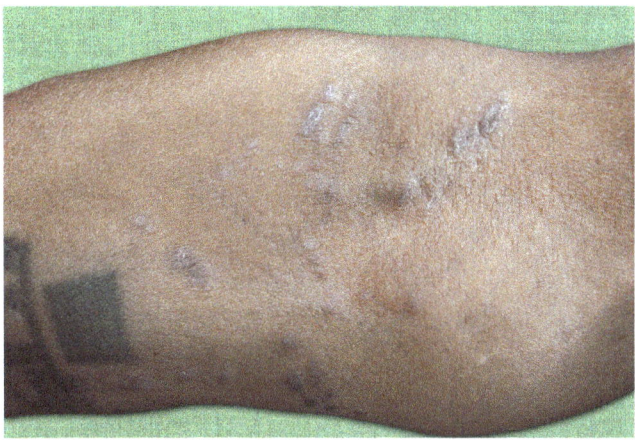

Fig. 13: Clinical photogrpah: Lichen planus

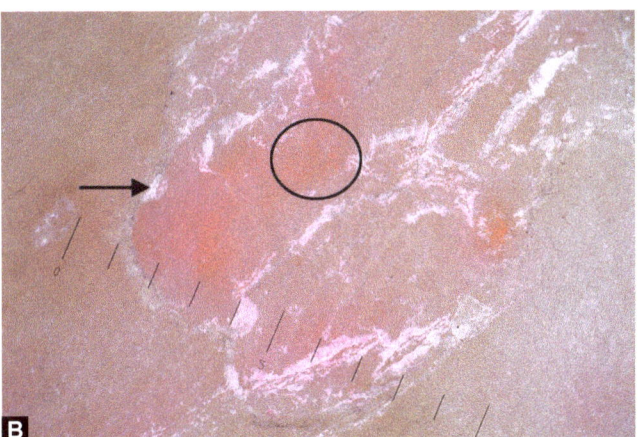

Figs 12A and B: (A) Clinical image: Palmoplantar psoriasis; (B) Palmoplantar psoriasis: Dermoscopy shows presence of thick white scales (black arrow), regular arrangement of dilated capillaries (black circle)

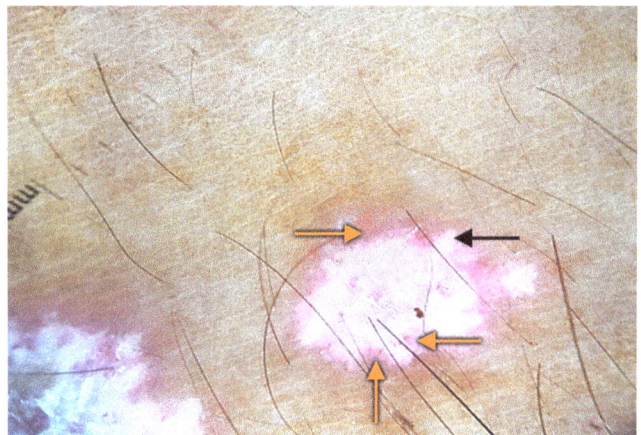

Fig. 14: Lichen planus: Dermoscopy shows violaceous hue and crossing white line on dull red back ground (Wickham's striae) (black arrow) and presence of peripheral dotted vessels (red arrow)

LICHEN PLANUS

Lichen planus is characterized by presence of Wickham's striae. It is a characteristic feature of lichen planus and histopathologically corresponds to wedge-shaped hypergranulosis. Wickham's striae is seen as white crossing lines on dull red background and peripheral dotted vessels and is a specific feature of lichen planus on dermoscopy.[3] Comedo-like opening, milia-like cysts are seen in lichen planus hypertrophicus (Figs 13 to 16).[3]

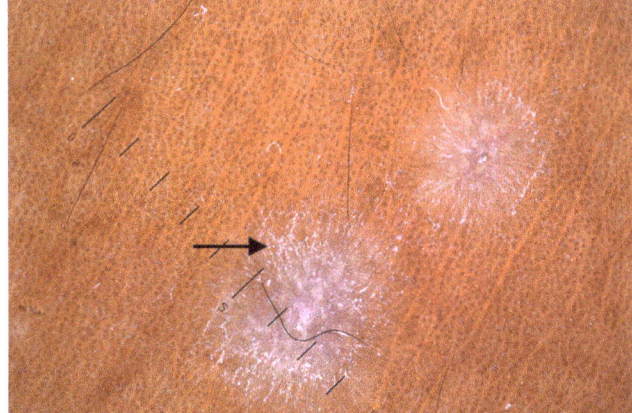

Fig. 15: Lichen planus: Dermoscopy shows Wickham striae (black arrow)

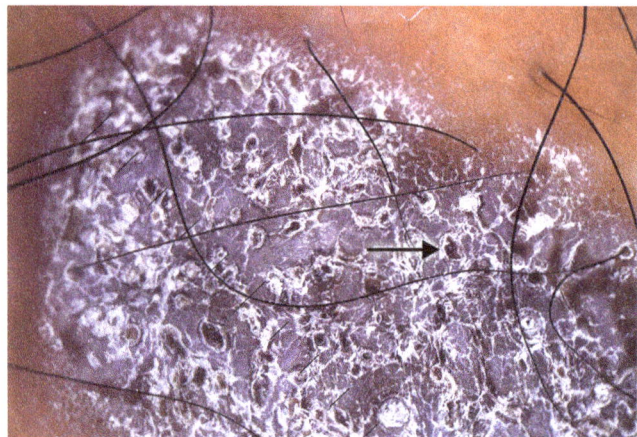

Fig. 16: Lichen planus hypertrophicus: Comedo-like opening can be seen (black arrow)

Oral Lichen Planus

Oral lichen planus also shows characteristic Wickham's striae and it can be used to differentiate it from other erosive lesions of oral mucosa. This finding is just an observation and needs to be corroborated by larger studies (Figs 17 and 18).

Lichen Planus Pigmentosus

Lichen planus pigmentosus is a variant of lichen planus characterized by brown to gray brown macules in sun-exposed areas of skin. Differential diagnosis of this condition includes erythema dyschromicum perstans, pigmented contact dermatitis and melasma. It has been discussed in detail in Chapter 5.

Lichen Striatus

It is an uncommon, self-limiting disorder of unknown etiology, characterized by presence of pink or skin-colored lichenoid papules in linear distribution on an extremity along line of Blaschko. Eruptions may become hypopigmented and nail involvement may occur rarely. Dermoscopy reveals deep white structures which resembles Wickham striae and brown, keratotic, cerebriform structure with pinpoint red dots surrounded by pale halo (Figs 19A and B).[10,11]

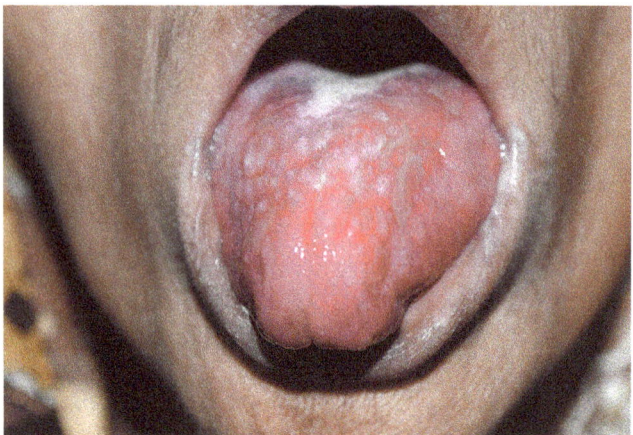

Fig. 17: Clinical photograph: Erosive lichen planus

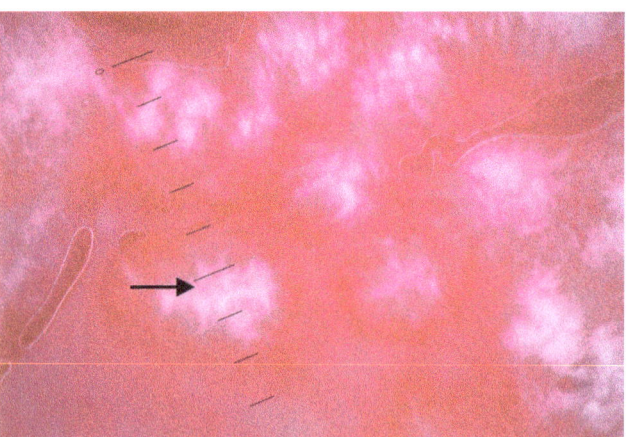

Fig. 18: Oral lichen planus: Dermoscopy shows Wickham striae (black arrow)

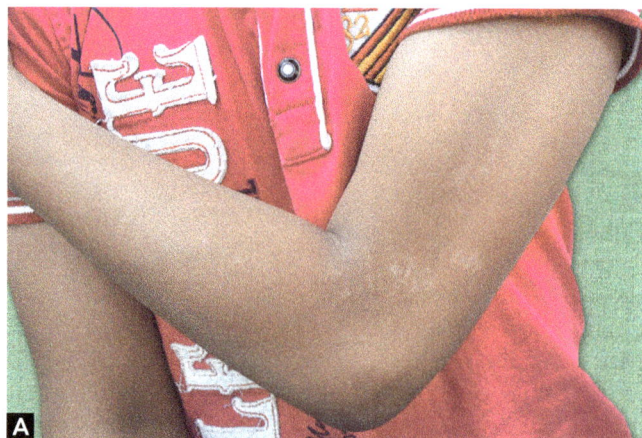

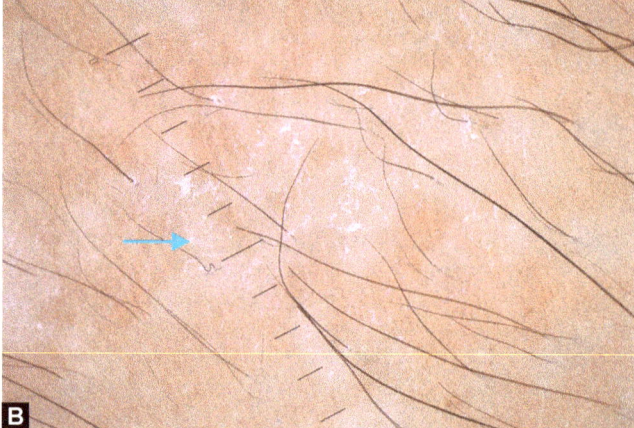

Figs 19A and B: (A) Lichen striatus: Clinical photograph; (B) Lichen striatus: Dermoscopy shows deep white structure resembling Wickham striae

PITYRIASIS ROSEA AND PITYRIASIS RUBRA PILARIS

Dermoscopy of pityriasis rosea is characterized by yellowish background color, peripheral arrangement of scales and patchy distribution of vessels (Fig. 20). Dermoscopy of juvenile pityriasis rubra pilaris has been described as presence of whitish keratotic plugs with surrounding linear vessels and central hair.[12]

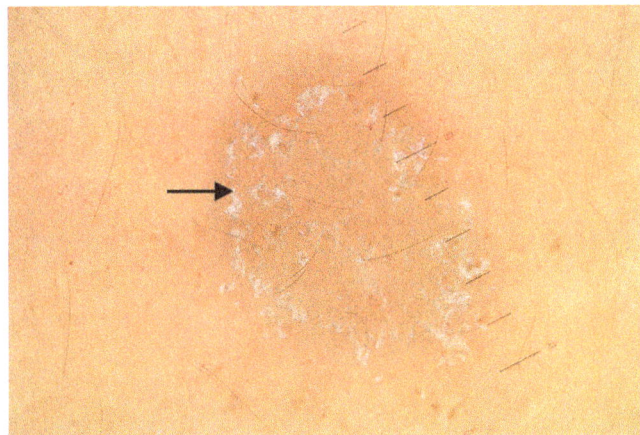

Fig. 20: Pityriasis rosea: Dermoscopy shows yellowish background and peripheral white scales (black arrow)

CONCLUSION

Dermoscopy is an important tool for diagnosis of inflammatory skin disorders especially papulosquamous disorders. It can mitigate need for biopsy in many cases and can give an important clue to diagnosis where clinical features are not typical.

REFERENCES

1. Lallas A, Giacomel J, Argenziano G, García-García B, González-Fernández D, Zalaudek I, et al. Dermoscopy in general dermatology: practical tips for the clinician. Br J Dermatol. 2014;170(3):514-26.
2. Fox BJ, Odom RB. Papulosquamous diseases: a review. J Am Acad Dermatol. 1985;12(4):597-624.
3. Vazquez-Lopez F, Manjon-Haces JA, Maldonado-Seral C, Raya-Aguado C, Pérez-Oliva N, Marghoob AA. Dermoscopic features of plaque psoriasis and lichen planus: new observations. Dermatology. 2003;207(2):151-6.
4. Pan Y, Chamberlain AJ, Bailey M, Chong AH, Haskett M, Kelly JW. Dermatoscopy aids in the diagnosis of the solitary red scaly patch or plaque-features distinguishing superficial basal cell carcinoma, intraepidermal carcinoma, and psoriasis. J Am Acad Dermatol. 2008;59(2):268-74.
5. Lallas A, Kyrgidis A, Tzellos TG, Apalla Z, Karakyriou E, Karatolias A, et al. Accuracy of dermoscopic criteria for the diagnosis of psoriasis, dermatitis, lichen planus and pityriasis rosea. Br J Dermatol. 2012;166(6):1198-205.
6. Lallas A, Apalla Z, Argenziano G, Sotiriou E, Di Lernia V, Moscarella E, et al. Dermoscopic pattern of psoriatic lesions on specific body sites. Dermatology. 2014;228(3):250-4.
7. Kim GW, Jung HJ, Ko HC, Kim MB, Lee WJ, Lee SJ, et al. Dermoscopy can be useful in differentiating scalp psoriasis from seborrhoeic dermatitis. Br J Dermatol. 2011;164(3):652-6.
8. Yadav TA, Khopkar US. Dermoscopy to detect signs of subclinical nail involvement in chronic plaque psoriasis: a study of 68 patients. Indian J Dermatol. 2015;60(3),272-5.
9. Piraccini BM, Bruni F, Starace M. Dermoscopy of non-skin cancer nail disorders. Dermatol Ther. 2012;25(6):594-602.
10. Taniguchi Abagge K, Parolin Marinoni L, Giraldi S, Carvalho VO, de Oliveira Santini C, Favre H. Lichen striatus: description of 89 cases in children. Pediatr Dermatol. 2004;21(4):440-3.
11. Coto-Segura P, Costa-Romero M, Gonzalvo P, Mallo-García S, Curto-Iglesias JR, Santos-Juanes J. Lichen striatus in an adult following trauma with central nail plate involvement and its dermoscopy features. Int J Dermatol. 2008;47(12):1324-5.
12. López-Gómez A, Vera-Casaño Á, Gómez-Moyano E, Salas-García T, Dorado-Fernández M, Hernández-Gil-Sánchez J, et al. Dermoscopy of circumscribed juvenile pityriasis rubra pilaris. J Am Acad Dermatol. 2015;72(1 Suppl):S58-9.

SECTION 4

Infectious Disorders

Manas Chatterjee

Section Outline

- Infectious Disorders

CHAPTER 10

Infectious Disorders

Shekhar Neema, Manas Chatterjee

INTRODUCTION

Dermoscopy of infestations is also known as entomodermoscopy. Dermoscopy of infections and infestations can help in the diagnosis of disease in difficult cases and it can also help in knowing whether a patient has been treated successfully. It can be used for diagnosis of bacterial, fungal, viral and parasitic infections. Dermoscopy of infectious disorders has a very important consideration of transmission of infection when same dermoscope is used in multiple patients; it can be an important source of nosocomial infection. Alcohol-based gels should be used as an interface for potentially infectious conditions and dermoscope lens should be cleaned with alcohol wipes before using it in another patient.[1]

SCABIES

Scabies is caused by mite *Sarcoptes scabiei var hominis*. Characteristic clinical sign of scabies is presence of burrow, which is a tunnel made by mite in dermis and visible as white line ranging from 1 mm to 10 mm in length and present on interdigital spaces of hand and flexural aspect of wrist, elbow, axilla, abdomen and genitalia. Dermoscopy is found to be more sensitive than skin scraping and adhesive tape test for diagnosis of scabies in resource poor setting.[2]

Dermoscopic feature of scabies is presence of dark triangular area at the end of wavy white line, also known as jet with contrail. Jet or the dark part corresponds to anterior part of mite while contrail corresponds to burrow (Fig. 1).

PEDICULOSIS

Pediculosis capitis is infestation caused by *Pediculus humanus capitis*. It is a very common infestation especially in school going children and causes itching and secondary infection.

Dermoscopy can be used for rapid diagnosis of pediculus infestation and effectiveness of treatment. With the help of dermoscope, one can identify mite, nits and differentiate

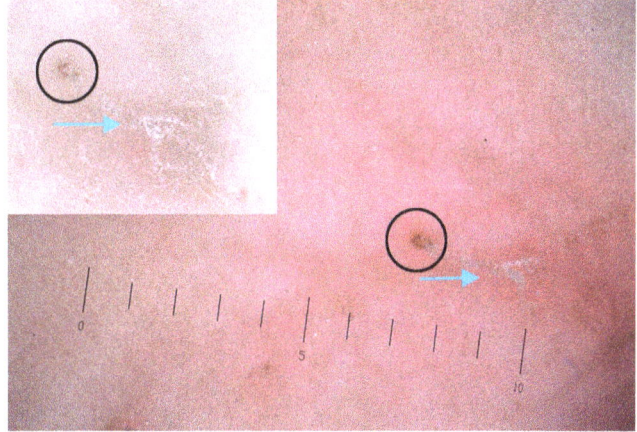

Fig. 1: Dark triangular structure (black circle) depicting mite and white wavy line (blue arrow) depicting burrow—jet with contrail structure

nits containing vital nymph from pseudonits (empty nits) and scales. Full nits appear as ovoid brown structures with convex extremity while empty nits appear as translucent structure. Presence of full nits signifies active infestation (Figs 2A and B).[3]

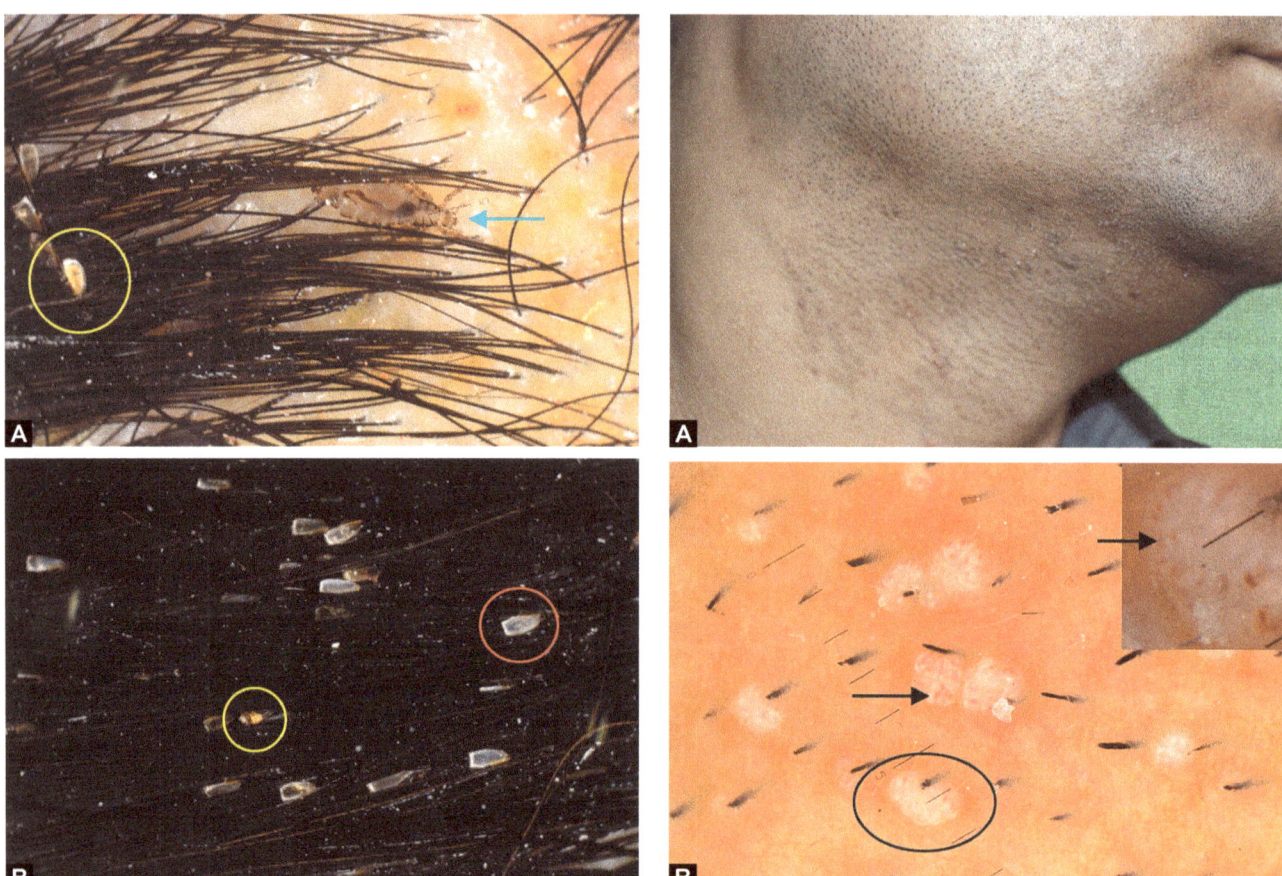

Figs 2A and B: (A) Shows adult mite (blue arrow) and nit (yellow circle) with live nymph; (B) Shows full nits (yellow circle) appearing as ovoid brown structure while pseudonits (red circle) which appears as amorphous whitish structure

Figs 3A and B: (A) Clinical photograph of verrucae vulgaris; (B) Dermoscopy shows homogenous white structure which obscures dermatoglyphics (black circle) and presence of dotted vessels (black arrow), inset shows digitally magnified image of dotted vessels

VIRAL INFECTIONS

Human Papillomavirus Infection

Human papillomavirus (HPV) infection causes warts, which can be classified depending on location and morphology as common warts, plantar warts, genital warts and plane warts. Dermoscopy can be useful in diagnosis of HPV infection as well as therapeutic response. Vessel morphology in lesion is an important feature for diagnosis of HPV infection (Figs 3 to 6).[4,5]

Molluscum Contagiosum

Molluscum contagiosum is a common viral infection especially in children and immunocompromised adults. It is diagnosed clinically and in difficult cases requires histopathology. Dermoscopy can help in rapid diagnosis of difficult cases where amorphous clods or white to yellowish amorphous structure are visible along with crown vessels (peripheral linear or branching vessels) (Figs 7A to C).[5,6]

FUNGAL INFECTIONS

Superficial fungal infections like dermatophytosis and pityriasis versicolor are conventionally diagnosed on clinical examination and diagnosis can be confirmed by 10% KOH (potassium hydroxide) mount. Dermoscopy can be used as an auxiliary tool when scales are not visible clinically as in pityriasis versicolor or dermatophytosis when its classical clinical picture has been altered by steroid application. Dermoscopy is a very important tool for diagnosis of onychomycosis and its differentiation from nail psoriasis and other nail conditions. It is also an important screening tool in patients with tinea capitis where rapid diagnosis in community setting can be made with the help of a dermoscope (Figs 8 to 11).[7-9]

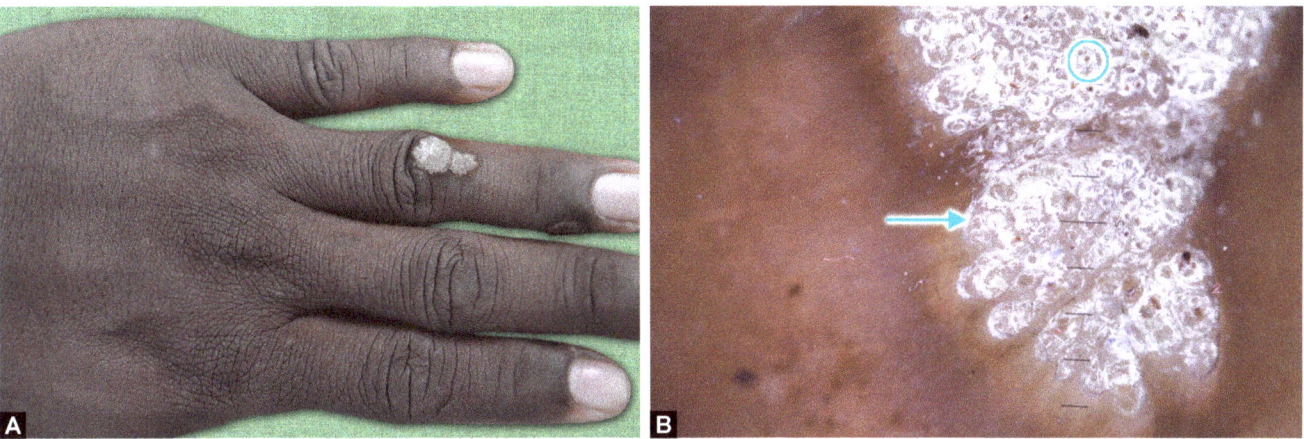

Figs 4A and B: (A) Clinical photograph shows hyperkeratotic wart; (B) Dermoscopy shows thick white scales (blue arrow) and dotted vessels (blue circle)

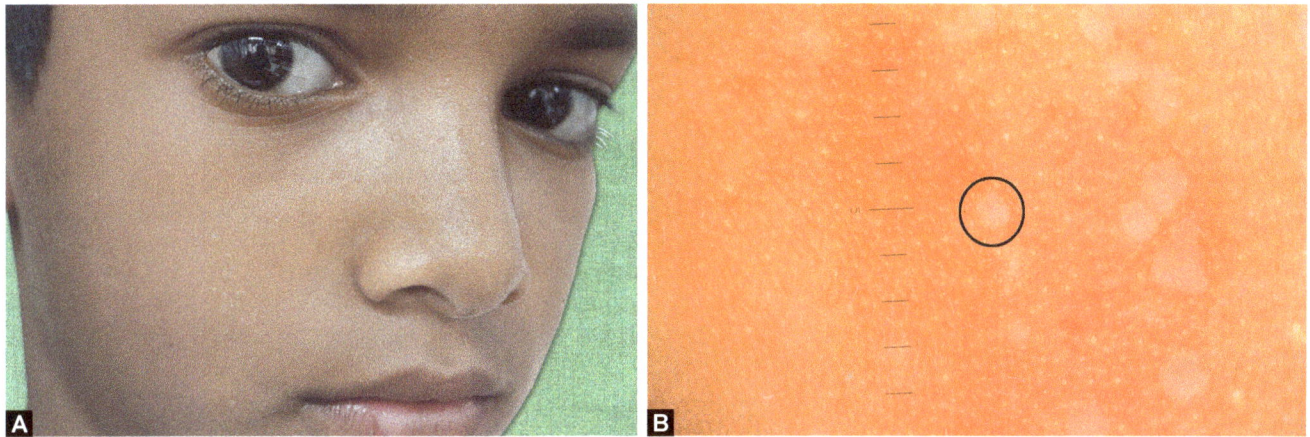

Figs 5A and B: (A) Clinical photograph of plane warts; (B) Homogenous white structure obscuring dermatoglyphics (black circle). In darker skin, vessels are difficult to visualize in handheld dermoscopy

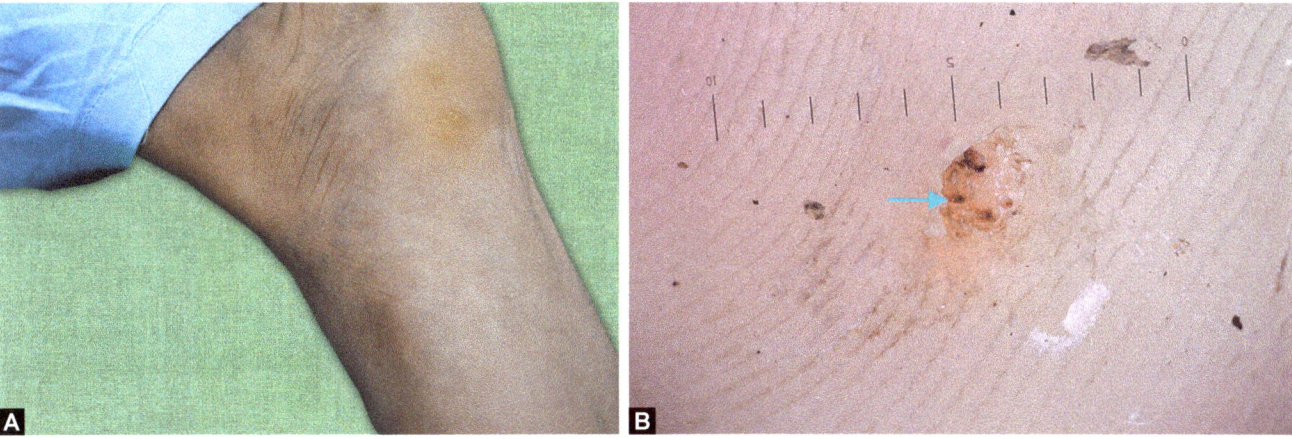

Figs 6A and B: (A) Clinical photograph of plantar warts; (B) Dermoscopy shows presence of dotted vessels and obscuration of dermatoglyphics (blue arrow). Callosity shows structureless areas as compared to plantar warts

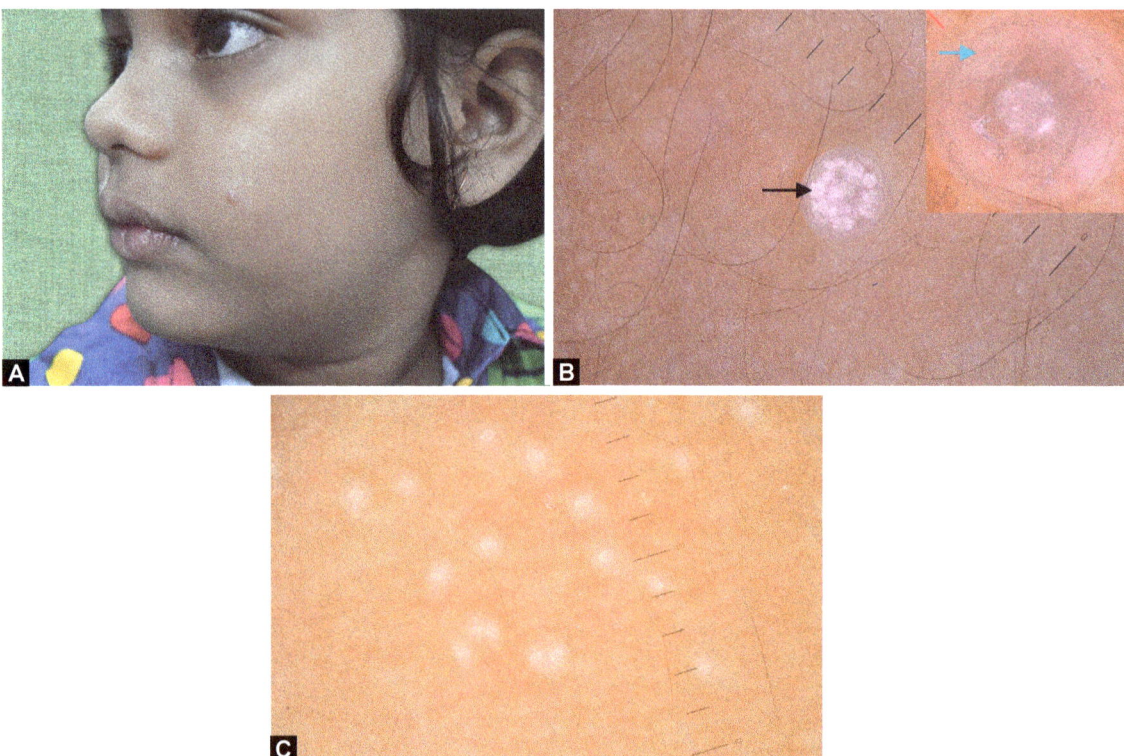

Figs 7A to C: (A) Clinical photograph of molluscum contagiosum; (B) Dermoscopy shows amorphous white clods (black arrow). Faint linear vessels are visible in digitally zoomed image in inset (blue arrow); (C) Dermoscopy shows "starry sky appearance" in multiple molluscum in forearm

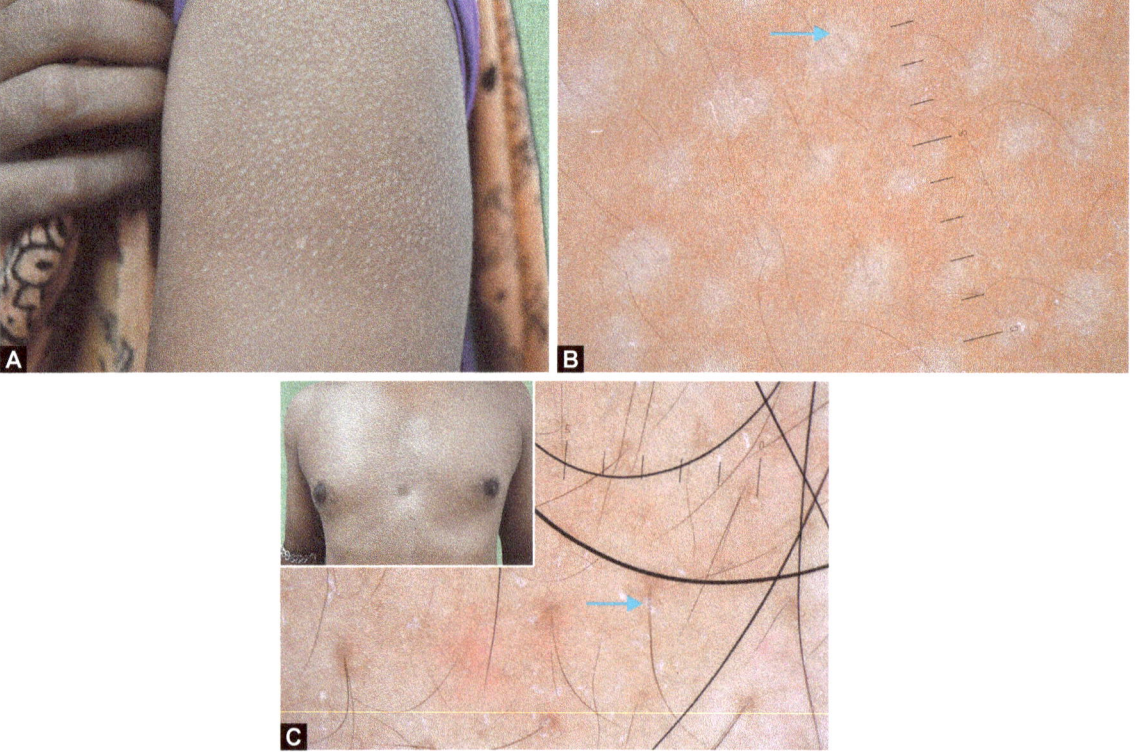

Figs 8A to C: (A) Clinical photograph of pityriasis versicolor; (B) Presence of perifollicular scales (blue arrow); (C) Presence of perifollicular scales (blue arrow) in a case of pityriasis versicolor with solitary lesion which appears clinically as seborrheic keratosis (inset)

Chapter 10 Infectious Disorders

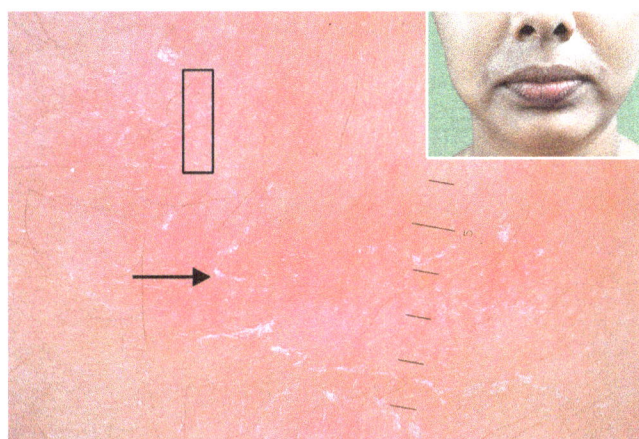

Fig. 9: Presence of scales (black arrow) and linear vessels, telangiectasia (black rectangle) are visualized in dermoscopy of steroid modified tinea faciei (clinical picture in inset)

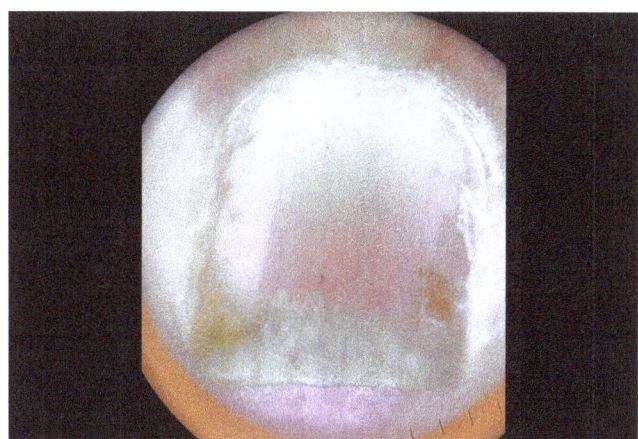

Fig. 10: Dermoscopy of onychomycosis shows jagged spike pattern

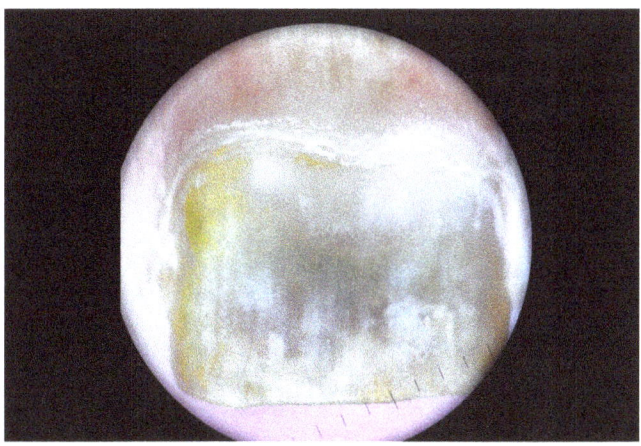

Fig. 11: Dermoscopy of onychomycosis shows jagged spike pattern and longitudinal striations

CONCLUSION

Entomodermoscopy is useful for rapid diagnosis of infection and infestations. It can also be used to know the adequacy of treatment.

REFERENCES

1. Kelly SC, Purcell SM. Prevention of nosocomial infection during dermoscopy? Dermatol Surg. 2006;32(4):552-5.
2. Walter B, Heukelbach J, Fengler G, Worth C, Hengge U, Feldmeier H. Comparison of dermoscopy, skin scraping, and the adhesive tape test for the diagnosis of scabies in a resource-poor setting. Arch Dermatol. 2011;147(4):468-73.
3. Zalaudek I, Giacomel J, Cabo H, Di Stefani A, Ferrara G, Hofmann-Wellenhof R, et al. Entodermoscopy: a new tool for diagnosing skin infections and infestations. Dermatology. 2008;216(1):14-23.
4. Tschandl P, Argenziano G, Bakos R, Gourhant JY, Hofmann-Wellenhof R, Kittler H, et al. Dermoscopy and entomology (entomodermoscopy). J Dtsch Dermatol Ges. 2009;7(7):589-96.
5. Lallas A, Giacomel J, Argenziano G, García-García B, González-Fernández D, Zalaudek I, et al. Dermoscopy in general dermatology: practical tips for the clinician. Br J Dermatol. 2014;170(3):514-26.
6. Mun JH, Ko HC, Kim BS, Kim MB. Dermoscopy of giant molluscum contagiosum. J Am Acad Dermatol. 2013;69(6):e287-8.
7. Zhou H, Tang XH, De Han J, Chen MK. Dermoscopy as an ancillary tool for the diagnosis of pityriasis versicolor. J Am Acad Dermatol. 2015;73(6):e205-6.
8. Rudnicka L, Olszewska M, Rakowska A, Slowinska M. Trichoscopy update 2011. J Dermatol Case Rep. 2011;5(4):82-8.
9. Piraccini BM, Balestri R, Starace M, Rech G. Nail digital dermoscopy (onychoscopy) in the diagnosis of onychomycosis. J Eur Acad Dermatol Venereol. 2013;27(4):509-13.

SECTION 5
Autoimmune and Granulomatous Disorders

Subrata Malakar

Section Outline

- Autoimmune Diseases
- Dermoscopy of Granulomatous Disorders

CHAPTER 11

Autoimmune Diseases

Rahul Arora, Shekhar Neema

INTRODUCTION

The term autoimmune diseases signifies the presence of specific immunoglobulins that react with one or more self-epitopes requiring prior activation of autoreactive B-cells by memory T-cells. Dermoscopy including nail fold capillaroscopy can help to recognize and differentiate the various autoimmune diseases.

DISCOID LUPUS ERYTHEMATOSUS

The dermoscopic patterns observed in discoid lupus erythematosus vary according to the stage of the disease. While the early lesions show predominance of follicular plugging, follicular whitish halo and white scales, late lesions are characterized by white structureless areas, telangiectatic vessels and pigmentary structures. Other recently described features include the presence of arborizing vessels and follicular red dots.[1] Dermoscopic evaluation of the scale may show the tin-tack sign. The capillaroscopic features include dilated and tortuous vessels in proximal nail fold (Figs 1 to 5).

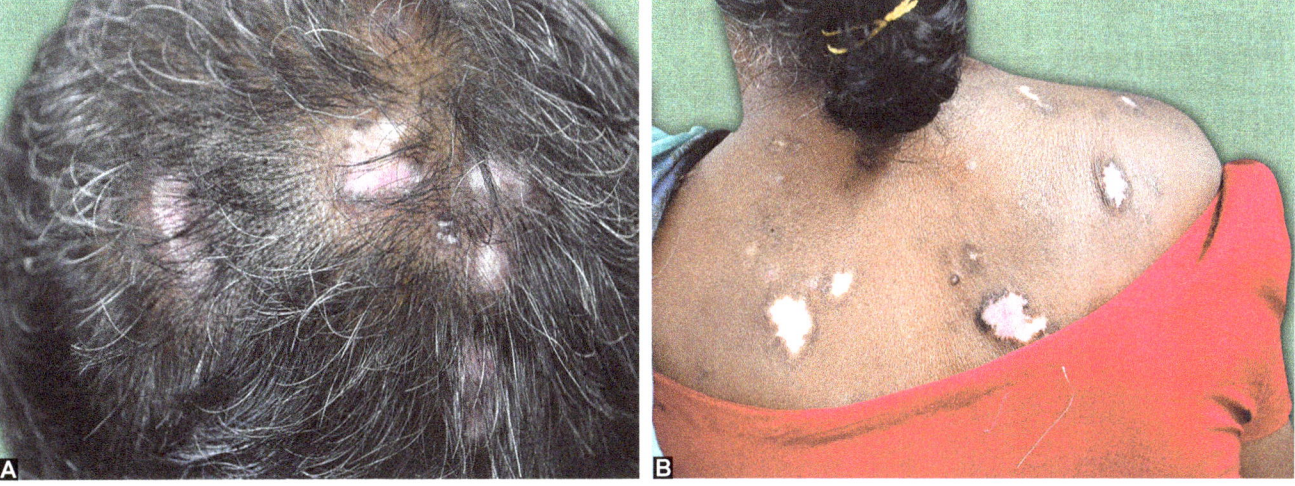

Figs 1A and B: Clinical photographs: Discoid lupus erythematosus

Section 5 Autoimmune and Granulomatous Disorders

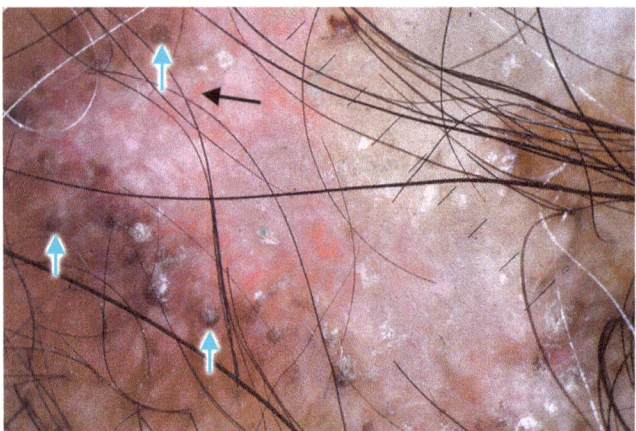

Fig. 2: Trichoscopy shows thick arborizing vessels (black arrow), yellow dots (blue arrow). Two types of vessels seen on dermoscopy of discoid lupus erythematosus are thin arborizing vessels and thick arborizing vessels. Thick arborizing vessels are thicker than hair shaft

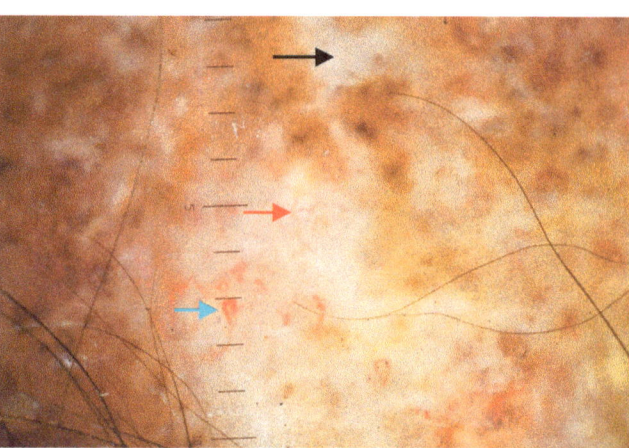

Fig. 5: Dermoscopy shows white structureless areas (black arrow) and thick (blue arrow) and thin arborizing vessels (red arrow). This dermoscopic picture is suggestive of late lesion of discoid lupus erythematosus

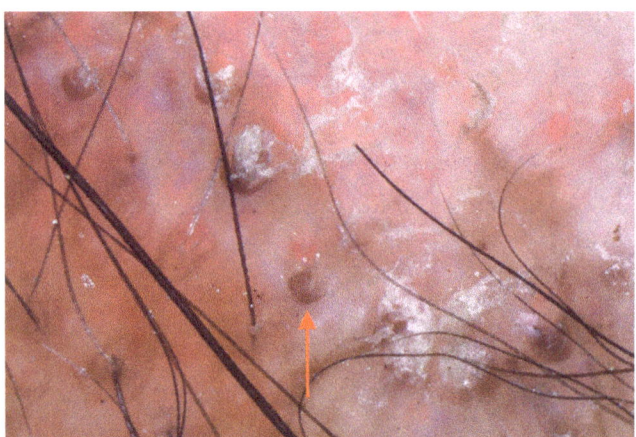

Fig. 3: Trichoscopy shows fine scaling and magnified view of yellow dots (red arrow). Yellow dots in discoid lupus erythematosus are bigger than alopecia areata and androgenetic alopecia, they have double margin. Yellow dots correspond to follicular hyperkeratotic plugs and are marker of active disease

LICHEN SCLEROSUS ET ATROPHICUS

Lichen sclerosus et atrophicus (LSA) is characterized by follicular plugging and lichenoid cell infiltrate. The characteristic dermoscopic findings of extragenital LSA include the comedo-like openings and the whitish patch[2] (Figs 6 and 7).[2] In addition, linear branching vessels, comma vessels and hairpin vessels can also be seen.[3] Comedo-like openings represent follicular plugging and white areas represent epidermal atrophy.

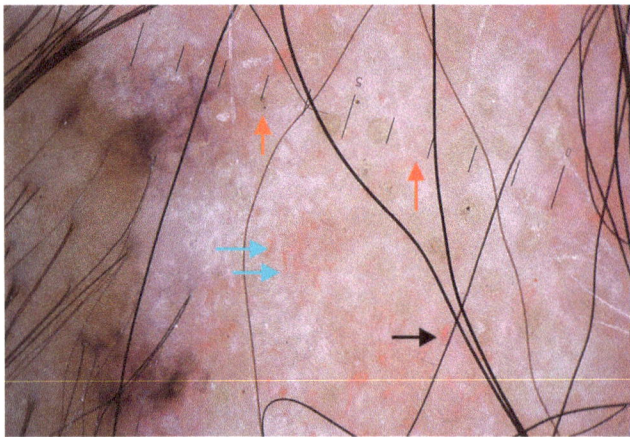

Fig. 4: Trichoscopy shows thin arborizing vessel (blue arrow), thick arborizing vessel (black arrow) and yellow dots (red arrow) suggestive of follicular plugging

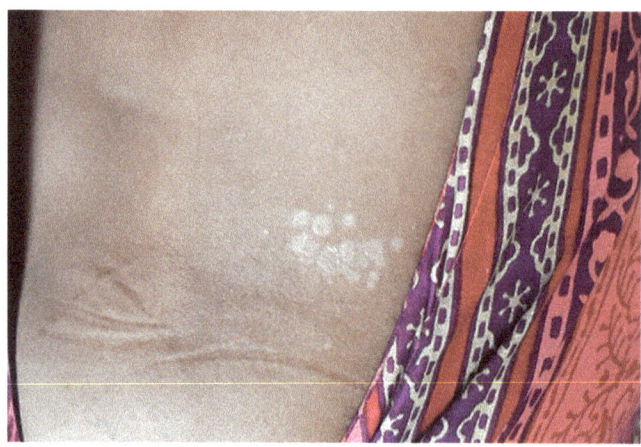

Fig. 6: Clinical photograph: lichen sclerosus et atrophicus

Chapter 11   Autoimmune Diseases

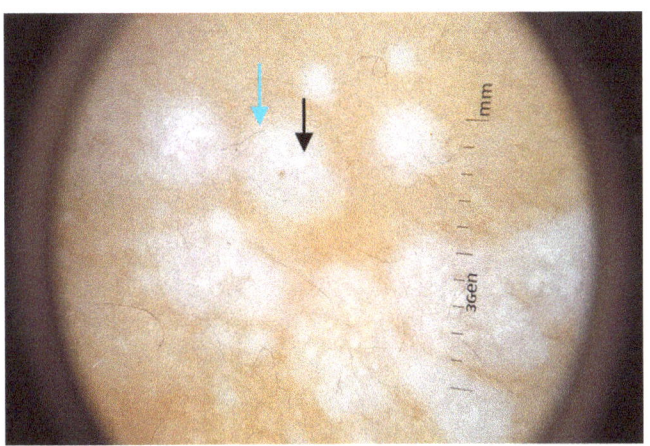

Fig. 7: Lichen sclerosus et atrophicus: dermoscopy shows white areas (blue arrow) and comedo-like openings (black arrow)

MORPHEA

Morphea is characterized by sclerosis of reticular dermis and loss of appendages. Campion, et al.[4] described the dermoscopic feature of morphea as accentuated fibrotic beams crossed by spreading telangiectasia with evidence of loss of appendages. In addition, pigment network-like structure can also be seen.[3]

SYSTEMIC SCLEROSIS

Systemic sclerosis is a connective tissue disease, characterized by vasomotor disturbance and fibrosis of skin. Cutaneous features includes Raynaud's phenomenon, sclerosis of skin, hyperpigmentation and hypopigmentation of skin and matt like telangiectasia (Figs 8 to 10).[5]

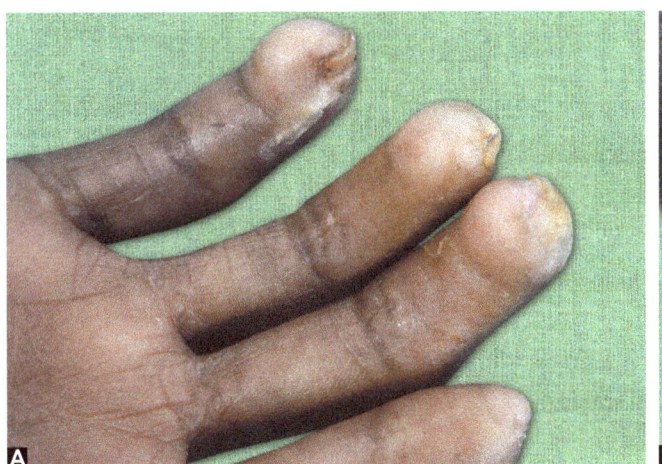
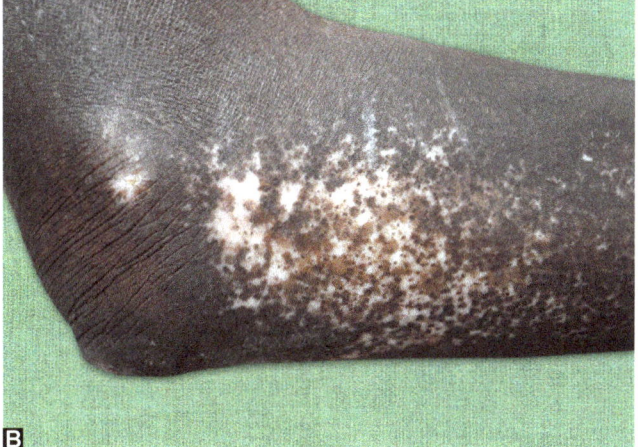

Figs 8A and B: Clinical photographs: Systemic sclerosis showing digital pitted scars and depigmented macules

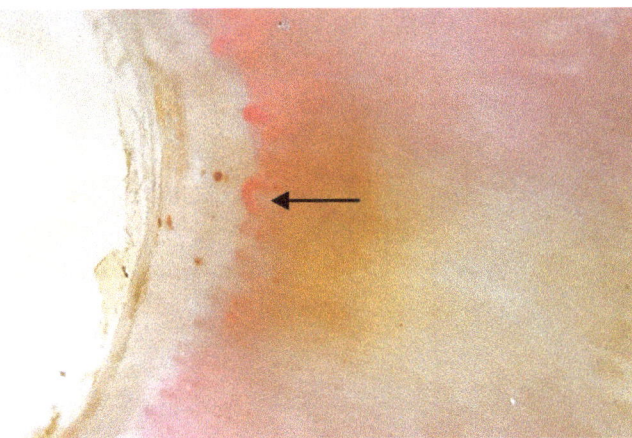

Fig. 9: Dermoscopy of nail fold showing dilatation of nail fold capillaries

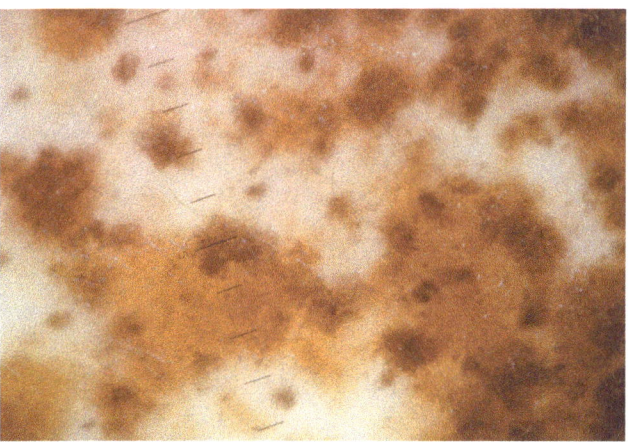

Fig. 10: Dermoscopy of depigmented areas shows vitiligo-like areas, with preservation of perifollicular pigment

REFERENCES

1. Lallas A, Apalla Z, Lefaki I, Sotiriou E, Lazaridou E, Ioannides D, et al. Dermoscopy of discoid lupus erythematosus. Br J Dermatol. 2013;168:284–8.
2. Garrido-Rios AA, Alvarez-Garrido H, Sanz-Munoz C, Aragoneses-Fraile H, Manchado-Lopez P, Miranda-Romero A. Dermoscopy of extragenital lichen sclerosus. Arch Dermatol. 2009;145:1468.
3. Shim WH, Jwa SW, Song M, Kim HS, Ko HC, Kim MB, et al. Diagnostic usefulness of dermatoscopy in differentiating lichen sclerous et atrophicus from morphea. J Am Acad Dermatol. 201r;66(4):690-1.
4. Campione E, Paterno EJ, Diluvio L, Orlandi A, Bianchi L, Chimenti S. Localized morphea treated with imiquimod 5% and dermoscopic assessment of effectiveness. J Dermatolog Treat. 2009;20(1):10-3.
5. Hasegawa M. Dermoscopy findings of nail fold capillaries in connective tissue diseases. J Dermatoy. 2011;38(1):66-70.

CHAPTER 12

Dermoscopy of Granulomatous Disorders

Uday Khopkar, Shubhangi Mahajan

INTRODUCTION

Granulomatous diseases, especially of infective etiology continue to pose diagnostic challenges to clinical dermatologists. At times, noninfective granulomas like sarcoidosis and granuloma annulare need to be differentiated from infective ones. Most cases are currently resolved by histopathologic differences. However, a noninvasive investigation like dermoscopy may still has place in clinician's reserves.

In 2004, Vázquez-López et al., for the first time, evaluated dermoscopic patterns in a large series of different nontumoral dermatoses and found linear and dotted vessels, appearing either alone (monomorphous) or together (mixed or polymorphous) as the most common vascular pattern.[1] In 2008, Brasiello et al. reported a case of lupus vulgaris with the findings of branched telangiectasia on orange-yellow background with milia-like cysts and whitish reticular streaks.[2] Llambrich et al. studied 26 cases of cutaneous leishmaniasis in 2009 and reported different dermoscopic features like generalized erythema (100%), yellow tears (53%), hyperkeratosis (50%), central erosion or ulceration (46%), erosion or ulceration associated with hyperkeratosis (38%), and white starburst-like pattern (38%). In addition, they reported comma-like and linear vessels as the most common vascular pattern in their series.[3] Pellicano et al. studied dermoscopic pattern in seven cases of cutaneous sarcoidosis and reported small grouped, translucent orange globular structures associated with linear vessels of variable diameter in all seven cases. In five cases, additional central scar-like areas resembling white structureless areas or white lines in between the translucent orange globules were seen.[4] Lallas et al. in 2013 included 24 patients of granuloma annulare with dotted in 19 (40.4%), short linear in 10 (21.3%) or linear arborizing vessels in 7 (14.9%) cases. The background color was a combination of red and white in 20 of the 47 lesions (42.6%), red only in 17 (36.2%), white only in 9 (19.1%) and a combination of white and yellow in 1 case (2.1%).[5]

In another study, Pellicano et al. in 2013 evaluated 12 patients of granuloma annulare and 12 patients of necrobiosis lipoidica. In all cases of granuloma annulare, dermoscopy revealed peripheral structureless orange-reddish borders without evident vessels except five cases which showed isolated unfocussed small vessels.[6] Yücel et al. in a series of cutaneous leishmaniasis in 2013 mentioned newer dermoscopic findings. Dermoscopy of total 145 lesions showed generalized erythema in all (100%), yellow tears (50%), central erosion or ulceration (46%), erosion or ulceration associated with hyperkeratosis (38%) and white starburst-like pattern (38%). Comma-shaped vessels and linear irregular vessels are the most common vascular patterns observed.[7] Lallas et al. made their dermoscopic observations in 2014 on a series of patients with inflammatory facial dermatoses. They could differentiate granulomatous conditions, like sarcoidosis and lupus vulgaris, from nongranulomatous conditions, like granuloma faciale, discoid lupus erythematosus and seborrheic dermatitis. They noted orange-yellow structureless areas with linear branching vessels on dermoscopy in both the above-mentioned conditions.[8]

LUPUS VULGARIS

We observed the characteristic orangish hue of the background skin with milia-like cysts and reticular streaks with arborizing telangiectasia in case of lupus vulgaris. At periphery of lesion accentuated reticular hyperpigmentation was seen. Healing lesions of lupus vulgaris showed prominence of reticular streaks suggestive of scaling (Figs 1A to C).

TUBERCULOSIS VERRUCOSA CUTIS

We also observed similar pinkish-orange hue on dermoscopy of a plaque present on thigh in case of tuberculosis verrucosa cutis. It also showed multiple patulous follicular openings with cribriform atrophic areas in periphery which are suggestive of scarring. Enlarged view of pinkish-orange area showed reticular white streaks and plugged dilated follicles while that of cribriform area showed wider reticular

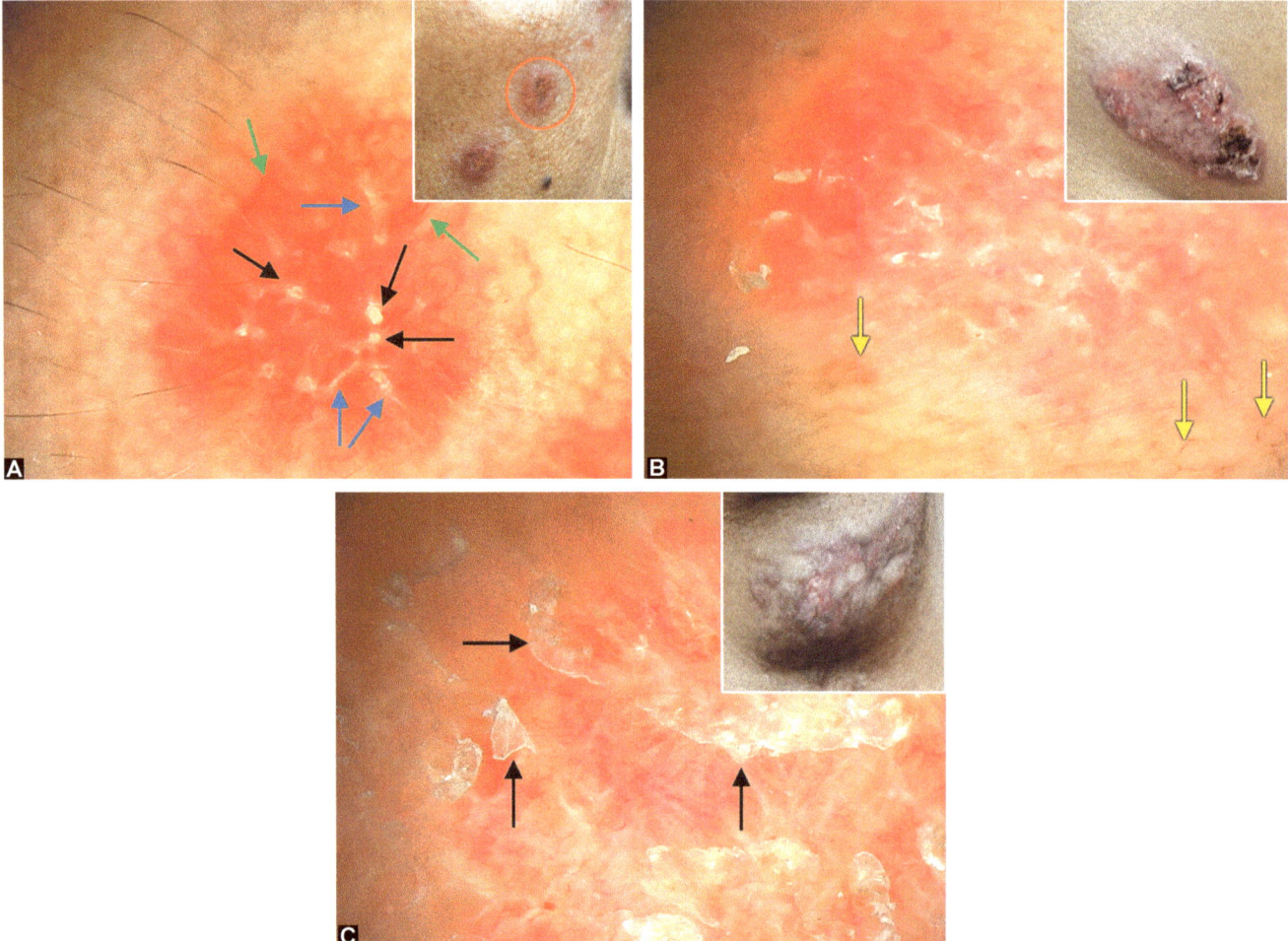

Figs 1A to C: Dermoscopic images of lupus vulgaris: (A) Diffuse orange white area with whitish reticular streaks (blue arrows) and milia-like cysts (black arrows) and arborizing telangiectasia (green arrows); (B) Prominent white reticular streaks on orange-yellow background with accentuation of normal pigmentation at the periphery of lesion (yellow arrows); (C) Healing lesion shows more of white area than orange area along with accentuation of reticular streaks suggestive of scaling (black arrows). Insets show clinical photographs of lesions

white streaks on hyperpigmented background with lack of appendages (Figs 2A to C).

POST-KALA-AZAR DERMAL LEISHMANIASIS

In case of post-kala-azar dermal leishmaniasis, dermoscopy of hypopigmented patch of forearm showed polygonal globular pattern with central white dots which correspond to follicular openings and peripheral reticulate hyperpigmentation. Dermoscopy of nodular lesion on lateral border of dorsum of left hand showed inflated balloon appearance with loss of follicular openings and increased peripheral reticulate pigmentation (Figs 3A and B).

BORDERLINE LEPROMATOUS HANSEN'S DISEASE

In case of borderline lepromatous Hansen's disease, dermoscopy of erythematous scaly plaque of left pinna showed orangish-white area with linear telangiectasia. Similar findings are seen in a flat-topped erythematous papule over right leg which on higher resolution showed wider and coalescing reticular white streaks and globular white structures along with linear telangiectasia (Figs 4A to C).

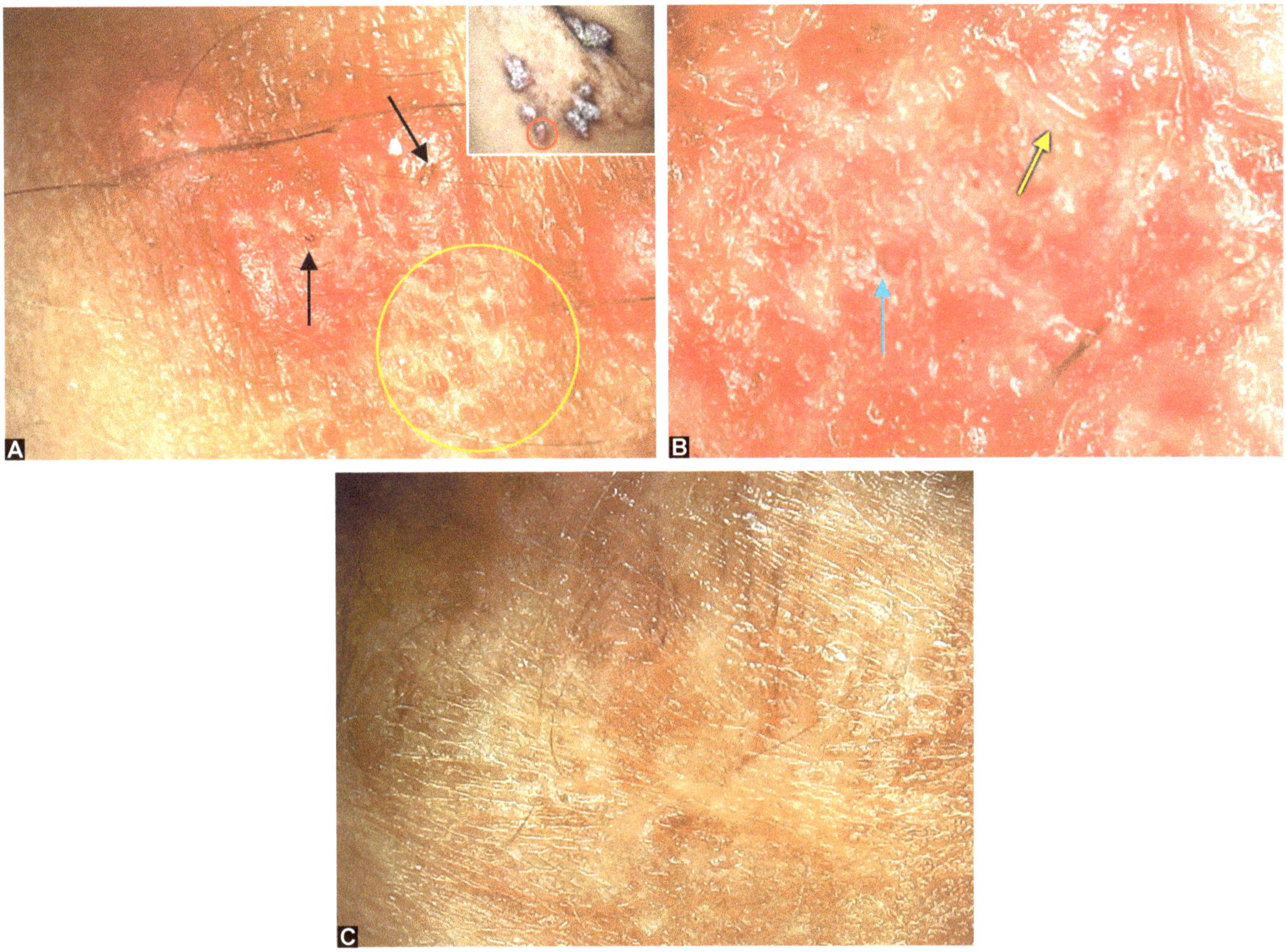

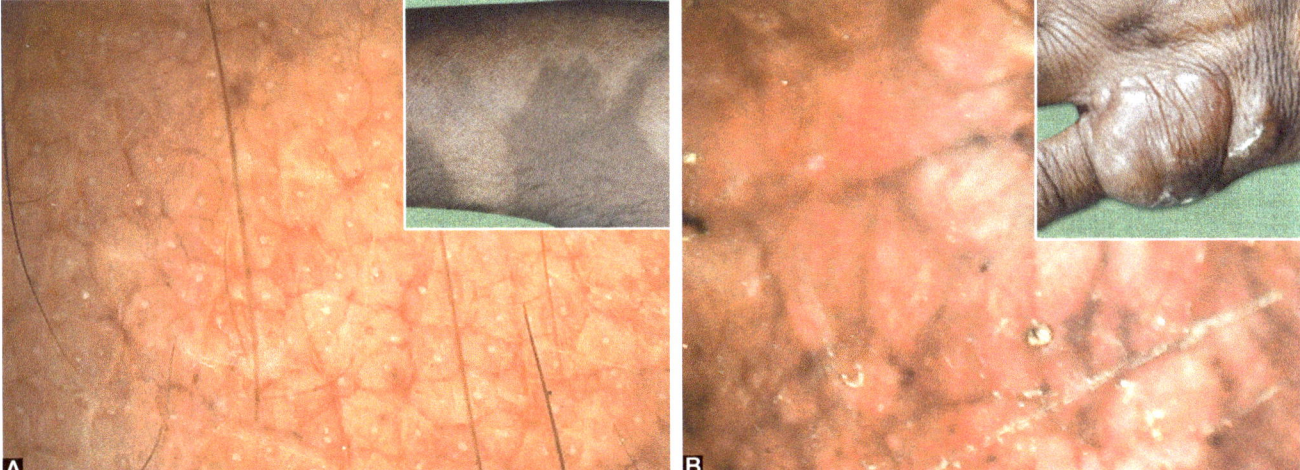

Figs 2A to C: Dermoscopy of a plaque of tuberculosis verrucosa cutis which is present on right thigh shows: (A) Low power-pink-orange hue with patulous follicular openings (black arrows) and cribriform atrophic areas; (B) Enlarged dermoscopic view of upper part shows reticular white streaks (yellow arrow) and plugged dilated follicles (blue arrow); (C) Higher magnification of cribriform scar shows wider reticulate white streaks on hyperpigmented background with lack of appendages. Insets show clinical photographs of lesions

Figs 3A and B: Dermoscopic images of post-kala-azar dermal leishmaniasis: (A) Hypopigmented patch on forearm shows polygonal globular pattern with central white dots (follicular openings) and peripheral reticulate hyperpigmentation; (B) Nodular lesion shows deflated balloon appearance or raisin-like appearance with loss of follicular openings and increased peripheral reticular pigmentation. Insets show clinical photographs of lesions

In borderline lepromatous Hansen's disease, dermoscopy of an erythematous plaque on abdomen showed partial loss of pigment network compared to peripheral normal skin. It also showed structureless white areas and irregularly branched red streaks which can be better appreciated on higher magnification (Figs 5A and B).

CONCLUSION

Dermoscopy is a promising noninvasive test that may be useful aid in the diagnosis of various granulomatous dermatoses. It is necessary to validate the diagnostic signs in brown colored skin of Indians by this investigation in many more patients.

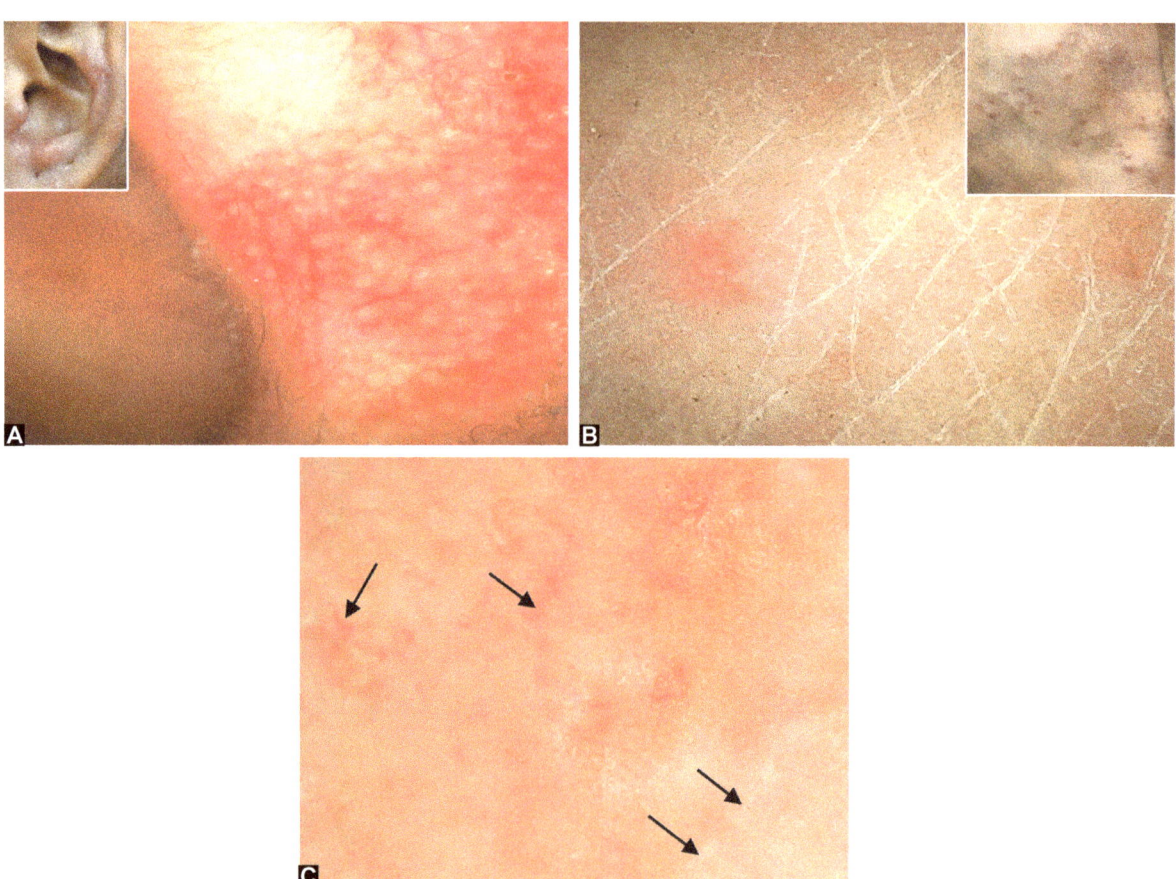

Figs 4A to C: Dermoscopic images of borderline lepromatous Hansen's disease: (A) Dermoscopy of erythematous scaly plaque of pinna showed orangish-white area with linear telangiectasia; (B) Dermoscopy from tiny flat-topped papule of left leg showed similar orangish-white area with linear telangiectasia; (C) On higher resolution, wider and coalescing reticular streaks with globular white structures and telangiectasia are seen. Inset shows clinical photographs

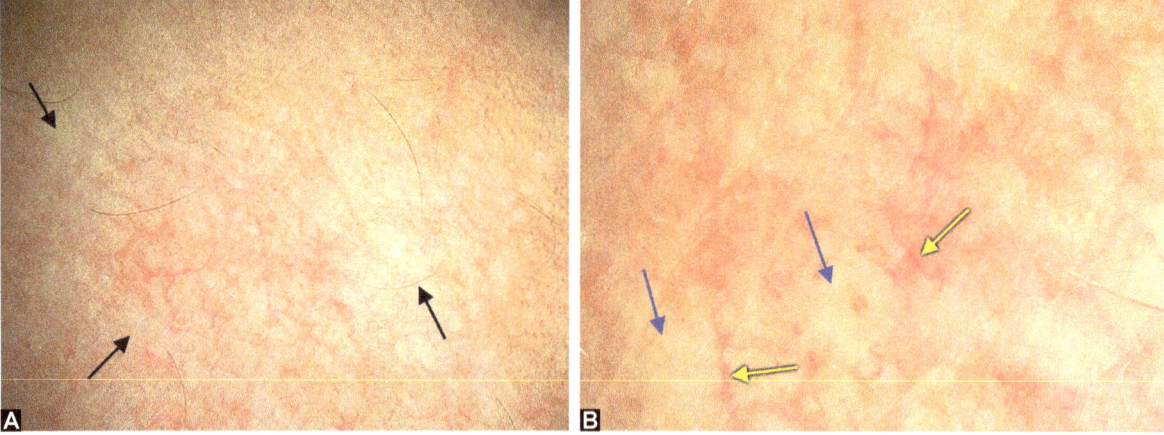

Figs 5A and B: Dermoscopic image of an erythematous plaque on abdomen in a case of borderline lepromatous Hansen's disease: (A) Low power shows partial loss of pigment network (black arrows) with structureless white areas and irregularly branched red streaks; (B) On higher magnification, structureless white areas (blue arrows) and irregularly branched red streaks (yellow arrows) are easily appreciated

REFERENCES

1. Vázquez-López F, Kreusch J, Marghoob AA. Dermoscopic semiology: further insights into vascular features by screening a large spectrum of nontumoral skin lesions. Br J Dermatol. 2004;150(2):226-31.
2. Brasiello M, Zalaudek I, Ferrara G, Gourhant JY, Capoluongo P, Roma P, et al. Lupus vulgaris: a new look at an old symptom–the lupoma observed with dermoscopy. Dermatology. 2009;218(2):172-4.
3. Llambrich A, Zaballos P, Terrasa F, Torne I, Puig S, Malvehy J. Dermoscopy of cutaneous leishmaniasis. B J Dermatol. 2009;160(4):756-61.
4. Pellicano R, Tiodorovic-Zivkovic D, Gourhant JY, Catricalà C, Ferrara G, Caldarola G, et al. Dermoscopy of cutaneous sarcoidosis. Dermatology. 2010;221(1):51-4.
5. Lallas A, Zaballos P, Zalaudek I, Apalla Z, Gourhant JY, Longo C, et al. Dermoscopic patterns of granuloma annulare and necrobiosis lipoidica. Clin Exp Dermatol. 2013;38(4):425-7.
6. Pellicano R, Caldarola G, Filabozzi P, Zalaudek I. Dermoscopy of necrobiosis lipoidica and granuloma annulare. Dermatology. 2013;226(4):319-23.
7. Yücel A, Günaşti S, Denli Y, Uzun S. Cutaneous leishmaniasis: new dermoscopic findings. Int J Dermatol. 2013;52(7):831-7.
8. Lallas A, Argenziano G, Apalla Z, Gourhant JY, Zaballos P, Di Lernia V, et al. Dermoscopic patterns of common facial inflammatory skin diseases. J Eur Acad Dermatol Venereol. 2014;28(5):609-14.

SECTION 6
Skin Tumors

Subrata Malakar

Section Outline

- Benign and Premalignant Tumors of Skin
- Dermoscopy of Malignant Cutaneous Tumors

CHAPTER 13

Benign and Premalignant Tumors of Skin

Subrata Malakar

INTRODUCTION

Dermoscopy has been proved useful for studying benign skin tumors. The application of dermoscope allows the assessment of important characteristics of tumor not evident on physical examination. The purpose of dermoscopy should be to provide additional information to the one already deduced by naked eyes.

DERMATOFIBROMA

Dermatofibroma (superficial benign fibrous histiocytoma) is a common benign skin tumor, most often seen on extremities especially the lower leg, usually as a solitary slightly pigmented firm papule (Figs 1 and 2).[1] The presence of Fitzpatrick's dimple sign (epidermal tethering to the underlying lesion on lateral compression) though considered to be characteristic of dermatofibroma, does not always confirm the lesion is dermatofibroma. In such situation, dermoscopy is useful in coming to diagnosis.[2]

Dermoscopy of dermatofibroma reveals a pseudo-network surrounding a central pale amorphous scar-like area, the pseudo-network is secondary to basal cell layer hyperpigmentation, and the central scar-like area reflects the collagenous stroma of dermatofibroma (Fig. 3).[3,4] This is the typical dermoscopic pattern of dermatofibroma. Apart from this typical pattern there are nine other patterns of dermatofibroma, which are as follows:[3]

1. Delicate pigment network distributed throughout the lesion
2. Peripheral pigment network surrounding a central white network
3. Peripheral homogenous pigmentation surrounding a central scar-like area
4. Areas of multifocal scar-like patches

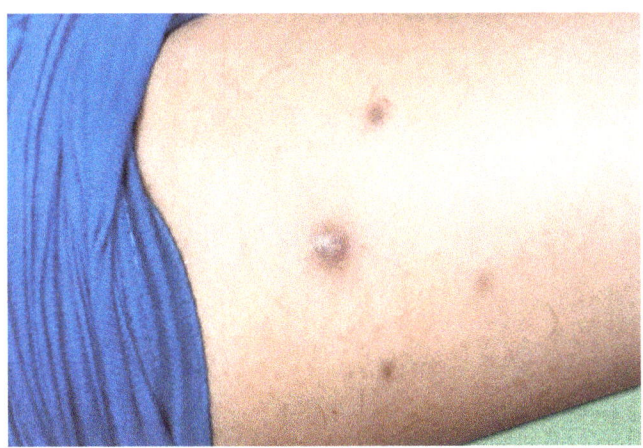

Fig. 1: Dermatofibroma over leg

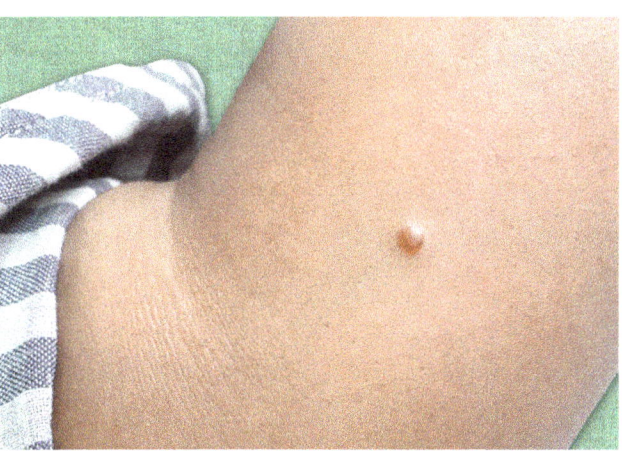

Fig. 2: Dermatofibroma over the forearm

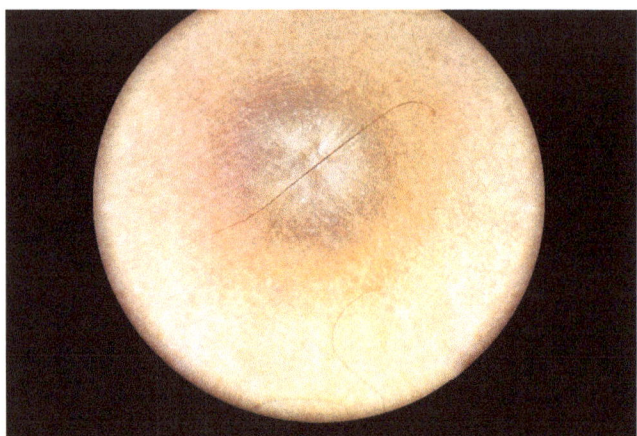

Fig. 3: Central scar-like structure and fine peripheral melanocytic network

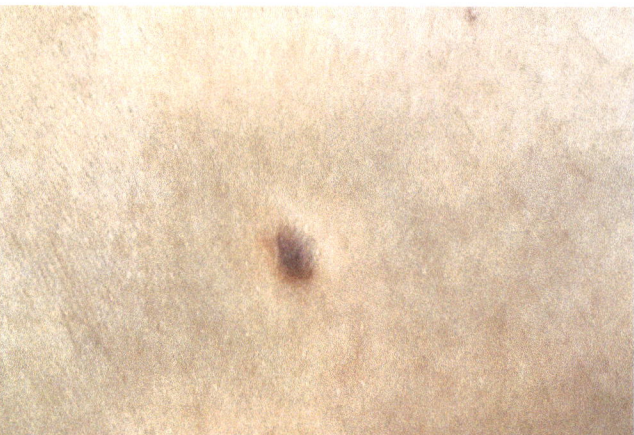

Fig. 5: Dermatofibroma

5. White scar-like patch throughout the lesion
6. Homogenous pigmentation throughout the lesion
7. Peripheral pigment network surrounding a central homogenous patch
8. White network throughout the lesion
9. Atypical pattern comprises combination of various features, some may exhibit bluish-red homogenous areas, white linear streaks (chrysalis-like structure), various vascular patterns [dotted vessels, coma vessels, hairpin vessels, glomerular vessels, telengiectasias (Fig. 4), linear irregular vessels, polymorphous or atypical vessels] and erythema (Figs 5 and 6).

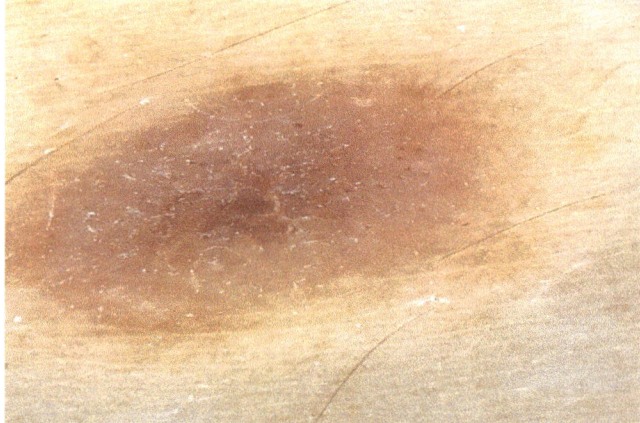

Fig. 6: Mosaic pigment network with comedo-like openings (author's observation)

ANGIOKERATOMA

Angiokeratomas are benign vascular lesions comprising subepidermal vascular ectasias which may produce overlying acanthosis and hyperkeratosis. Angiokeratomas present as hyperkeratotic, dark red to purple or black, slightly compressible papules (Fig. 7). Angiokeratoma lesions are of clinical importance as they often mimic a malignant melanoma and pigmented basal cell carcinoma.[5-7]

The typical dermoscopic features of angiokeratoma include dark lacunae, whitish veil, erythema, red lacunae and hemorrhagic crusts (Fig. 8). Dark lacunae corresponds

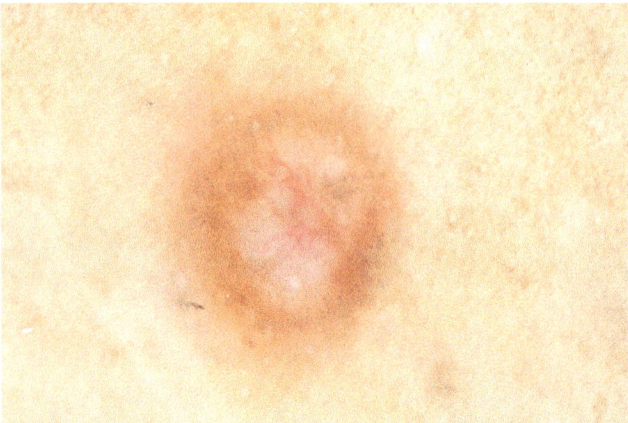

Fig. 4: Telangiectatic vessels across the typical pattern of dermatofibroma

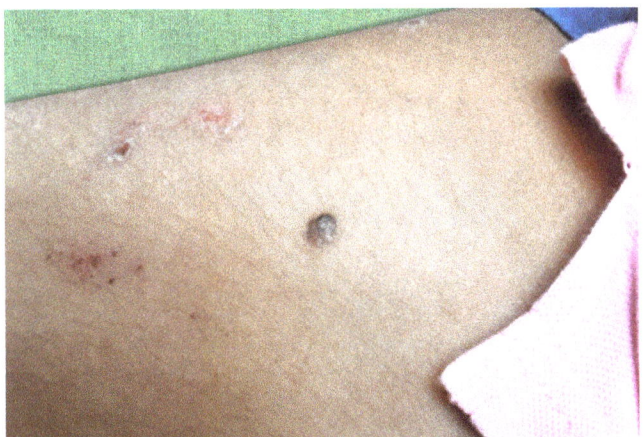

Fig. 7: Angiokeratoma

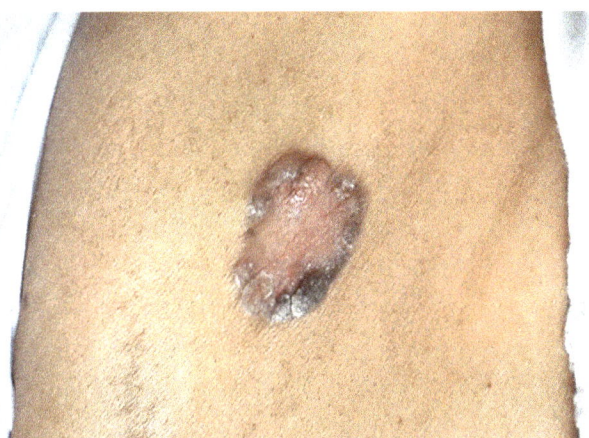

Fig. 9: Bowen's disease

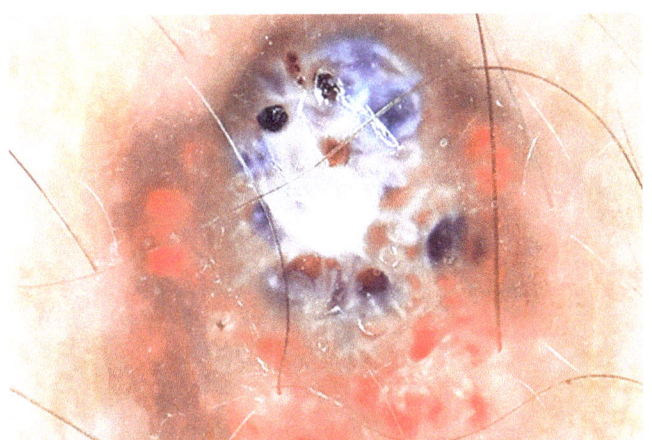

Fig. 8: Red lacuna, blue lacuna, white veil

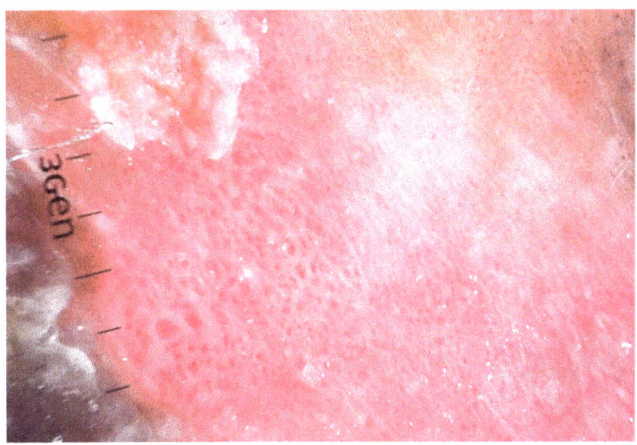

Fig. 10: Glomerular vessels arranged in clusters with scaling

to the partially or completely thrombosed dilated vessels. Whitish veil corresponds to hyperkeratosis and acanthosis, hemorrhagic crust corresponds to area of bleeding, and erythema reflects inflammation. Dark lacunae has been reported to exhibit a sensitivity of 93.8% and specificity of 99.1%, a feature which is absent in both malignant melanoma and pigmented basal cell carcinoma.[7] Dermoscopy appears to be a very useful noninvasive tool in establishing the diagnosis of angiokeratoma.

BOWEN'S DISEASE

Bowen's disease also known as squamous cell carcinoma (SCC) in situ, often presents with an asymptomatic, slowly enlarging, erythematous, well-demarcated scaly patch or plaque (Fig. 9). It may occur anywhere on the mucocutaneous surface. Dermoscopic features are typically characterized by glomerular vessels (tortuous vessels simulating renal glomerulus) arranged in clusters and a scaly surface (Fig. 10).[8,9]

KERATOACANTHOMA

They are solitary dome-shaped nodules with a smooth shiny surface and a central crateriform ulceration or keratin plug; usually appear on sun-exposed areas (Fig. 11). They are low-grade tumors that closely resemble SCC, some are of the view that they are a variant of invasive SCC. However, recent reports suggest them to be distinct entity on the basis of gene expression and cutaneous marker.[10,11]

Dermoscopic features of keratoacanthoma include central yellowish structureless keratin, surrounded by arborising vessels and/or hairpin vessels (Fig. 12). Though keratoacanthoma and SCC both share dermoscopic features,

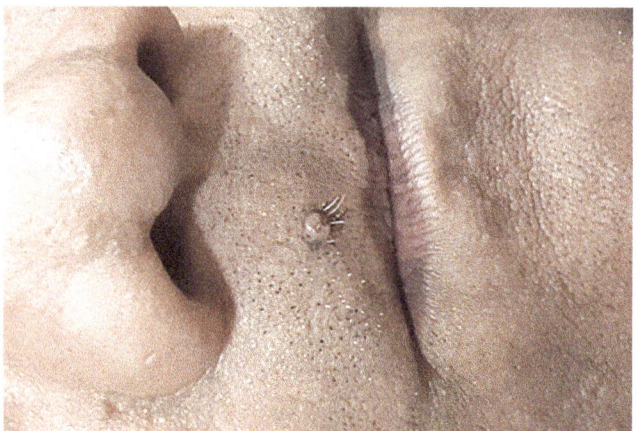

Fig. 11: Keratoacanthoma

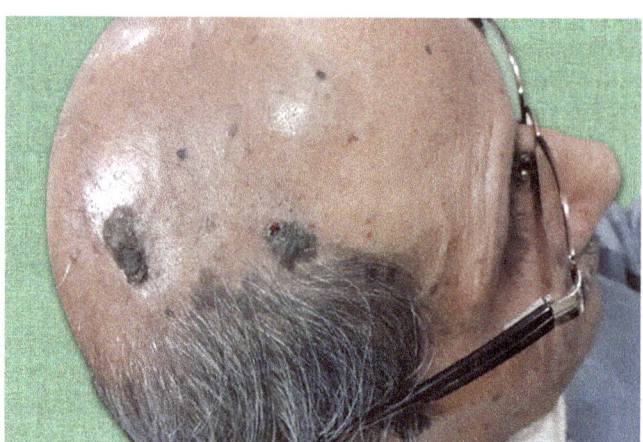

Fig. 13: Seborrheic keratoses

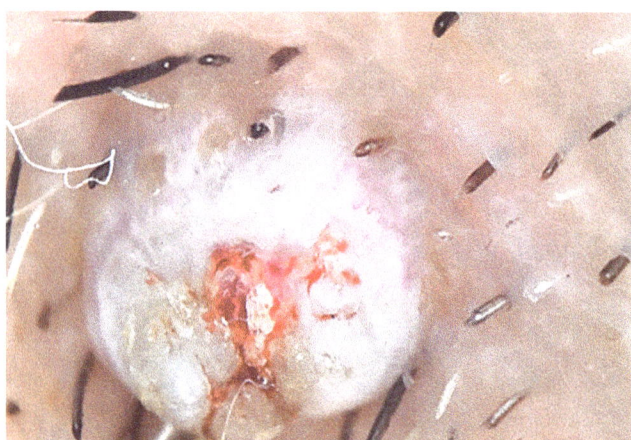

Fig. 12: Central crater, whitish structureless area and hairpin vessels in keratoacanthoma

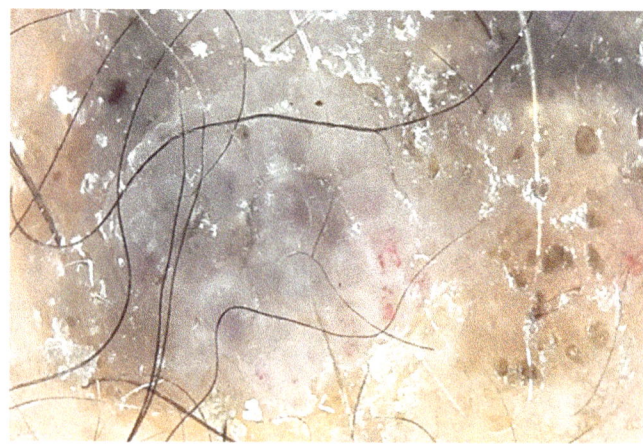

Fig. 14: Cerebriform structures, milia-like cysts, hairpin vessels, comedo-like openings, moth-eaten appearance

central keratin is more common in keratoacanthoma than in SCC.[12]

SEBORRHEIC KERATOSIS

Seborrheic keratoses usually begin as sharply defined, light brown, flat macules that develop into verrucous surface, with multiple plugged follicles and a lackluster appearance. The lesions may be sparse or numerous (Fig. 13). Dermoscopic features are usually specific for its diagnosis.

Typical dermoscopic features include the following (Figs 14 to 16):[13-15]

- *Milia-like cyst*: These are intraepidermal keratin cysts which appear as multiple bright white-yellowish structures. They are visualized better on nonpolarized dermoscopy.

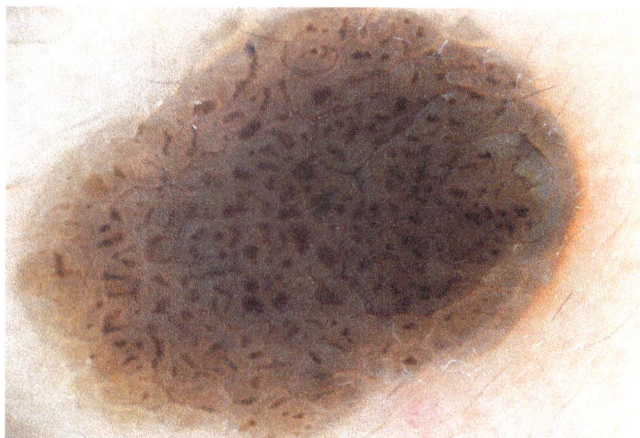

Fig. 15: Presence of multiple sulci and gyri may produce cerebriform pattern seen in seborrheic keratosis. *Courtesy:* Shekhar Neema, Command Hospital, Kolkata

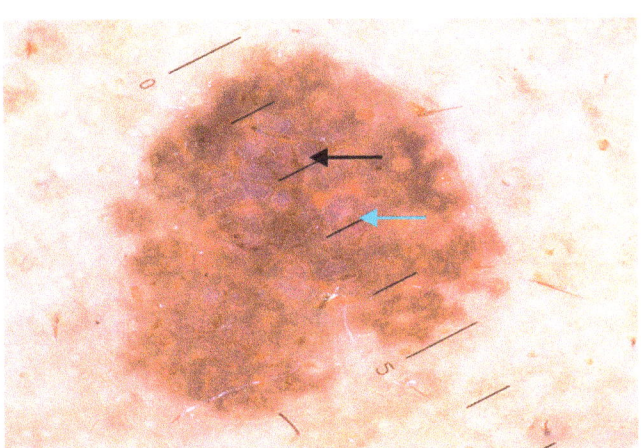

Fig. 16: Comedo-like opening (black arrow) and fissure (blue arrow)
Courtesy: Shekhar Neema, Command Hospital, Kolkata

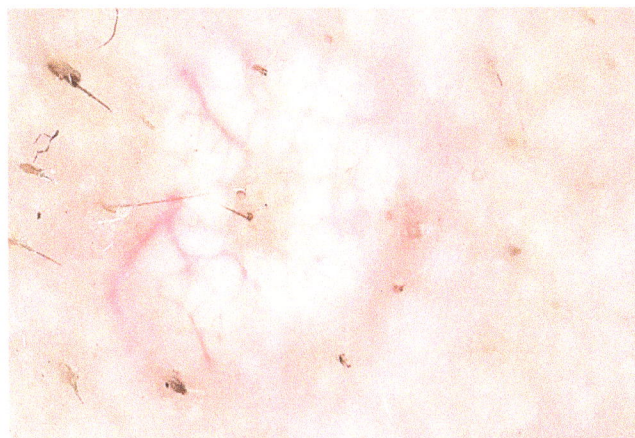

Fig. 18: Central follicular opening with pale yellow lobules and "crown vessels"

- *Comedo-like openings*: They are black to brown keratin plugs within dilated follicular openings.
- *Cerebriform pattern*: Multiple fissures (linear and curvilinear) and ridges resulting in cerebriform pattern are seen. Fissures are keratin-filled deep invaginations of the epidermis.
- Fingerprint structures and moth-eaten border.
- *Hairpin vessels*: They are "U"-shaped vessels twisted upon themselves with a whitish halo. Hairpin vessels may also be seen in melanomas, were it is surrounded by a pink halo.

SEBACEOUS HYPERPLASIA

The classic appearance of sebaceous hyperplasia is whitish-yellow or skin-colored papules varying in size from 2 mm to 9 mm, over the face (Fig. 17). Some papules may be associated with characteristics similar to basal cell carcinoma, such as telangiectasia.

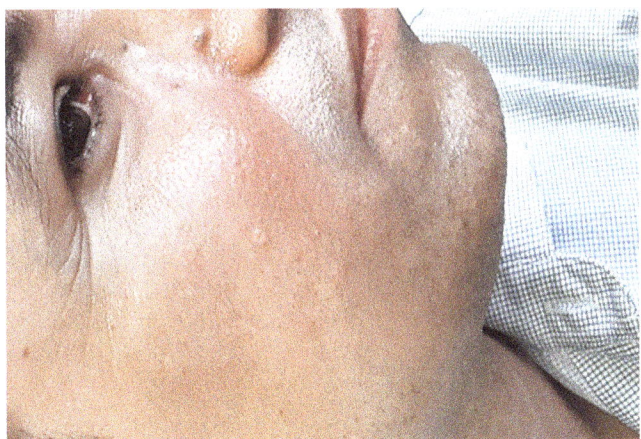

Fig. 17: Clinical picture: Sebaceous hyperplasia

Dermoscopy is useful in distinguishing between nodular basal cell carcinoma and sebaceous hyperplasia. Sebaceous hyperplasia is distinguished by pale yellow lobules surrounding a central follicular opening. There are curvilinear vessels at the periphery radiating towards the center (without crossing the center) termed as "crown vessels" (Fig. 18). [16-18]

REFERENCES

1. Naversen DN, Trask DM, Watson FH, Burket JM. Painful tumors of the skin: "LEND AN EGG". J Am Acad Dermatol. 1993;28(2 Pt 2):298-300.
2. Meffert JJ, Peake MF, Wilde JL. 'Dimpling' is not unique to dermatofibromas. Dermatology. 1997;195(4):384-6.
3. Zaballos P, Puig S, Llambrich A, Malvehy J. Dermoscopy of dermatofibromas: a prospective morphological study of 412 cases. Arch Dermatol. 2008;144(1):75-83.
4. Camara MF, Pinheiro PM, Jales RD, da Trindade Neto PB, Costa JB, de Sousa VL Multiple dermatofibromas: dermoscopic patterns. Indian J Dermatol. 2013;58(3):243.
5. Ozdemir R, Karaaslan O, Tiftikcioglu YO, Kocer U. Angiokeratoma circumscriptum. Dermatol Surg. 2004;30(10):1364-6.
6. Das A, Mondal AK, Saha A, Chowdhury SN, Gharami RC. Angiokeratoma circumscriptum neviforme: An entity, few and far between. Indian Dermatol Online J. 2014;5(4):472-4.
7. Zaballos P, Daufí C, Puig S, Argenziano G, Moreno-Ramírez D, Cabo H, et al. Dermoscopy of solitary angiokeratomas: a morphological study. Arch Dermatol. 2007;143(3):318-25.
8. Bugatti L, Filosa G, De Angelis R. The specific dermoscopical criteria of Bowen's disease. J Eur Acad Dermatol Venereol. 2007;21(5):700-1.
9. Zalaudek I, Argenziano G, Leinweber B, Citarella L, Hofmann-Wellenhof R, Malvehy J, et al. Dermoscopy of Bowen's disease. Br J Dermatol. 2004;150(6):1112-6.

10. Ra SH, Su A, Li X, Zhou J, Cochran AJ, Kulkarni RP, et al. Keratoacanthoma and squamous cell carcinoma are distinct from a molecular perspective. Mod Pathol. 2015;28(6):799-806.
11. Kanzaki A, Kudo M, Ansai S, Peng WX, Ishino K, Yamamoto T, et al. Insulin-like growth factor 2 mRNA-binding protein-3 as a marker for distinguishing between cutaneous squamous cell carcinoma and keratoacanthoma. Int J Oncol. 2016;48(3):1007-15.
12. Rosendahl C, Cameron A, Argenziano G, Zalaudek I, Tschandl P, Kittler H. Dermoscopy of squamous cell carcinoma and keratoacanthoma. Arch Dermatol. 2012;148(12):1386-92.
13. Braun RP, Rabinovitz HS, Krischer J, Kreusch J, Oliviero M, Naldi L, et al. Dermoscopy of pigmented seborrheic keratosis: a morphological study. Arch Dermatol. 2002;138(12):1556-60.
14. Soyer HP, Kenet RO, Wolf IH, Kenet BJ, Cerroni L. Clinicopathological correlation of pigmented skin lesions using dermoscopy. Eur J Dermatol. 2000;10(1):22-8.
15. Marghoob AA, Braun RP, Kopf AW. Re: Differentiating vessels from globules on dermoscopy. Dermatol Surg. 2005;31(1):120; author reply 120.
16. Argenziano G, Zalaudek I, Corona R, Sera F, Cicale L, Petrillo G, et al. Vascular structures in skin tumors: a dermoscopy study. Arch Dermatol. 2004;140(12):1485-9.
17. Bryden AM, Dawe RS, Fleming C. Dermatoscopic features of benign sebaceous proliferation. Clin Exp Dermatol. 2004;29(6):676-7.
18. Zaballos P, Ara M, Puig S, Malvehy J. Dermoscopy of sebaceous hyperplasia. Arch Dermatol. 2005;141(6):808.

CHAPTER 14

Dermoscopy of Malignant Cutaneous Tumors

Laxmisha Chandrashekar, Biswanath Behera

INTRODUCTION

Dermoscopy is a noninvasive outpatient procedure that has been conventionally used to differentiate benign moles from malignant melanomas. In recent times, the use of dermoscopy has increased in various areas of dermatology ranging from infectious, inflammatory and neoplastic disorder. The use of dermoscopy in cutaneous tumors is many folds; it gives a clue to the diagnosis of the neoplasm, helps in differentiating benign from malignant cutaneous neoplasms, differentiating between epithelial, melanocytic and adnexal neoplasms and also has a prognostic and therapeutic use. In this chapter, the dermoscopic features of various epithelial premalignant and malignant tumors and melanoma are being described.

DERMOSCOPY OF BASAL CELL CARCINOMA

The dermoscopic criteria proposed by Menzies et al.[1] in order to increase the diagnostic accuracy of basal cell carcinoma (BCC), especially to differentiate pigmented BCC from malignant melanoma is absence of pigment network and presence of one of the positive feature (ulceration, multiple blue-gray globules, leaf-like areas, large blue-gray ovoid nests, spoke wheel areas and arborizing telangiectasia) of BCC. Over the time, several diagnostic dermoscopic criteria have been put forward and updated. The dermoscopic features vary depending upon the patient's skin color and histopathological subtype. The various dermoscopic features described for BCC are:
- Arborizing vessels (Fig. 1)
- Superficial fine telangiectasia (Fig. 2)
- Blue-gray ovoid nests
- Multiple blue-gray globules
- In-focus dots
- Maple leaf-like areas (Fig. 3)
- Spoke wheel areas (Fig. 4)
- Concentric structures, ulceration (Fig. 5)
- Multiple small erosions
- Shiny white-red structureless areas (Fig. 2) and short white streaks (chrysalis).[2]

Dermoscopy can also predict the histologic subtype of BCC, thus can aid in guiding the mode of therapy needed. A translucent pinkish background with prominent arborizing vessels and ulceration is frequently seen in the case of nonpigmented nodular BCC, while pigmented BCC are typified by multiple blue-gray dots or globules, blue-grey ovoid nests and usually associated with arborizing vessels. Maple leaf-like area, spoke wheel areas and concentric structures are typically present at the periphery or superficial part of nodular BCC. Superficial BCC is characterized by superficial fine telangiectasia with few ramifications, shiny white or red structureless areas and multiple small erosions. Morpheaform BCC can have a whitish background while infiltrative

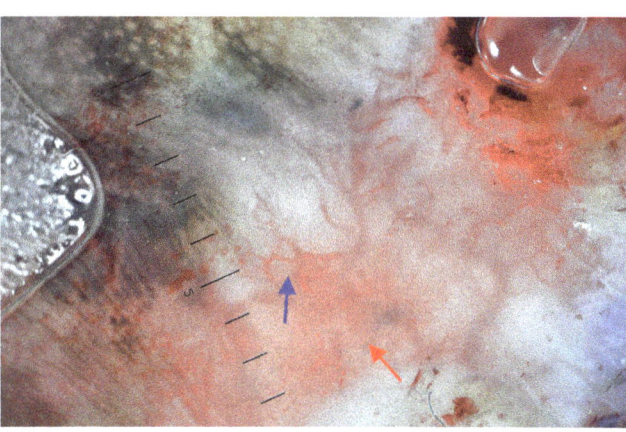

Fig. 1: Milky-red structureless areas (red arrow), arborizing vessels (blue arrow), hemorrhage and out of focus blue-gray ovoid nest

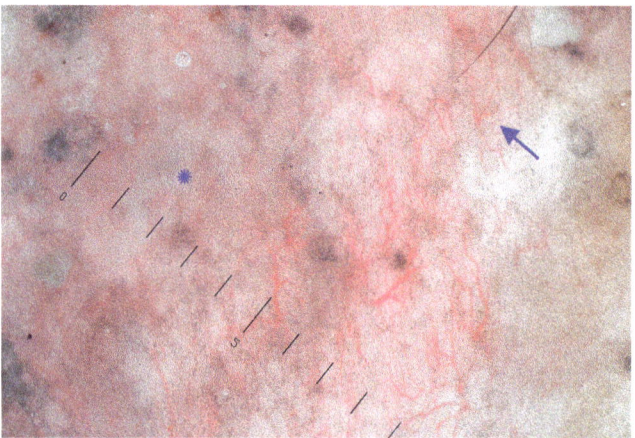

Fig. 2: Shiny white-red structureless areas (asterix) and arborizing telangiectasias (arrow)

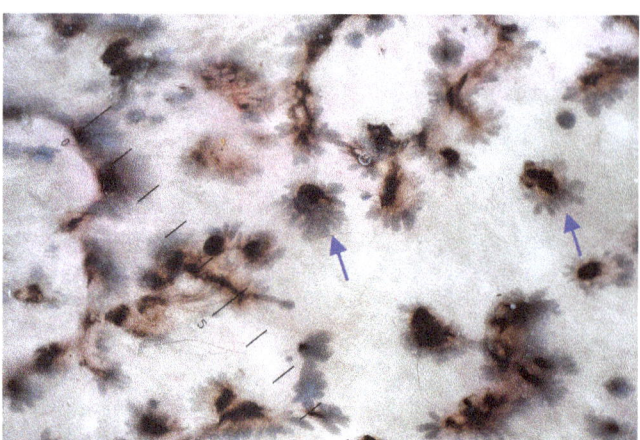

Fig. 4: Multiple spoke wheel areas (arrows)

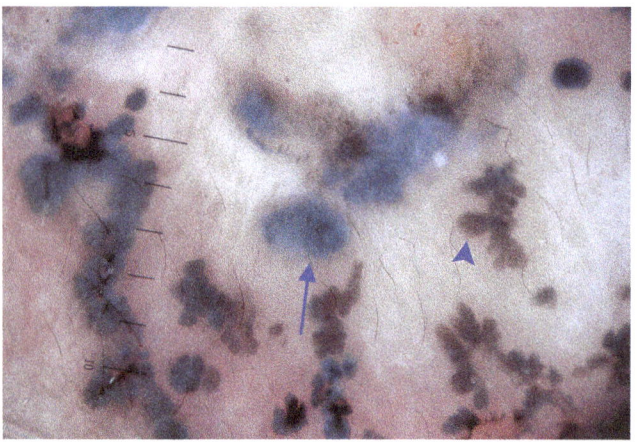

Fig. 3: Maple leaf-like areas (arrow head) and large blue-gray ovoid nest (arrow) over a reddish-pink background

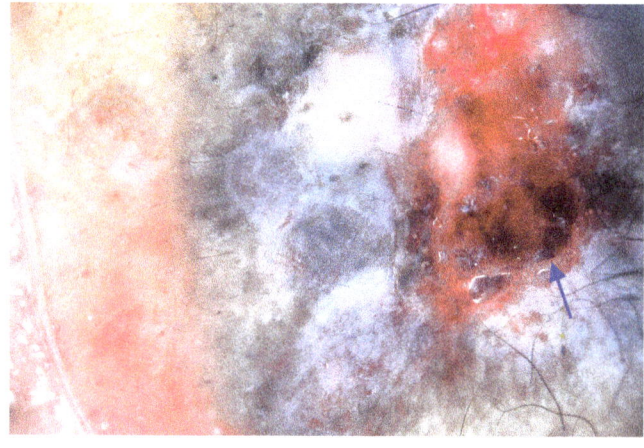

Fig. 5: Maple leaf-like areas, reddish-pink areas and ulceration (arrow)

variant demonstrates white or red structureless areas.[3,4] Fibroepithelioma of Pinkus is characterized by a white-pinkish background color with fine arborizing vessels in the center and dotted vessels at the periphery.[5] The rare type basosquamous variant will have features of both BCC and squamous cell carcinoma (SCC) such as unfocused (peripheral) arborizing vessels, white structureless areas, superficial scale, keratin masses, ulceration or blood crusts, blue-grey blotches and blood spots in keratin masses (Table 1).[6]

DERMOSCOPY OF SQUAMOUS CELL CARCINOMA AND KERATOACANTHOMA

The various dermoscopic features described for SCC or keratoacanthoma (KA) are keratin crust or scale, central keratin mass, white circles, white structureless area, keratin pearl, blood spots and polymorphous vessels including glomerular, linear irregular, atypical and hairpin vessels (Figs 6 and 7).[7]

DERMOSCOPY OF MALIGNANT MELANOMA

Out of various morphological and histological subtype of malignant melanoma, the acral melanomas (acral lentiginous melanoma and melanoma of nail apparatus) are common in Indian population. The dermoscopic features described for acral lentiginous melanoma are irregular diffuse pigmentation (Fig. 8) and the parallel-ridge pattern (in contrast to parallel furrow pattern in benign lesions; Fig. 9). The dermoscopic features for nail apparatus melanoma are irregular lines with variegations in colors, spacing,

Chapter 14 Dermoscopy of Malignant Cutaneous Tumors

Table 1: Dermoscopic features of basal cell carcinoma with histopathological correlation

Dermoscopic feature	Corresponding histopathological findings
Arborizing vessels	Dilated vessels in the dermis
Superficial fine telangiectasia	Telangiectatic vessels located in the papillary dermis
Blue-gray ovoid nests	Relatively large well-defined tumor nests with pigment aggregates, invading the dermis
Multiple blue-gray globules	Papillary and/or reticular dermal located small, roundish tumor nests with central pigmentation
In-focus dots	Small aggregate of pigmented neoplastic cells or free pigment deposition along the dermoepidermal junction and/or melanophages
Maple leaf-like areas	Interconnected multifocal tumor nests containing pigment aggregates
Spoke wheel areas (characterized by centrally located pigmentation with finger-like projections)	Tumor nests arising and connected to the epidermis
Ulceration	Loss of the epidermis
Shiny white-red structureless areas	Diffuse dermal fibrosis or fibrotic tumoral stroma
Short white streaks (chrysalis) (only under polarized dermoscopy)	Collagenous stroma and fibrosis in the dermis

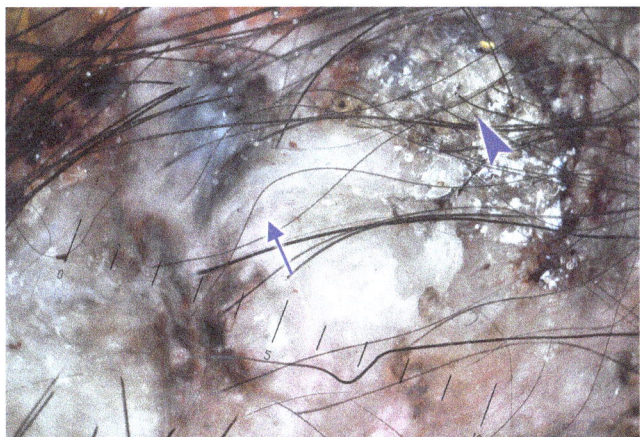

Fig. 6: Squamous cell carcinoma of scalp demonstrating white keratin (arrow head), white structureless area, hairpin vessel (arrow) and linear irregular vessel

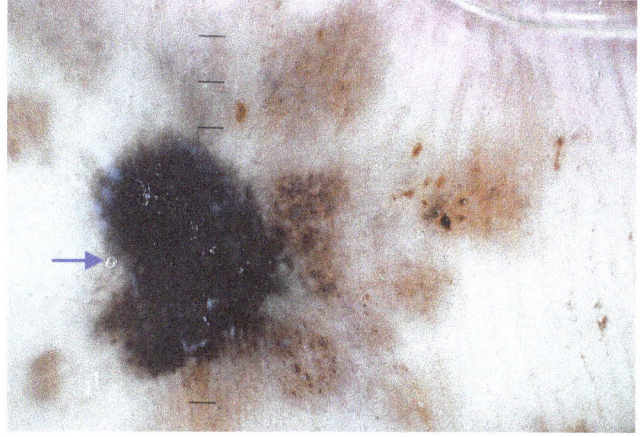

Fig. 8: Acral lentiginous melanoma showing irregular diffuse pigmentation (arrow)

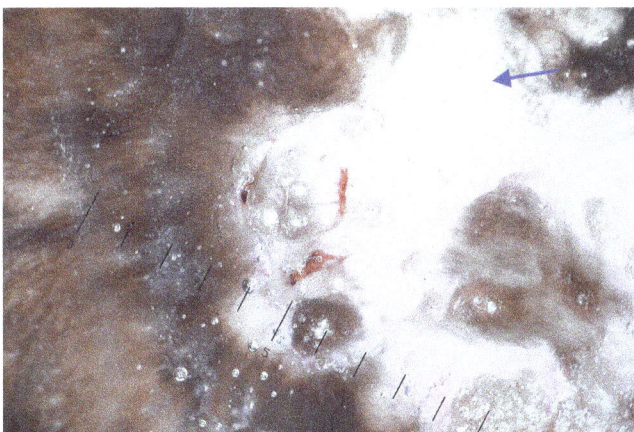

Fig. 7: Dermoscopy of a squamous cell carcinoma demonstrating white structureless area (arrow) and hairpin and dotted vessels

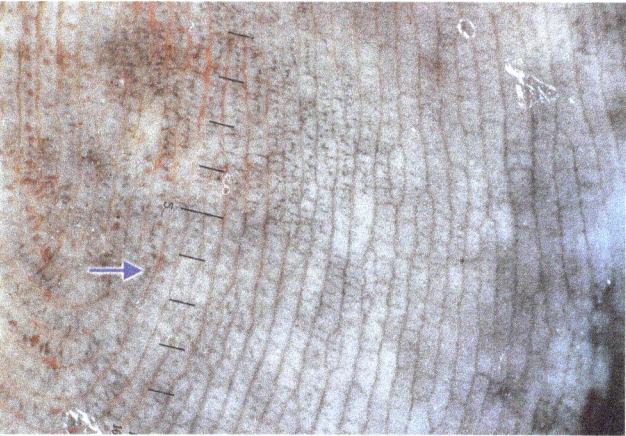

Fig. 9: Acral lentiginous melanoma demonstrating parallel ridge pattern (arrow)

width and disruption of parallelism. The dermoscopic features of acral amelanotic melanoma is dominated by retention of microscopic pigmentation, milky-red areas and polymorphous vascular pattern consisting linear irregular vessels, dotted vessels and hairpin vessels.[8,9]

DERMOSCOPY OF BOWEN'S DISEASE

Dermoscopic features of Bowen's disease (BD) described for the Asian population is typified by the presence of a scaly surface (Fig. 10) and vascular structures, out of which glomerular vessels are frequently observed and others being dotted, linear irregular, atypical and arborizing vessels.[10] The other dermoscopic features described are white structureless area, linear brown or gray dots, streaks, squamous or verrucous surface, irregularly distributed patches of pigmentation, pigmented pseudo-network, homogeneous grayish-brown pigmentation and bleeding (Figs 11 and 12).[11,12]

DERMOSCOPY OF ACTINIC KERATOSIS

The nonpigmented actinic keratosis (AK) is characterized by presence of "strawberry pattern" which consists of whitish surface scales (Fig. 13), hyperkeratotic follicles and an interfollicular erythematous pseudo-network.[13] The pigmented AKs under dermoscopy reveal multiple slate-

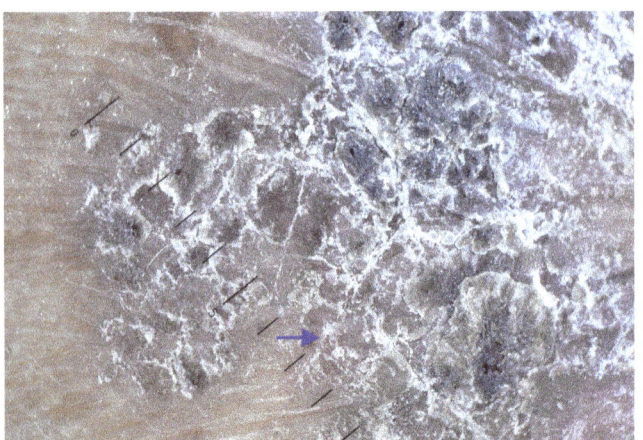

Fig. 10: Bowen disease: Diffuse scaling (arrow) and verrucous surface

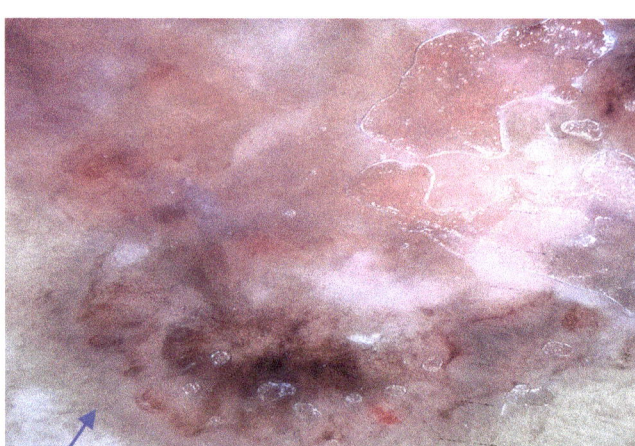

Fig. 12: Bowen disease: Prominent peripheral streak (arrow) and gray-brown dots

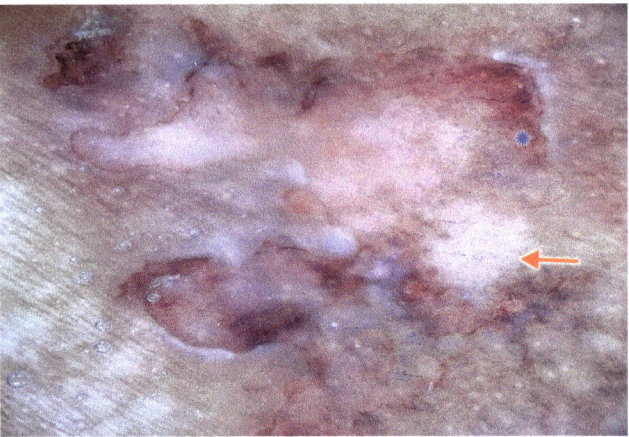

Fig. 11: Bowen dsease: White structureless area (arrow), patchy irregular gray-brown pigmentation (star), gray-brown dots and peripheral streaks

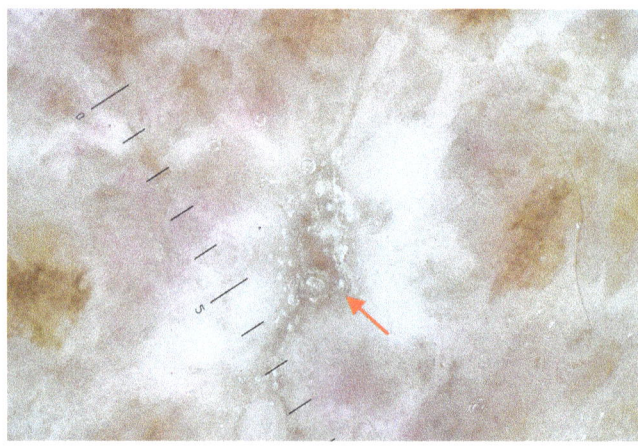

Fig. 13: Actinic keratoses: White structureless area, scaling (arrow) and multiple red dots

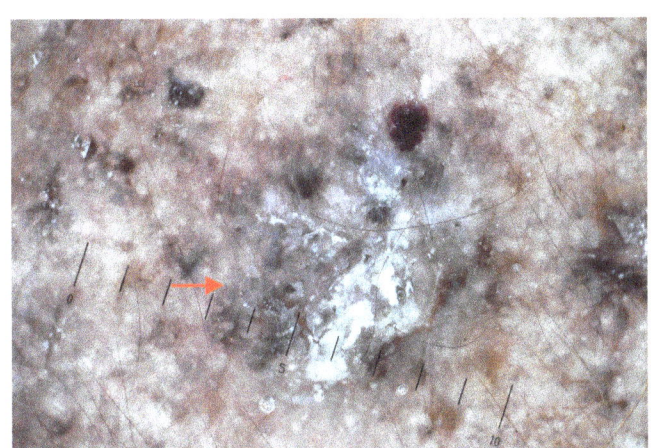

Fig. 14: Actinic keratoses: Central scaling and peripheral pseudo-pigment network (arrow)

gray to dark-brown dots and globules around the follicular ostia, annular-granular pattern and brown to gray pseudo-network (Fig. 14).[14]

REFERENCES

1. Menzies SW, Westerhoff K, Rabinovitz H, Kopf AW, McCarthy WH, Katz B. Surface microscopy of pigmented basal cell carcinoma. Arch Dermatol. 2000;136(8):1012-6.
2. Lallas A, Apalla Z, Argenziano G, Longo C, Moscarella E, Specchio F, et al. The dermatoscopic universe of basal cell carcinoma. Dermatol Pract Concept. 2014;4(3):11-24.
3. Lallas A, Argenziano G, Zendri E, Moscarella E, Longo C, Grenzi L, et al. Update on non-melanoma skin cancer and the value of dermoscopy in its diagnosis and treatment monitoring. Expert Rev Anticancer Ther. 2013;13(5):541-58.
4. Zaludek I, Kreusch J, Giacomel J, Ferrara G, Catricalà C, Argenziano G. How to diagnose nonpigmented skin tumors: a review of vascular structures seen with dermoscopy: part II. Nonmelanocytic skin tumors. J Am Acad Dermatol. 2010;63(3):377-88.
5. Longo C, Lallas A, Kyrgidis A, Rabinovitz H, Moscarella E, Ciardo S, et al. Classifying distinct basal cell carcinoma subtype by means of dermatoscopy and reflectance confocal microscopy. J Am Acad Dermatol. 2014;71(4):716-24.
6. Boyd AS, Stasko TS, Tang YW. Basaloid squamous cell carcinoma of the skin. J Am Acad Dermatol. 2011;64(1):144-51.
7. Lin MJ, Pan Y, Jalilian C, Kelly JW. Dermoscopic characteristics of nodular squamous cell carcinoma and keratoacanthoma. Dermatol Pract Concept. 2014;4(2):9-15.
8. Saida T, Miyazaki A, Oguchi S, Ishihara Y, Yamazaki Y, Murase S, et al. Significance of dermoscopic patterns in detecting malignant melanoma on acral volar skin: results of a multicenter study in Japan. Arch Dermatol. 2004;140(10):1233-8.
9. Phan A, Dalle S, Touzet S, Ronger-Savlé S, Balme B, Thomas L. Dermoscopic features of acral lentiginous melanoma in a large series of 110 cases in a white population. Br J Dermatol. 2010;162(4):765-71.
10. Mun JH, Kim SH, Jung DS, Ko HC, Kwon KS, Kim MB. Dermoscopic features of Bowen's disease in Asians. J Eur Acad Dermatol Venereol. 2010;24(7):805-10.
11. Chung E, Marchetti MA, Pulitzer MP, Marghoob AA. Streaks in pigmented squamous cell carcinoma in situ. J Am Acad Dermatol. 2015;72(1 Suppl):S64-5.
12. Bugatti L, Filosa G, De Angelis R. Dermoscopic observation of Bowen's disease. J Eur Acad Dermatol Venereol. 2004;18(5): 572-4.
13. Giacomel J, Lallas A, Argenziano G, Bombonato C, Zalaudek I. Dermoscopic "signature" pattern of pigmented and nonpigmented facial actinic keratoses. J Am Acad Dermatol. 2015;72(2):e57-9.
14. Moscarella E, Rabinovitz H, Zalaudek I, Piana S, Stanganelli I, Oliviero MC, et al. Dermoscopy and reflectance confocal microscopy of pigmented actinic keratoses: a morphological study. J Eur Acad Dermatol Venereol. 2015;29(2):307-14.

SECTION 7
Onychoscopy

Nirmal B

Section Outline

- Onychoscopy

Onychoscopy

Nirmal B

INTRODUCTION

Nail dermoscopy requires good knowledge of nail anatomy, physiology and pathogenesis of nail diseases. Nailfold capillaroscopy (NFC) is widely utilized by rheumatologists and dermatologists to monitor evolution and response to treatment of connective tissue diseases. The nail unit is in fact not visible as a whole at one time. Dermoscope has to be moved forth and down and from side to side to get an idea of the whole nail. Performing nail dermoscopy and taking good quality images requires practice.

RELEVANT ANATOMY OF NAIL UNIT[1]

Proximal Nail Fold

Cuticle is visible as a transparent transverse band that seals the plate to proximal nail fold (PNF). Each capillary vessel resembles a hairpin, being formed by two arms that make a distal convex loop. They have uniform morphology and are homogeneously aligned. Normal density is 30 linear capillaries per 5 mm (Fig. 1).

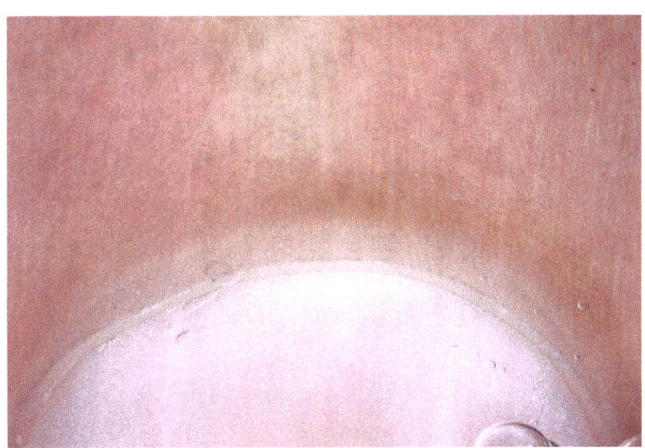

Fig. 1: Normal nailfold capillaroscopy (NFC) pattern observed in the nondominant fourth finger showing uniform hairpin-shaped morphology and homogenous arrangement
Courtesy: Department of Dermatology, Christian Medical College, Vellore

Nail Plate

Normal nail plate surface is smooth and shiny.

Nail Bed

Nail bed is visible below the transparent plate and appears pale pink. Distal nail bed shows longitudinally arranged capillaries that parallel that of dermal ridges.

Hyponychium

Capillaries in hyponychium appear as tiny red dots.

INDICATIONS OF ONYCHOSCOPY IN DERMATOLOGY

All nail disorders can be observed by dermoscopy. In most cases, it only permits better visualization already evident to naked eye except for few diseases in which the technique really adds vital information to clinical examination. The indications include the following:
- Traumatic disorders
  - Traumatic onycholysis
  - Transverse leukonychia of toe nails
  - Subungual hematoma
- Infective disorders
  - Wart
  - Pseudomonas superinfection
  - Onychomycosis

- Inflammatory disorders
  - Psoriasis
  - Lichen planus
  - Pyogenic granuloma
- Nail melanonychia
- Nailfold capillaroscopy.

SUBUNGUAL HEMATOMA

The color of subungual hematoma reflects the age of the lesion. Recent lesions are purple or black whereas older lesions are more brownish (Fig. 2). The proximal end of the hemorrhage is round and the distal end is characterized by a streaks-like or filamentous pattern due to longitudinal ridges present in the nail bed.[2]

PSEUDOMONAS SUPERINFECTION

Pseudomonas cannot infect healthy nails, but can colonize subungual space and nail plate when they are damaged. Dermoscopy shows deep green pigmentation involving only parts of the nail plate with irregular surface (Fig. 3).

ONYCHOMYCOSIS

The dermoscopic findings that are exclusive for onychomycosis[3] include the following:
- Jagged edge of proximal margin of onycholysis, with sharp structures (spikes) directed to PNF (Fig. 4)
- White-yellow longitudinal striae in the onycholytic nail plate (Fig. 5)
- Overall appearance of affected nail plate in parallel bands of different colors, resembling aurora borealis (Fig. 6).

PSORIASIS

The onychoscopic findings of psoriasis include coarse pits on the nail plate, regular onycholysis, oil drop sign, dilated globose vessels, splinter hemorrhages and streaky capillaries (Fig. 7). Dermoscopy in psoriasis of nail unit is of value in detection of subclinical cases.[4]

NAIL MELANONYCHIA

In the nail unit, melanocytes are found both in nail matrix and nail bed. Those in the nail matrix produce melanin, but those in the latter do not. Hence, melanomas originating from the nail bed tend to be amelanotic. Childhood longitudinal melanonychia of a single digit is most commonly nevus whereas adult-onset melanonychia of a single digit should be carefully evaluated and often needs a biopsy. Pigmentation of nail is not necessarily due to melanin and other causes include exogenous pigmentation, fungal melanonychia and green nails. If melanonychia involves several digits, the causes include ethnic pigmentation (Fig. 8), systemic drugs (Fig. 9), friction, pregnancy, endocrine disorders and onychotillomania.

Melanoma in the nail unit can be identified by brown to black band width breadth of 3 mm or more with variegated borders, irregular margins, irregular color, non-parallel lines and noncontinuous lines, with extension of pigment onto the proximal and/or lateral nail fold (Hutchinson's sign).[5]

NAILFOLD CAPILLAROSCOPY

Nailfold capillaries were first observed in 17th century with primitive magnifying equipment. Research in second

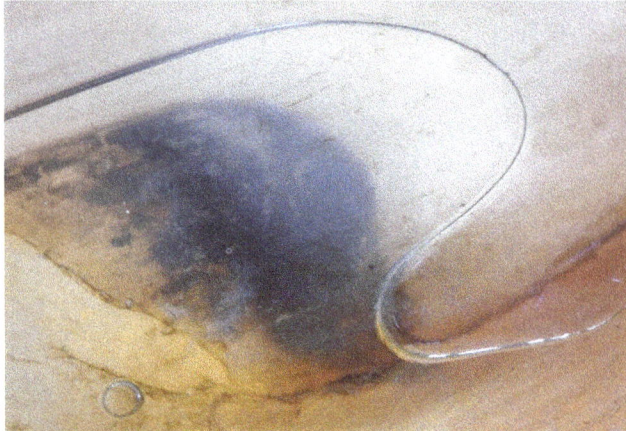

Fig. 2: Subungual hematoma: Early lesion showing purple-black homogenous areas with proximal rounded edge and distal globules and streaky pattern
Courtesy: Department of Dermatology, Christian Medical College, Vellore

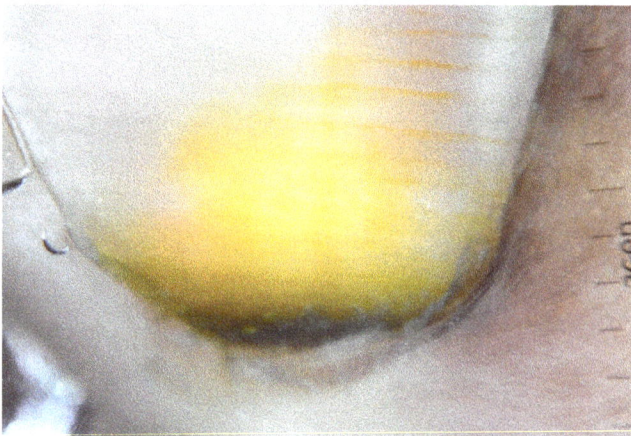

Fig. 3: Pseudomonas superinfection of nail unit showing irregular greenish pigmentation of nail plate
Courtesy: Department of Dermatology, Christian Medical College, Vellore

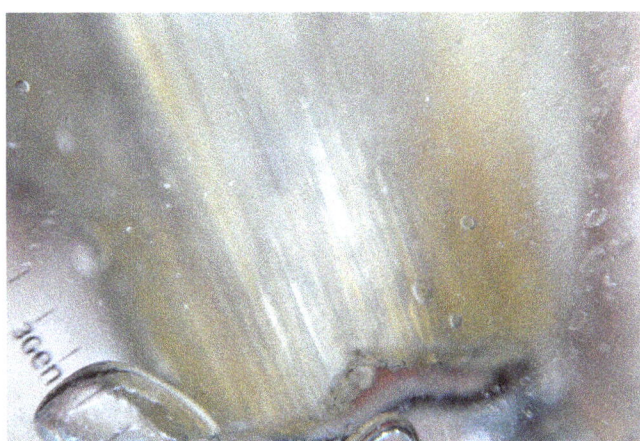

Fig. 4: Onychomycosis showing jagged proximal edge of onycholysis
Courtesy: Department of Dermatology, Christian Medical College, Vellore

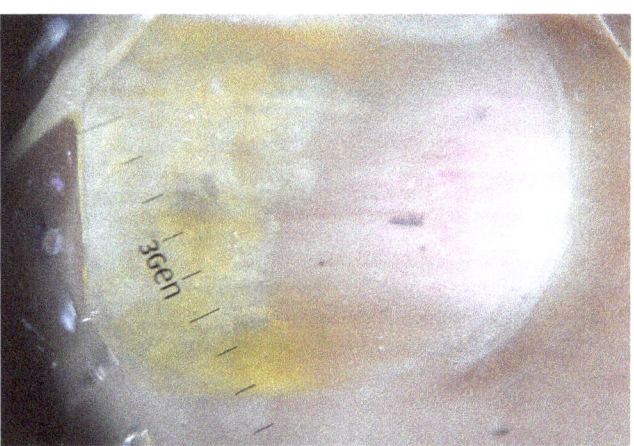

Fig. 7: Nail psoriasis showing dilated fusiform vessels surrounded by a prominent halo, splinter hemorrhages and linear onycholysis
Courtesy: Department of Dermatology, Christian Medical College, Vellore

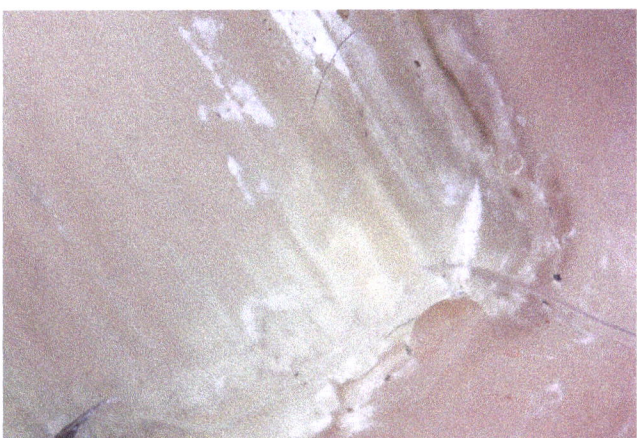

Fig. 5: Onychomycosis showing longitudinal yellowish white striae
Courtesy: Department of Dermatology, Christian Medical College, Vellore

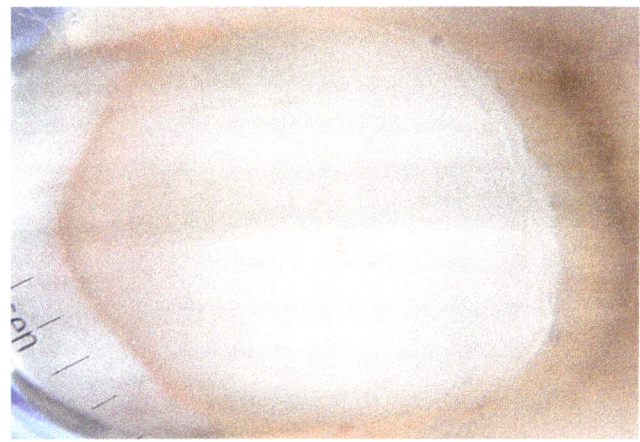

Fig. 8: Ethnic pigmentation showing brown streaks in several digits
Courtesy: Department of Dermatology, Christian Medical College, Vellore

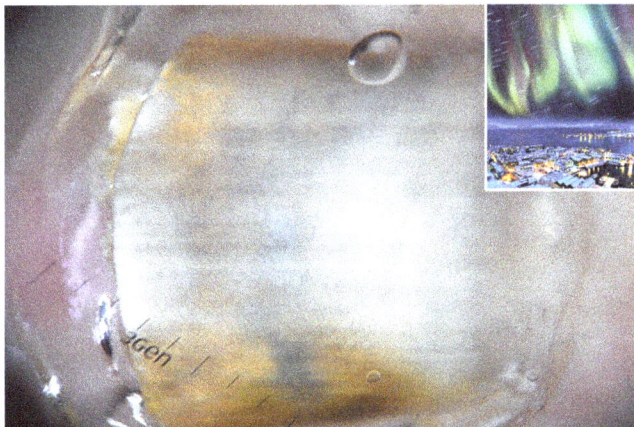

Fig. 6: Onychomycosis showing parallel bands of different colors called "Aurora borealis" pattern. Inset: Aurora borealis—a natural phenomenon showing multiple colors on the sky in the North Pole
Courtesy: Department of Dermatology, Christian Medical College, Vellore

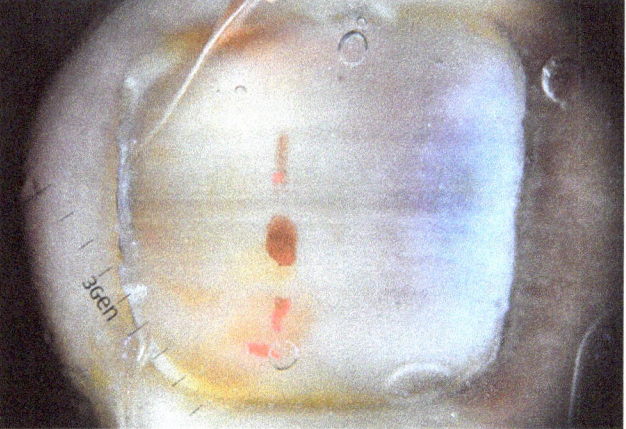

Fig. 9: Blue lunula due to oral hydroxychloroquine sulfate
Courtesy: Department of Dermatology, Christian Medical College, Vellore

half of the 19th century established direct link between capillary abnormalities and disease conditions. There has been a great recognition of its significance with the advent of videocapillaroscopes.

Two basic nailfold capillaroscopy (NFC) patterns[6] are recognized in connective tissue disorders:
1. *Systemic lupus erythematosus (SLE) pattern*: Showing widened tortuous meandering loops resembling a renal glomerulus. Vessel dilation and avascular dropouts are minimal in this pattern (Fig. 10).
2. *Scleroderma-dermatomyositis pattern (Figs 11 to 13)*: Showing at least two of the following in at least two nail folds (Maricq criteria):[7]

- Enlargement of capillary loops
- Capillary hemorrhages (more than two punctuate hemorrhages per finger or confluent hemorrhage areas)
- Loss of capillary loops (avascular areas)
- Disorganization of capillary loops
- Budding or bushy capillaries
- Enlarged twisted capillaries

Although NFC can be performed with highly specialized videocapillaroscopy, dermoscopes suffice for distinguishing between normal and abnormal NFC.[8] As dermoscopy is an operator-dependent technique with large intra- and inter-observer discrepancies, adequate training is needed to perform accurate NFC.

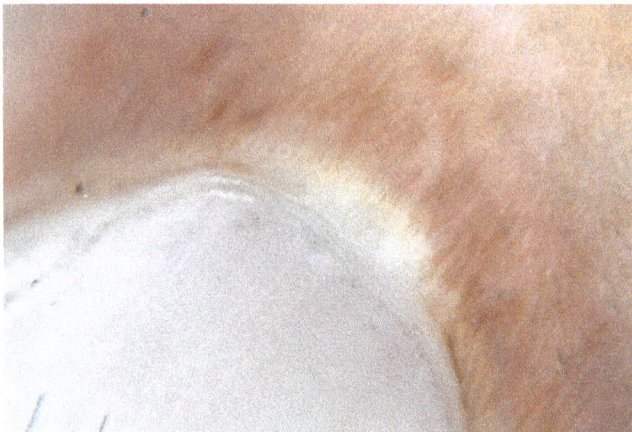

Fig. 10: Systemic lupus erythematosus (SLE) pattern showing elongated capillary loops
Courtesy: Department of Dermatology, Christian Medical College, Vellore

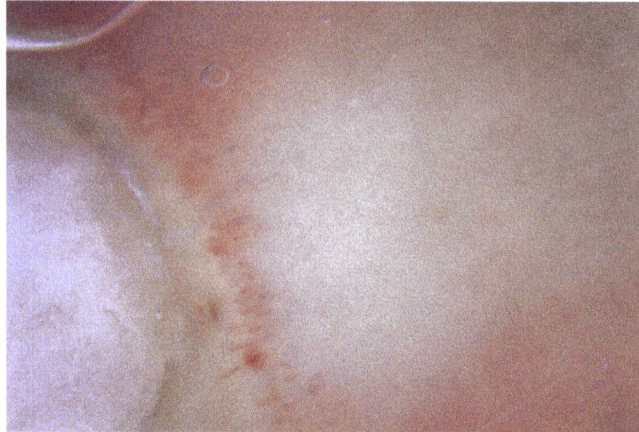

Fig. 12: Active systemic sclerosis-dermatomyositis (SSc-DM) pattern showing many enlarged capillaries and confluent hemorrhage, with few ramified capillaries and mild capillary distribution alteration. There are a few avascular areas and background is hazy
Courtesy: Department of Dermatology, Christian Medical College, Vellore

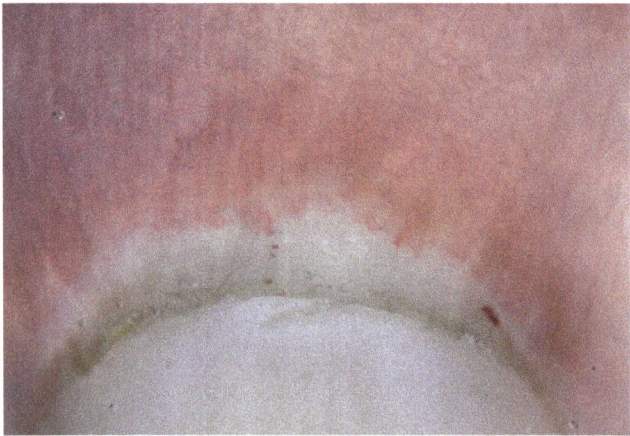

Fig. 11: Early systemic sclerosis-dermatomyositis (SSc-DM) pattern showing few enlarged capillaries and hemorrhage, with preserved capillary distribution and architecture. There are no avascular areas and background is clear
Courtesy: Department of Dermatology, Christian Medical College, Vellore

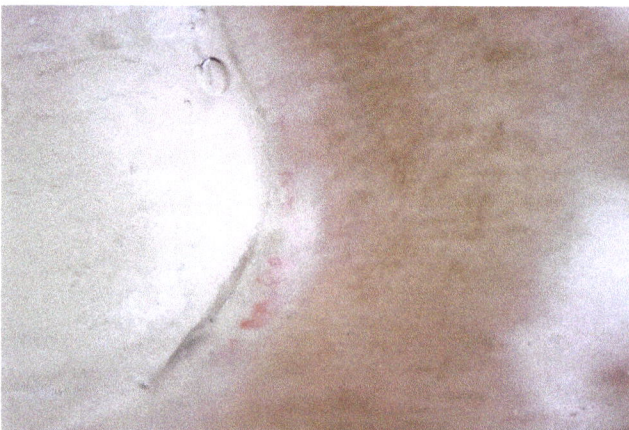

Fig. 13: Late systemic sclerosis-dermatomyositis (SSc-DM) pattern showing few giant capillaries with few bushy capillaries and disorganized capillary distribution. There are many avascular areas and background is very hazy
Courtesy: Department of Dermatology, Christian Medical College, Vellore

REFERENCES

1. Piraccini BM, Bruni F, Starace M. Dermoscopy of non-skin cancer nail disorders. Dermatol Ther. 2012;25:594-602.
2. Mun JH, Kim GW, Jwa SW, Song M, Kim HS, Ko HC, et al. Dermoscopy of subungual haemorrhage: its usefulness in differential diagnosis from nail-unit melanoma. Br J Dermatol. 2013;168:1224-9.
3. Jesús-Silva MA, Fernández-Martínez R, Roldán-Marín R, Arenas R. Dermoscopic patterns in patients with a clinical diagnosis of onychomycosis—results of a prospective study including data of potassium hydroxide (KOH) and culture examination. Dermatol Pract Concept. 2015;5:39-44.
4. Yadav TA, Khopkar US. Dermoscopy to detect signs of subclinical nail involvement in chronic plaque psoriasis: A study of 68 patients. Indian J Dermatol. 2015;60:272-5.
5. Piraccini BM, Dika E, Fanti PA. Tips for diagnosis and treatment of nail pigmentation with practical algorithm. Dermatol Clin. 2015;33:185-95.
6. Connective tissue diseases. In: Baran R, de Berker DA, Holzberg M, Thomas L (Eds). Diseases of the Nails and their Management, 4th edition. West Sussex: Wiley-Blackwell; 2012. pp. 369-70.
7. Bergman R, Sharony L, Schapira D, Nahir MA, Balbir-Gurman A. The handheld dermatoscope as a nail-fold capillaroscopic instrument. Arch Dermatol. 2003;139:1027-30.
8. Dogan S, Akdogan A, Atakan N. Nailfold capillaroscopy in systemic sclerosis: is there any difference between videocapillaroscopy and dermatoscopy? Skin Res Technol. 2013;19:446-9.

SECTION 8

Trichoscopy

BS Chandrashekhar

Section Outline

- Trichoscopy
  - Normal Scalp
  - Trichoscopy of Nonscarring Alopecias
  - Trichoscopy of Scarring Alopecias
  - Trichoscopy of Scaly Scalp Conditions
  - Tinea Capitis

CHAPTER 16

Trichoscopy

BS Chandrashekhar, Samipa S Mukherjee

NORMAL SCALP

BS Chandrashekhar, Samipa S Mukherjee

INTRODUCTION

Lidia Rudnicka and Malgorzata Olszewska coined the term "Trichoscopy" for dermoscopy of hair and the scalp.[1] Trichoscopy is a noninvasive tool useful for detection of scalp and hair disorders. In order to understand what is abnormal, one must first understand what is normal. Repeated training of the eyes to see the normal helps to rapidly pick up the abnormalities in the picture. While examining a scalp for the evidence of dermatological disorders the following needs to be observed:
- Hair
- Interfollicular space
- Pigmentary pattern
- Vascular pattern
- Presence and position of scales.

The permutation and combination of changes in the above five parameters help to arrive at a conclusive diagnosis.

HAIR

While looking at the hair under a dermoscope, one must observe the follicular units, the uniform diameter of the hair, the pigmentation of the hair and surface or structural changes, if any, of the hair. A normal hair in a pigmented skin is uniform in diameter with uniform pigmentation and the follicular units are most commonly composed of at least two hair (Fig. 1).

INTERFOLLICULAR SPACE

The interfollicular space (Figs 2A and B) needs to be assessed for the presence of dots: white, yellow or black, vasculature and pigmentation.[2] In a normal scalp the interfollicular area has pinpoint white dots, which correspond to the eccrine gland openings; empty follicles which progressively increase in different alopecias, honeycomb pigmentary pattern; and vasculature which may not be visible on a pigmented scalp. The leave-on products and environmental dust particles may often present as dots or pseudoscales.

PIGMENTARY PATTERN

Honeycomb pigmentary pattern is the characteristic of a normal scalp in pigmented skin.[3] The pigmented lines correspond to the rete ridge melanocytes which surround the hypochromic area. Perifollicular and interfollicular erythema is common (Figs 3A to C).

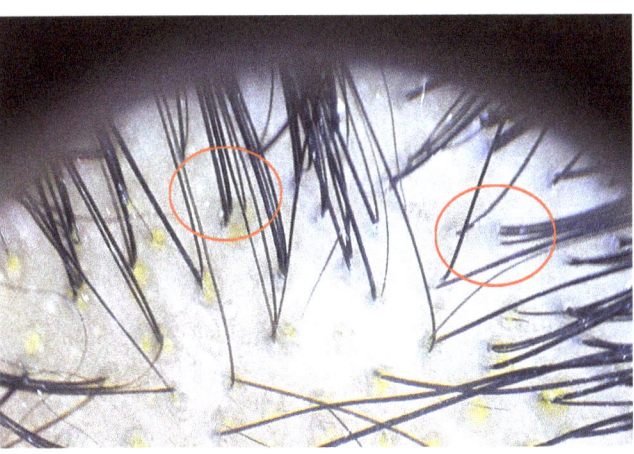

Fig. 1: Follicular unit

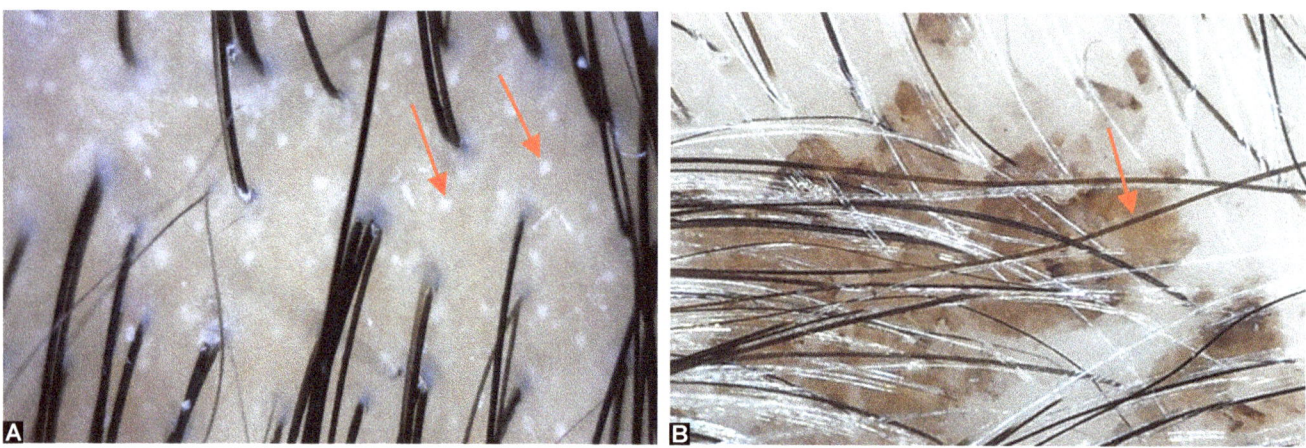

Figs 2A and B: (A) White dots; (B) Pseudoscales

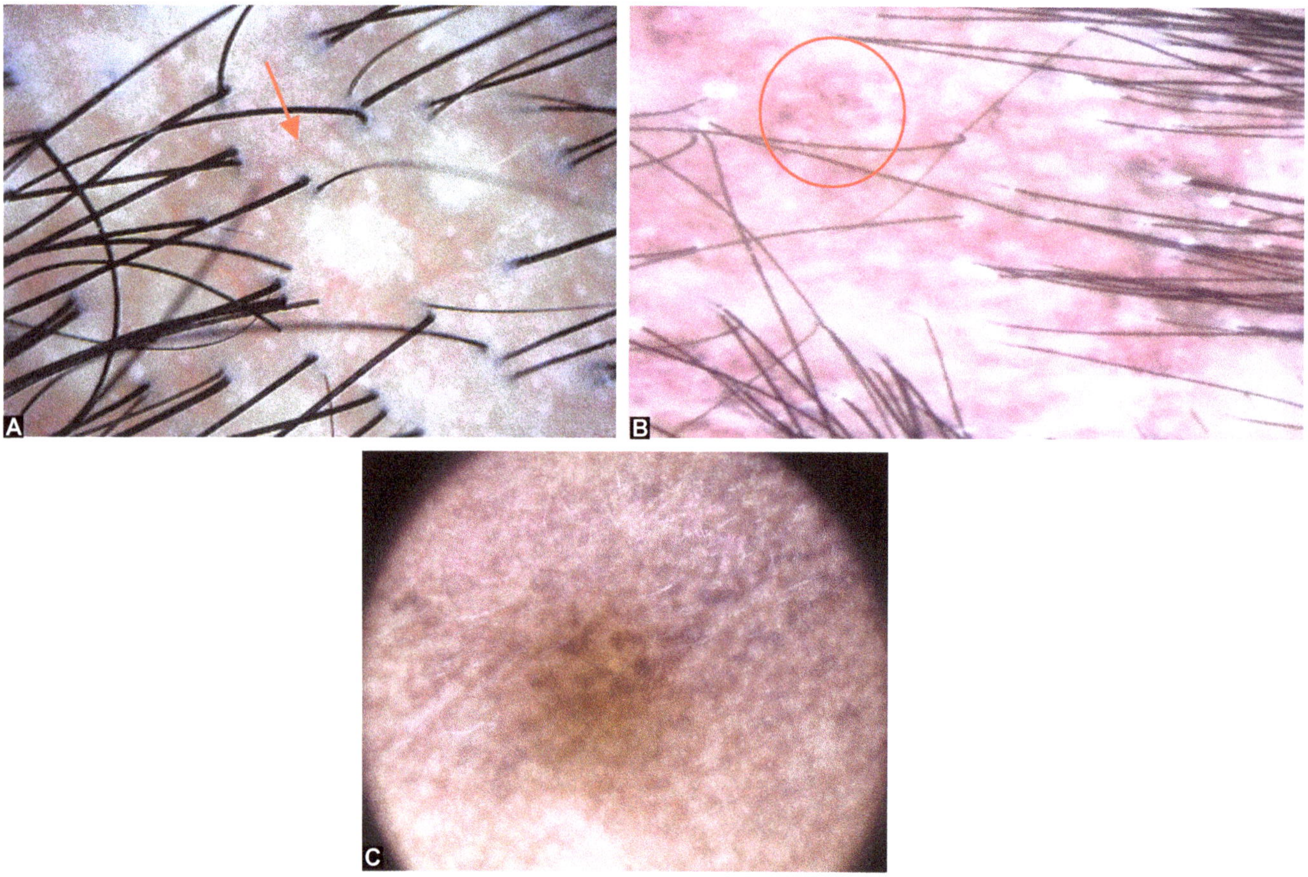

Figs 3A to C: (A) Honeycomb pattern; (B) Perifollicular erythema; (C) Interfollicular pigmentary pattern

VASCULAR PATTERN

Interfollicular space shows the presence of regularly arranged vascular loops and arborizing vessels which may not be seen in skin of color.[2] Vessels are best seen with video dermoscopy. Firm pressure on the vessels will lead to blanching, thereby obscuring the finding. Interfollicular vascular loops appear like regularly arranged fine hairpin-shaped structures. Arborizing red lines correspond to the subcapillary vascular plexus and are vessels of larger caliber (Fig. 4).

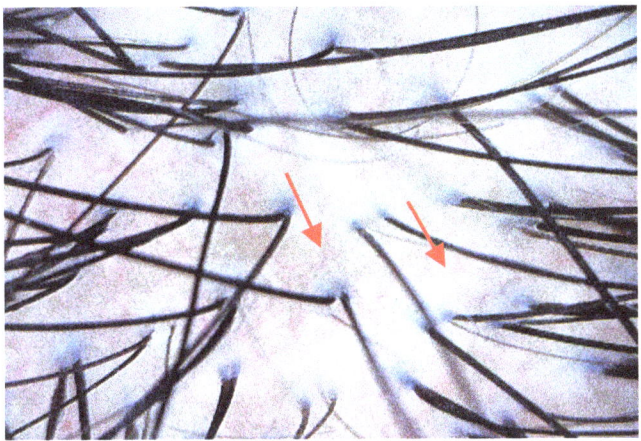

Fig. 4: Vascular loops

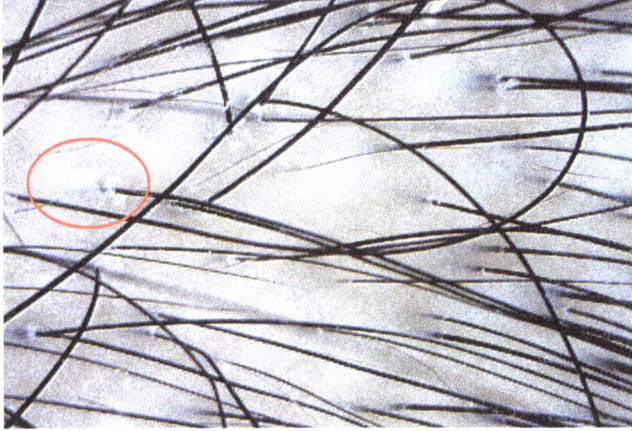

Fig. 5: Scales

SCALES

The presence of scales may be in the interfollicular space or around the hair follicles. The presence of minimal scaling is seen on normal scalp but becomes more important when it is diffuse, thick and is micaceous or greasy (Fig. 5).

CONCLUSION

It is important to know normal hair trichoscopy, to diagnose abnormal presentations of various hair disorders. It requires little bit practice and frequent use of trichoscopy.

REFERENCES

1. Rudnicka L, Olszewska M, Rakowska A, Kowalska-Oledzka E, Slowinska M. Trichoscopy: a new method for diagnosing hair loss. J Drugs Dermatol. 2008;7:651-4.
2. Tosti A, Duque-Estrada B. Dermoscopy in hair disorders. J Egypt Women Dermatol Soc. 2010;7:1-4.
3. Tosti A. Hair shaft disorders. In: Tosti A (Ed). Dermoscopy of Hair and Scalp: Pathological and Clinical Correlation, Illustrated edition. USA: CRC Press; 2007. pp. 51-3.

TRICHOSCOPY OF NONSCARRING ALOPECIAS

BS Chandrashekhar, Samipa S Mukherjee

INTRODUCTION

Nonscarring alopecias are a group of hair disorders which manifests with hair loss without presence of any scarring. They form one of the most common groups of hair disorders with good prognosis and response to treatment. Differentiating various types of nonscarring alopecias especially in a female patient may be difficult. Dermoscopy helps in evaluating various parameters to delineate common forms of nonscarring alopecia-like patterned hair loss, alopecia areata and chronic telogen effluvium, thus obviating the need for invasive procedures like biopsy.

PATTERNED HAIR LOSS [1-3]

Male patterned hair loss affects almost about 80% males during their lifetime and is characterized by progressive recession of frontotemporal hair line and vertex corresponding to the Hamilton and Norwood scaling. It is characterized by reduction in length, diameter and pigmentation of hair.

Points to be looked for are as follows:
- *Hair diameter diversity*: It is defined as the variation in the caliber of hair corresponding to the process of miniaturization in patterned hair loss (Fig. 6). A hair diameter diversity of more than 20% is considered as diagnostic of androgenetic alopecia.
- *Short vellus hair*: It is a sign of severe miniaturization and is more prominent in the vertex and temporal areas (Figs 7 to 10).
- *Pinpoint white dots*: They represent the eccrine openings of the sweat gland on the scalp (Fig. 8).
- *Scalp pigmentation in normal reticulate pattern*: Accentuation of the reticular pattern of pigmentation of the scalp is generally a finding on the scalp with hair loss as a consequence of sun exposure.
- *Yellow dots*: They represent the follicular ostia filled with debris and sebum (Fig. 9).
- *Peripilar sign*: This sign is characterized by the presence of a brown depressed halo at the follicular ostia around the emerging hair shaft (Fig. 10). The peripilar sign may be about just 1 mm and is associated with perifollicular inflammation. Thus, this sign may be seen in early stages of androgenetic alopecia. The prognostic significance of this sign is still questionable, however, since it is present in the early stages of androgenetic alopecia it may provide a clue regarding the true duration of the disease.

ALOPECIA AREATA [4-6]

Alopecia areata is another common noncicatricial alopecia affecting about 2% of the general population. It is an autoimmune condition mediated by T cells in genetically and immunologically predisposed individuals. It presents with patchy oval-shaped hair loss which may be unifocal, multifocal or diffuse. Although focal alopecia areata does not cause a diagnostic dilemma most of the times, diffuse variant of alopecia areata can mimic both diffuse unpatterned hair loss and chronic telogen effluvium.

Points to be noted are as follows:
- *Yellow dots*: They are representative of keratin to sebum-filled infundibula and present as round to polycyclic yellow-pink dots devoid of hair follicles or have only miniaturized fine hair. They are rarely seen on black or pigmented scalp.
- *White dots*: Pigmented scalp may show pinpoint white dots instead of yellow dots (Fig. 11B).
- *Black dots*: They represent the shafts that have fractured before emanating from the scalp (cadaverized hair) (Figs 12A and B).

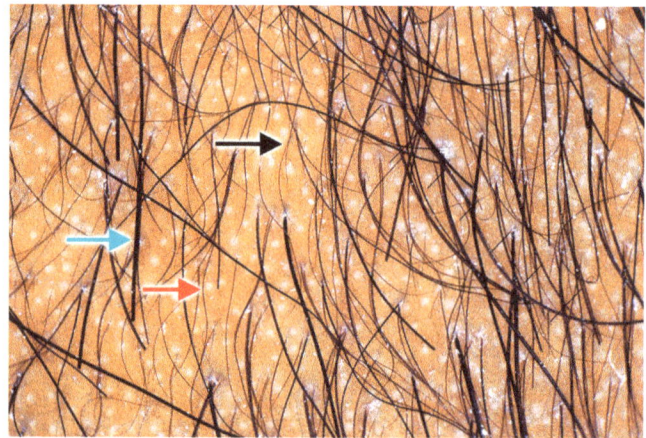

Fig. 6: Dry trichoscopy shows variable hair shaft thickness, presence of thick terminal hair (blue arrow) and thin miniaturized hairs (black arrow). Pinpoint white dots (red arrow) corresponds to empty hair follicle opening and opening of eccrine sweat ducts, it is a common find in dark skin individuals. Majority of follicular units showing single hair shafts
Courtesy: Dr Shekhar Neema, Command Hospital, Kolkata

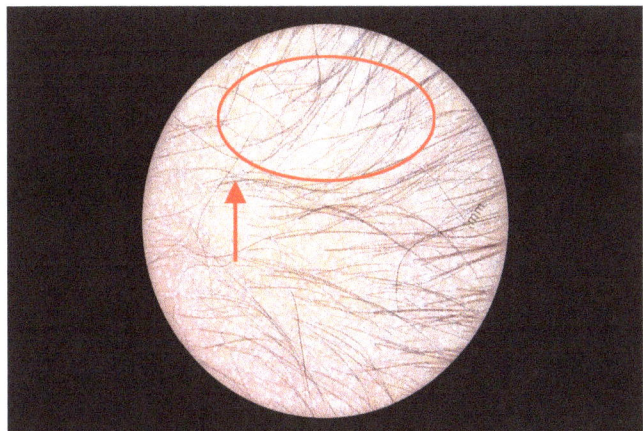

Fig. 7: Multiple vellus hairs (red circle) and white dots (red arrow)

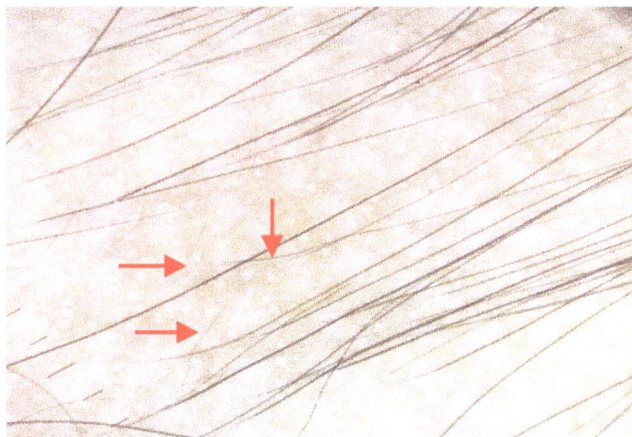

Fig. 8: Variation in hair diameter diversity, vellus hair and presence of white dots

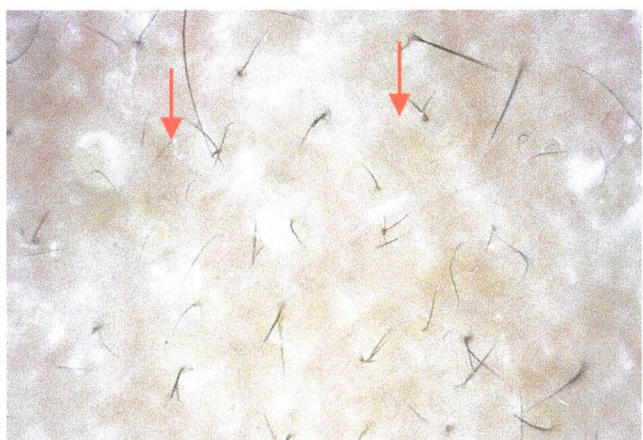

Fig. 9: Yellow dots in androgenetic alopecia. It contains predominantly sebaceous material mixed with variable amount of keratin. Sebaceous gland in hair follicle continue to secrete sebum even after miniaturization, resulting in formation of yellow dots

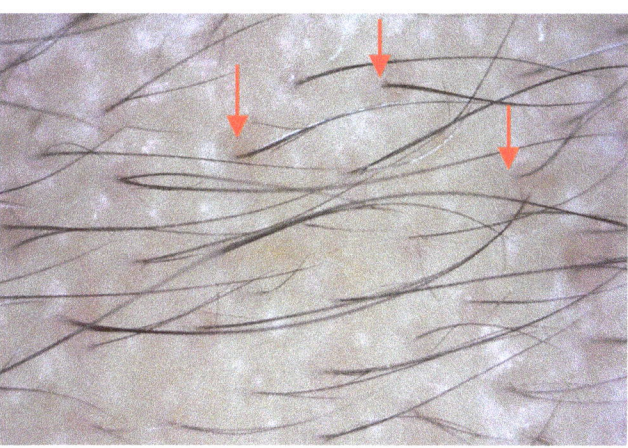

Fig. 10: Peripilar sign: Dark depressed halo at follicular ostia. Suggestive of early androgenetic alopecia

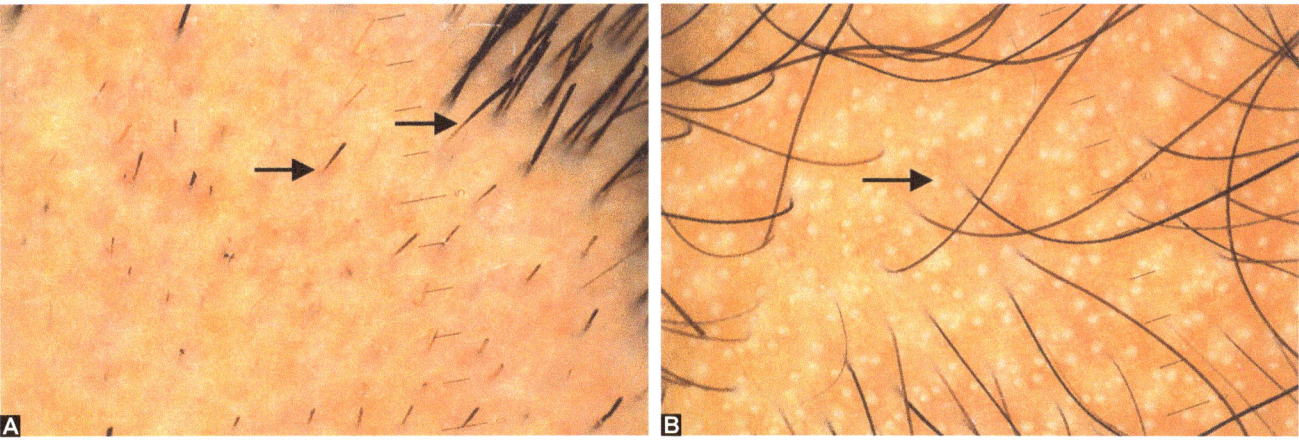

Figs 11A and B: (A) Presence of microexclamation mark hairs in alopecia areata (black arrow): They have thin proximal end and thicker at distal end. Normal exclamation mark hairs which can be visualized with naked eyes are approximately 1 cm long, however, trichoscopy allows visualization of hairs as small as 1–2 mm in size and are known as microexclamation mark hairs; (B) White dots in alopecia areata (black arrow)
Courtesy: Dr Shekhar Neema, Command Hospital, Kolkata

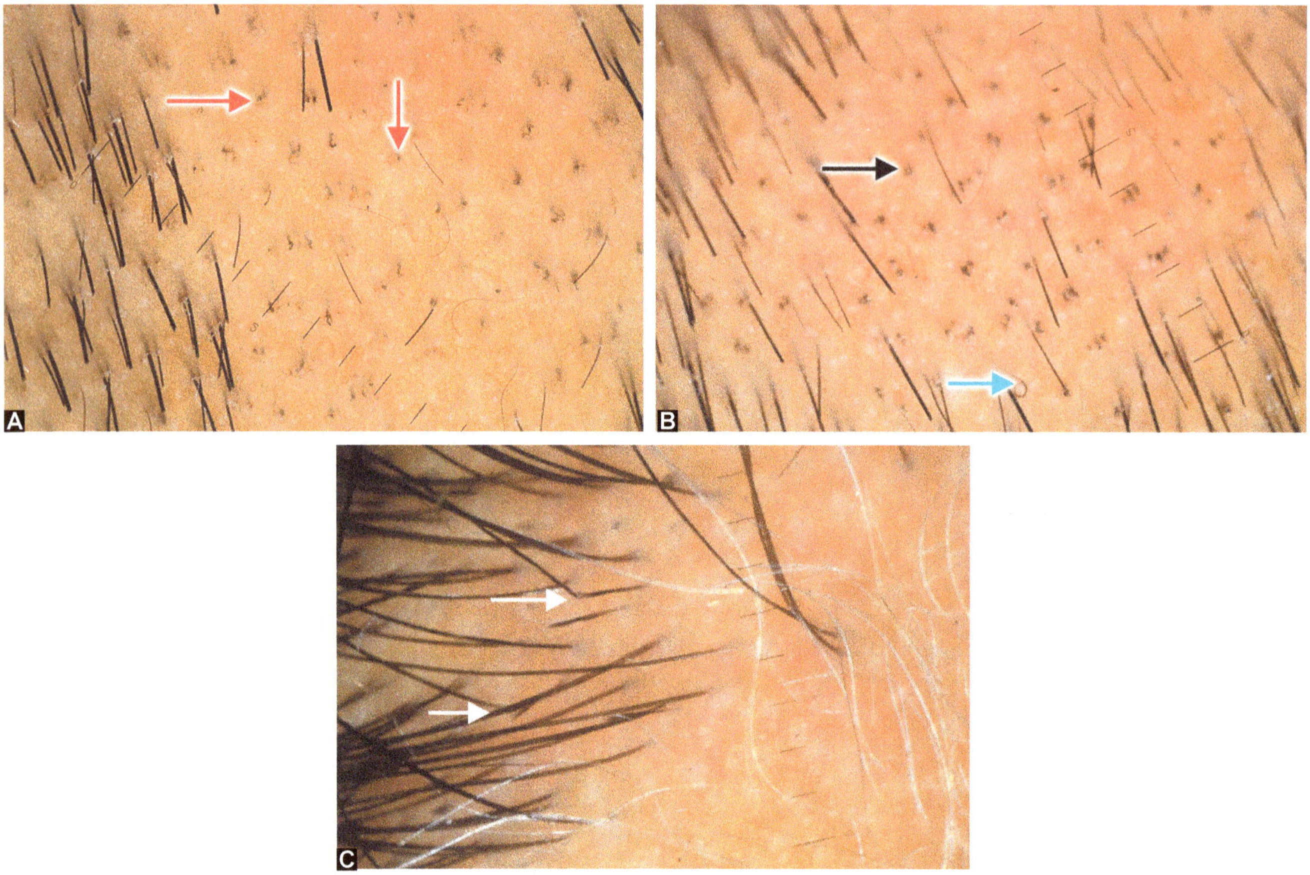

Figs 12A to C: (A) Presence of black dots in alopecia areata (red arrow). Black dots are residue of hairs broken at the level of the scalp and are indicator of active disease; (B) Presence of black dots (black arrow) and pig tail hair (blue arrow) in alopecia areata; (C) Broken hairs in alopecia areata (white arrow)
Courtesy: Dr Shekhar Neema, Command Hospital, Kolkata

- *Broken hair and pseudomonilethrix hair*: This may not be an exclusive feature as it is also seen in trichotillomania, broken hairs present with broken dark pigmented tips (Fig. 12C). In acute alopecia areata, broken and exclamation mark hair are abundant. Beaded appearance may be observed known as pseudomonilethrix pattern.
- *Coudability*: Coudability hairs are normal-looking hairs which are tapered at proximal end. This dermoscopic feature is typically seen at the periphery of enlarging patches, useful marker of disease activity and is a surrogate marker for hair-pull test (Fig. 13).
- *Circle hair also known as pigtail hair*: The presence of numerous circle hair is suggestive of alopecia areata. They represent the miniaturized nanogen hair. It is a common feature of both acute and chronic alopecia areata (Fig. 12B).
- *Exclamation mark hair*: This can be seen when the proximal end of hair is tapered and the distal end is thicken giving rise to the exclamation mark appearance (Figs 12A and B).
- *Other features*: Zigzag hairs, tulip hairs and upright regrowing hairs are also trichoscopic features in alopecia areata.

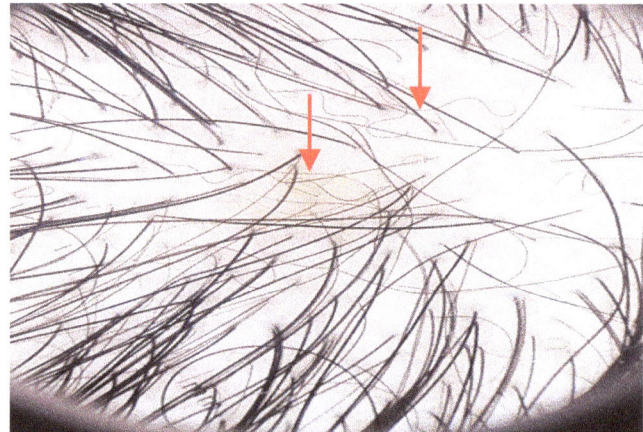

Fig. 13: Coudability hair: Proximal tapering of normal hair suggestive of active alopecia areata

ALOPECIA AREATA INCOGNITO[7]

It is an under-recognized entity. It presents with diffuse hair thinning rather than the typical presentation of alopecia areata with patches. Although literature says that this

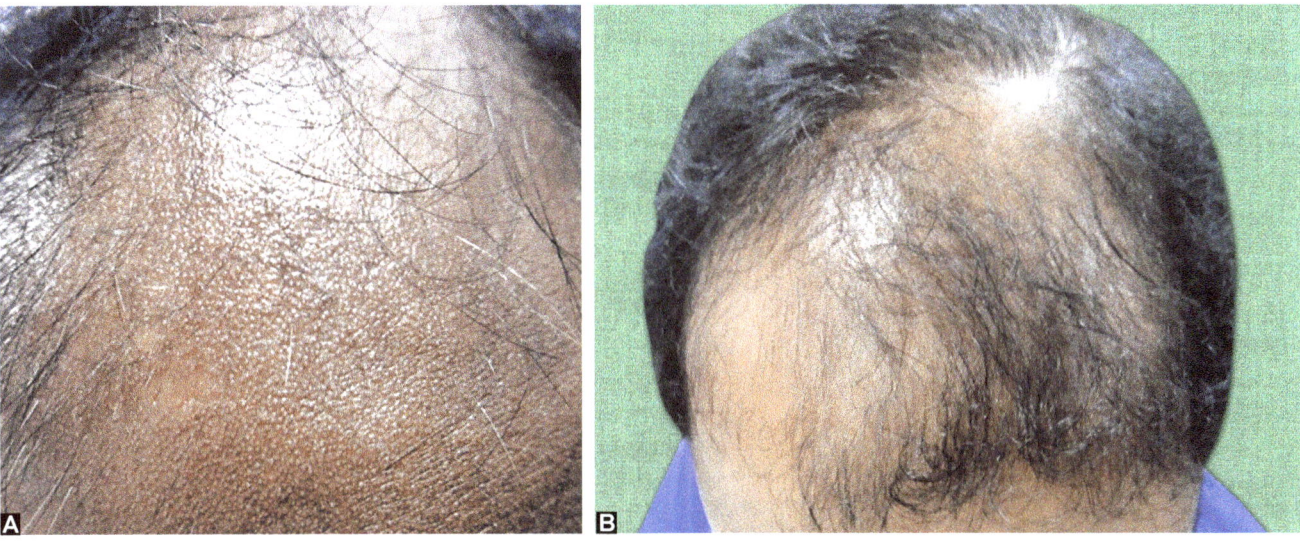

Figs 14A and B: Androgenetic alopecia overlap with alopecia areata incognito

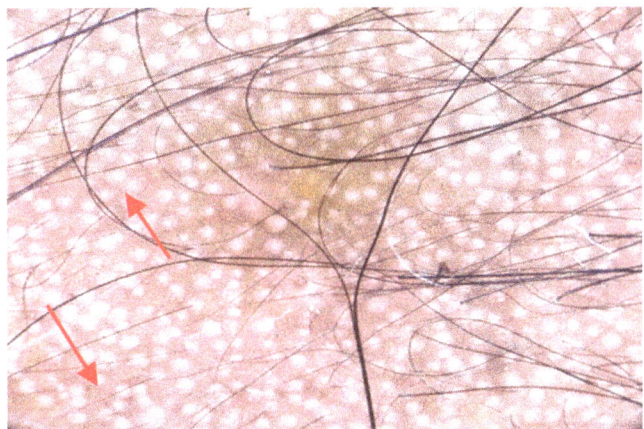

Fig. 15: Target sign or Bull's eye sign

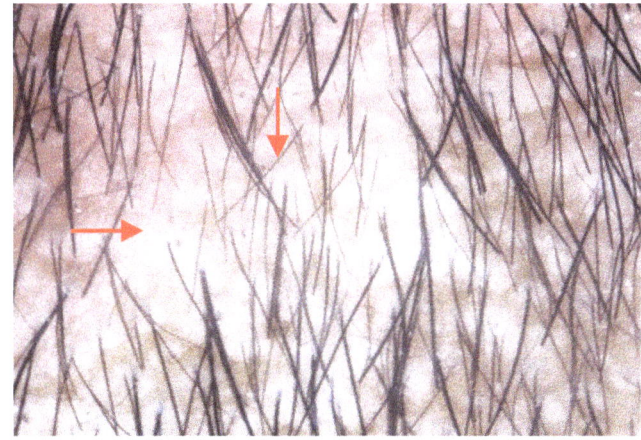

Fig. 16: Short regrowing tips of miniaturized hair

condition usually affects women, in author's experience a large number of male patients have a similar condition. As in females, it affects androgen-dependent areas of the scalp even in males. The authors believe that this could be a subset of androgenetic alopecia where there is intense inflammatory reaction in the perifollicular area. The presence of dermoscopic sign of Bull's eye or target sign has been elaborated as well. Also this subset responds better when a topical corticosteroid is added along with topical minoxidil for hair growth. During response, there is a disappearance of the classical bull's eye replaced by a flare. Clinical clues towards diagnosing this condition of overlap with androgenetic alopecia in males include asymmetrical distribution of patterned hair loss and markedly patulous follicular opening visible to the naked eye (Figs 14A and B).

Points to be noted are as follows:
- *Target sign or bull's eye sign*: This has been the nomenclature of the authors in their personal experience and it is defined by a bull's eye formation around the emerging hair follicle in the form of alternating whitish band and a pigmented ring simulating the target or a bull's eye. The postulate behind its existence has been clarified as the white band representing sebum and keratin which is surrounded by a pigmented ring representative of the inflammatory infiltrate histologically (Fig. 15). These patients post-treatment with routine minoxidil and addition of mid-potent topical corticosteroid show the well-defined bull's eye sign being replaced by an ill-defined flare (Fig. 16).
- *Short regrowing tips of miniaturized hair*: They represent the miniaturized nanogen hair and can also become coiled hair in few cases.

TELOGEN EFFLUVIUM: ACUTE AND CHRONIC[8]

Chronic Telogen Effluvium

Chronic telogen effluvium is an idiopathic, self-limiting condition with increased telogen shedding lasting at least 6 months in duration but not associated with the widening of the central part and miniaturization of hair follicles upon scalp biopsy. The most common age group of presentation is around 30–50 years with females predominantly presenting as diffuse hair loss. The female predominance of chronic telogen effluvium can be well explained by the newer insights into the pathogenesis which states that NK1 receptor expression in females is more than males which is one of the significant targets in the pathogenetic pathway.

Points to be noted are as follows (Figs 17 and 18):
- *No hair diameter diversity*: There is no evidence of hair diameter diversity
- Miniaturization does not occur
- All hair more or less of same diameter
- Short regrowing hair of uniform diameter may be present.

Acute Telogen Effluvium

Acute telogen effluvium is characterized by acute hair shedding with or without visible hair thinning. Although five functional types of acute telogen effluvium has been described in literature, the most commonly encountered are due to immediate anagen release as in poststress/postfever/postsurgery and delayed anagen release as seen in postpartum hair loss. Dermoscopy is not very useful in this particular condition as it may not show any specific features. However, most commonly there is presence of short regrowing hair which is evident and important to convince the patient regarding the nature of the disease. Hair shaft variability may be noted in patients with additional androgenetic alopecia.

TRICHOTILLOMANIA[9,10]

Trichotillomania is described as a chronic compulsive disorder presenting most commonly in childhood. It presents with single or multiple patches of nonscarring alopecia in accessible areas of the scalp or eyebrows or eyelashes and sometimes body hair. Clinical sign that provides a clue towards this entity is the feel of the patch with bare palm where the broken ends of the hair seems to poke the skin as opposed to the smooth patches of alopecia areata. Dermoscopy forms an important tool not only in the diagnosis of this particular disorder but also in improving patient compliance and acceptability towards the diagnosis.

Points to be noted area as follows:
- *Flame hair*: These are wavy, cone-shaped residues with flame appearance pathologically corresponding to pigment casts. These are the most characteristic finding of trichotillomania (Figs 19 to 21).
- *Broken hair*: They occur due to vigorous pulling or rubbing of hair. Irregularly broken hairs in trichotillomania are most common finding, however, it is not specific finding as it is also seen in alopecia areata and tinea capitis (Figs 20 and 21).
- *Hair dust*: Complete damage to hair shaft by mechanical manipulation may result in development of "hair dust" or "hair powder" (Fig. 22).
- *Perifollicular hemorrhage*: It represents pulling of hair, leading to trauma or due to secondary scratching which leads to tiny erosions and bleeding points.

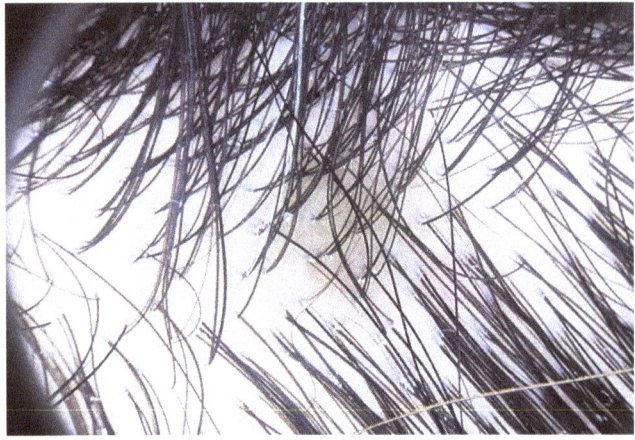

Fig. 17: Chronic telogen effluvium: No hair diameter diversity

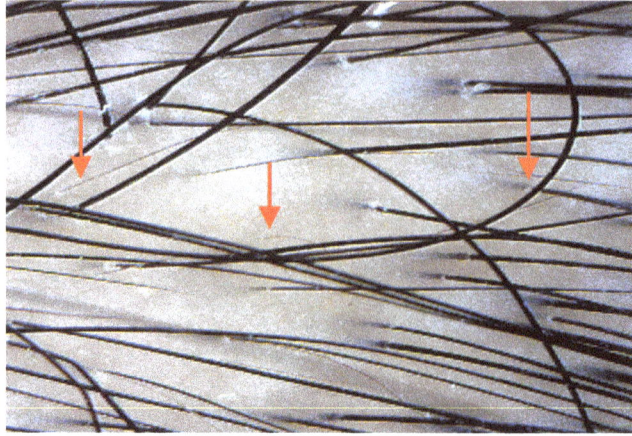

Fig. 18: Chronic telogen effluvium: Short regrowing hairs can be seen (red arrow)

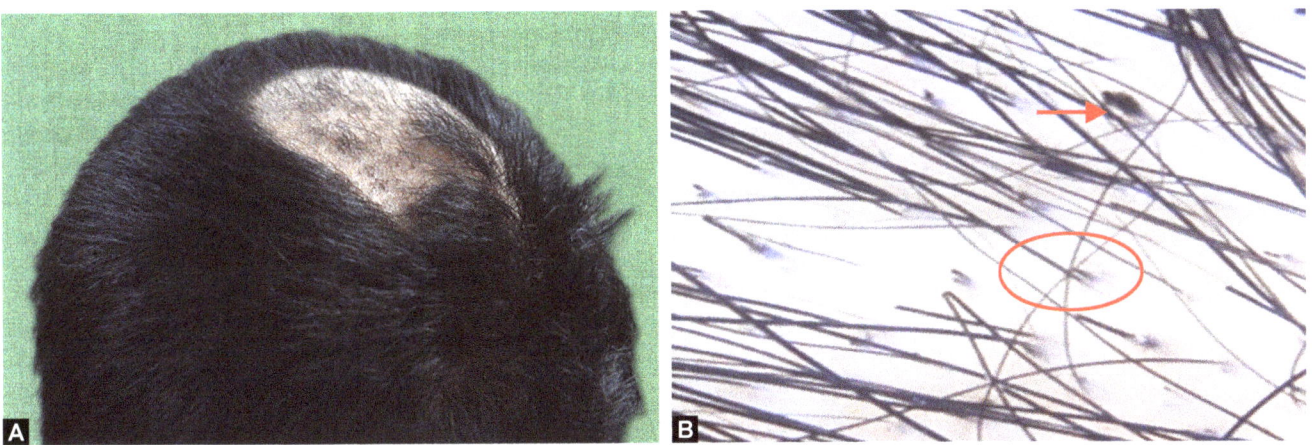

Figs 19A and B: (A) Clinical picture: Trichotillomania (*Courtesy*: Dr Shekhar Neema, Command Hospital, Kolkata); (B) Flame hair: Results from mechanical trauma to hair shaft. Red arrow—flame hair, red circle—broken hair

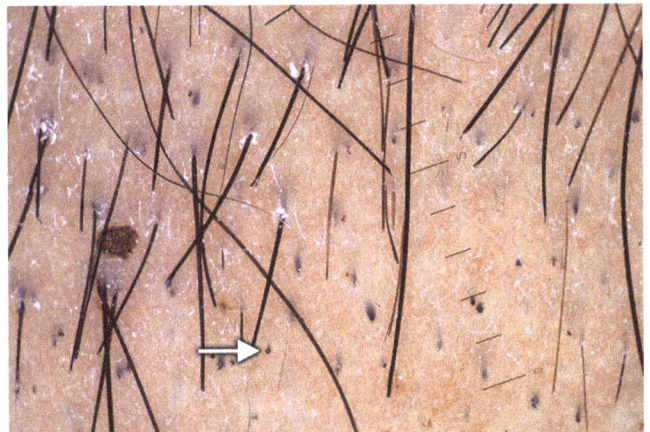

Fig. 20: Trichoscopy shows broken hairs of different length and morphology and presence of black dots (white arrow)
Courtesy: Dr Shekhar Neema, Command Hospital, Kolkata

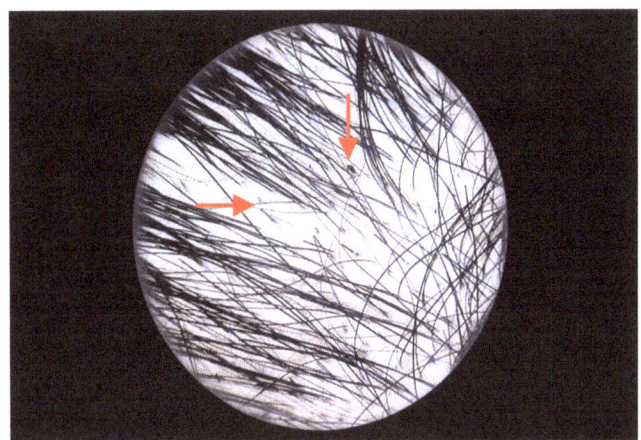

Fig. 21: Flame hairs and broken hairs

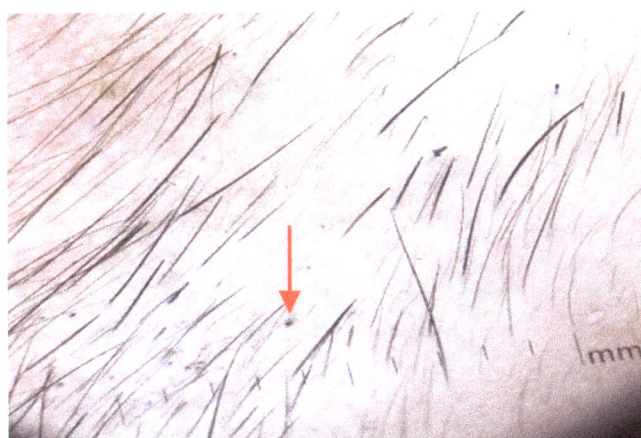

Fig. 22: Hair dust: Severe mechanical trauma leads to complete damage to hair shaft

- *Black dots*: It represents the broken stubs of hair on the skin surface (Fig. 20).
- *Other features*: V sign, tulip hairs, trichoptilosis (split ends) and microexclamation mark hairs (Figs 23A to C).

NUTRITIONAL DEFICIENCY

We commonly come across patients complaining of diffuse hair loss on the background of no apparent triggering factor. Few of them give history of crash dieting, having food fads, however, the vast majority seems to have hair loss without a definite cause.

Since hair is one of the most metabolically active tissues in the body, nutritional deficiency does have a role in loss of hair. In the author's opinion nutritional deficiency-induced hair loss could be one of the underdiagnosed entities.

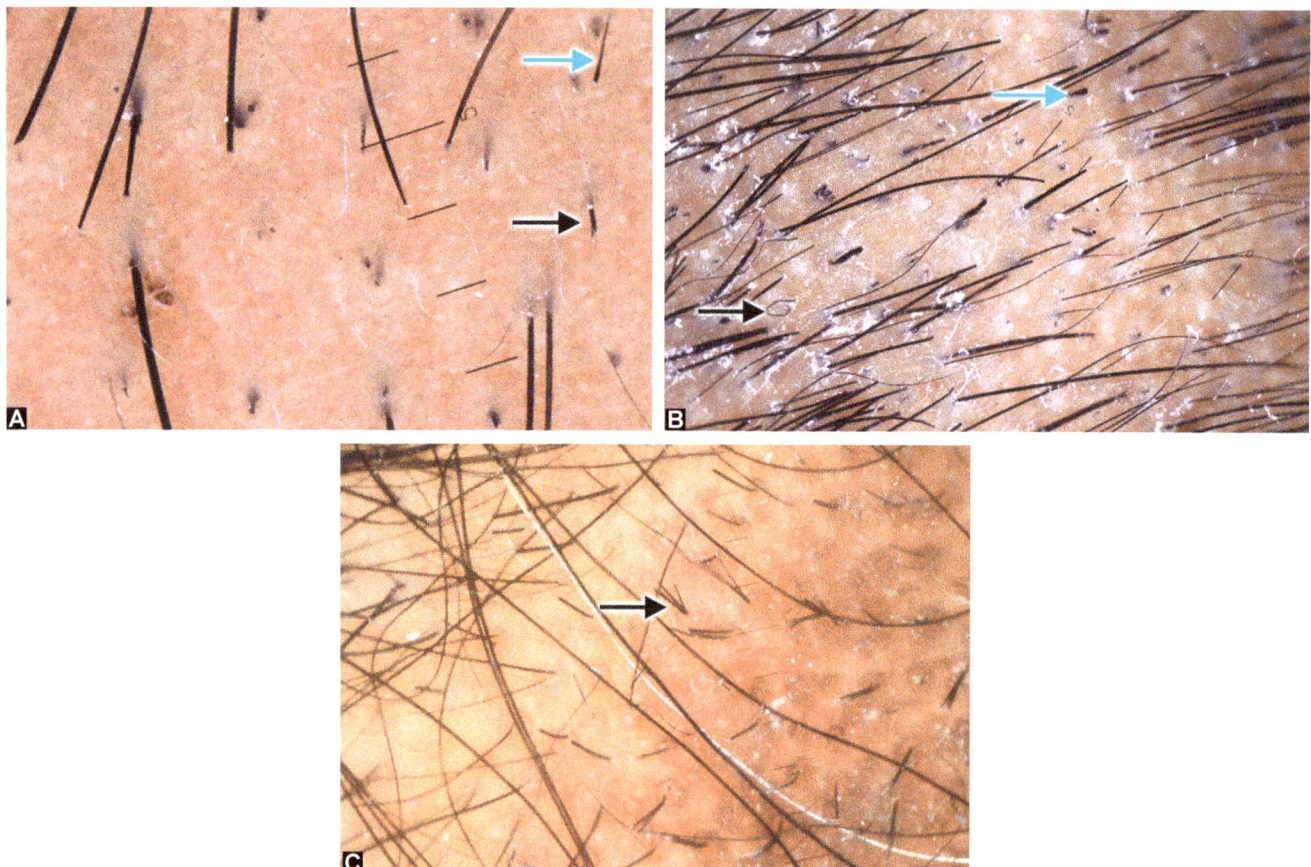

Figs 23A to C: (A) Trichoscopy shows presence of microexclamation mark hair (blue arrow) and trichoptilosis: Split ends (black arrow); (B) Trichoscopy shows coiled hairs (black arrow) and tulip hair (blue arrow). Tulip hairs are short hairs with dark tulip shaped ends. These hairs are characteristic of trichotillomania, but may also be seen in alopecia areata; (C) V sign in trichotillomania: V sign appears when person with trichotillomania pulls hair shaft appearing from single follicular unit simultaneously (black arrow). Other features of trichotillomania which can be seen are irregular broken hairs, trichoptilosis and microexclamation mark hair
Courtesy: Dr Shekhar Neema, Command Hospital, Kolkata

Although dermoscopy does not have any specific features in this kind of hair loss, a uniform reduction in the hair diameter in the absence of miniaturization could be an important pointer (Fig. 24).

CONGENITAL ATRICHIA WITH PAPULAR ERUPTION

Atrichia congenita with papular lesions represents a complex and heterogeneous group of genodermatoses characterized by irreversible complete hair loss soon after birth, and associated with the development of keratin-filled cysts over the body. Diagnosis of this particular genotrichoses is important for planning and counseling the patient. The dermoscopic feature of this particular entity has not been described in literature so far. According to the authors, the feature noted consistently in these patients is a cluster of star appearance which may be defined as aggregates of pinpoint white dots on the scalp in clusters of 8–10 arranged in a regular pattern all over the scalp. In the view of the authors, this appearance may be the result of the stranded hair bulbs and dermal papilla in the dermis which probably undergo fibrosis in due course of time and appear as white dots (Fig. 25).

CONGENITAL TRIANGULAR ALOPECIA

Congenital triangular alopecia also known as temporal triangular alopecia is nonscarring alopecia charcaterized by presence of alopecic patches in frontotemporal region of the scalp. It mostly appears during birth to first 9 years of life. Trichoscopy is helpful in diagnosis of this condition, especially when it occurs in atypical location and in adults. Trichoscopic features are presence of multiple vellus hairs (Figs 26 and 27).

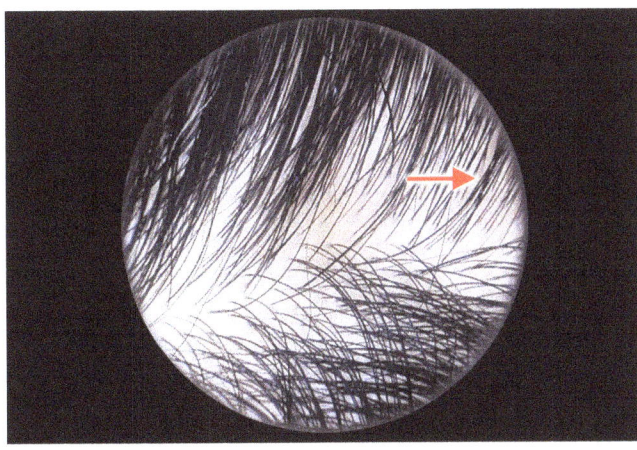

Fig. 24: Reduction in hair diameter on dermoscopy. Better appreciated on videodermoscopy where hair shaft measurements can be done

Fig. 25: Cluster of star appearance suggestive of congenital atrichia with papular eruption

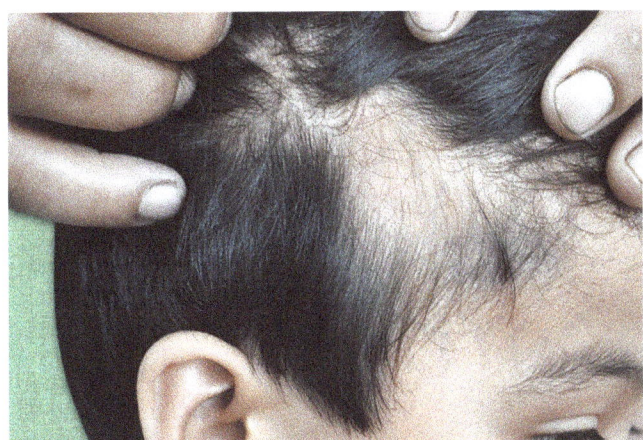

Fig. 26: Clinical picture: Congenital triangular alopecia
Courtesy: Dr Shekhar Neema, Command Hospital, Kolkata

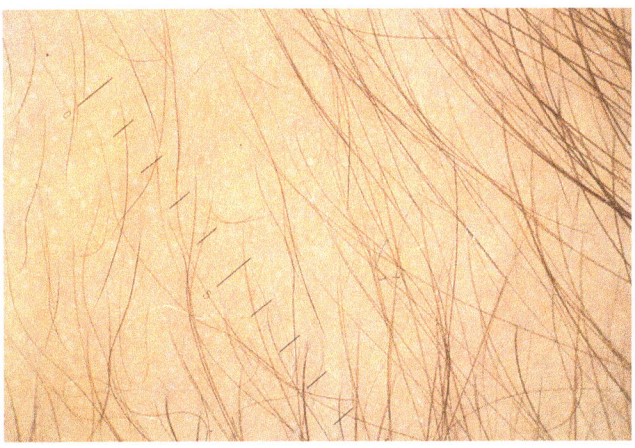

Fig. 27: Trichoscopy shows presence of multiple vellus hairs
Courtesy: Dr Shekhar Neema, Command Hospital, Kolkata

CONCLUSION

Patients with nonscarring alopecias get frequently misdiagnosed due to their similar presentation. Trichoscopic diagnosis of various types of non-scarring alopecias will be of immense help in prognostication and treatment of these disorders.

REFERENCES

1. Inui S, Nakajima T, Itami S. Scalp dermoscopy of androgenetic alopecia in Asian people. J Dermatol. 2009;36:82-5.
2. Deloche C, de Lacharriere O, Misciali C, Piraccini BM, Vincenzi C, Bastien P, et al. Histological features of peripilar signs associated with androgenetic alopecia. Arch Dermatol Res. 2004;295:422-8.
3. Ross EK, Vincenzi C, Tosti A. Videodermoscopy in the evaluation of hair and scalp disorders. J Am Acad Dermatol. 2006;55:799-806.
4. Inui S, Nakajima T, Nakagawa K, Itami S. Clinical significance of dermoscopy in alopecia areata: Analysis of 300 cases. Int J Dermatol. 2008;47:688-93.
5. Inui S, Nakajima T, Itami S. Dry dermoscopy in clinical treatment of alopecia areata. J Dermatol. 2007;34:635-9.
6. Inui S, Nakajima T, Itami S. Coudability hairs: A revisited sign of alopecia areata assessed by trichoscopy. Clin Exp Dermatol. 2010;35:361-5.
7. Tosti A, Whiting D, Iorizzo M, Pazzaglia M, Misciali C, Vincenzi C, et al. The role of scalp dermoscopy in the diagnosis of alopecia areata incognita. J Am Acad Dermatol. 2008;59:64-7.
8. Jain N, Doshi B, Khopkar U. Trichoscopy in alopecias: diagnosis simplified. Int J Trichology. 2013;5:170-8.
9. Lee DY, Lee JH, Yang JM, Lee ES. The use of dermoscopy for the diagnosis of trichotillomania. J Eur Acad Dermatol Venereol. 2009;23:731-2.
10. Rakowska A, Slowinska M, Olszewska M, Rudnicka L. New trichoscopy findings in trichotillomania: flame hairs, V-sign, hook hairs, hair powder, tulip hairs. Acta Derm Venereol. 2014;94(3):303-6.

TRICHOSCOPY OF SCARRING ALOPECIAS

BS Chandrashekhar, Samipa S Mukherjee

INTRODUCTION

Primary scarring alopecias or cicatricial alopecias are a group of hair disorders where there is permanent destruction of the hair follicle due to destruction of the stem cells in the bulge areas causing permanent scarring. Early detection of these disorders is of immense importance in treatment initiation and stopping the progression of the condition, since in many of these conditions the etiology is autoimmune. Dermoscopy forms an important screening tool for the diagnosis of these conditions and also helps in selecting an optimum biopsy site. Not just the diagnosis, dermoscopy can help monitor the disease progression, response to therapy and reactivation of the disorder.

Although in depth discussion of all the conditions may not be within the scope of this chapter, important points regarding well-established entity has been discussed.

LICHEN PLANOPILARIS

Lichen planopilaris (LPP) is one of the more common scarring alopecias which may be encountered in clinical practice. It may present by itself or as a part of syndrome in association with lichen planus of other areas of the body. When it presents on the scalp it is generally preceded by itching and most commonly tends to affect the middle-aged females. Clinically, it presents as patchy loss of hair with follicular papules, scalp erythema and scaling with varying grades of pruritus (Figs 28A and B).

The dermoscopic features of LPP include perifollicular scaling, tubular cast, perifollicular inflammation, loss of follicular openings, violaceous areas and white dots.[1] White dots in both discoid lupus erythematosus (DLE) and LPP probably correspond to impending fibrosis around follicle whereas white area, characteristic feature of DLE and not LPP is due to tissue fibrosis involving areas between the follicles in the dermis.[2] Other dermoscopic findings include broken hair, pili torti and blue-gray dots (Figs 29 and 30).

FRONTAL FIBROSING ALOPECIA

This entity was first described by Kossard in 1994 which is characterized by cicatricial hair loss in a fronto-temporo-parietal recession pattern with perifollicular erythema in areas of hair loss along with loss of eyebrows and loss of sidelocks (Figs 31A and B). Dermoscopy of the alopecic band[3,4] reveals perifollicular scaling, perifollicular blue-gray dots and a very faint erythema (Fig. 32). Absence of follicular openings, homogenous ivory colored background and follicular openings with lone hair at hair-bearing margin are other trichoscopic features of frontal fibrosing alopecia.

DISCOID LUPUS ERYTHEMATOSUS

Discoid lupus erythematosus of the scalp is not uncommon and may be associated with other cutaneous manifestation of the disease. Clinical examination generally reveals single or multiple patches of alopecia with central atrophy, erythema, follicular plugging and telangiectasia. Dermoscopy shows

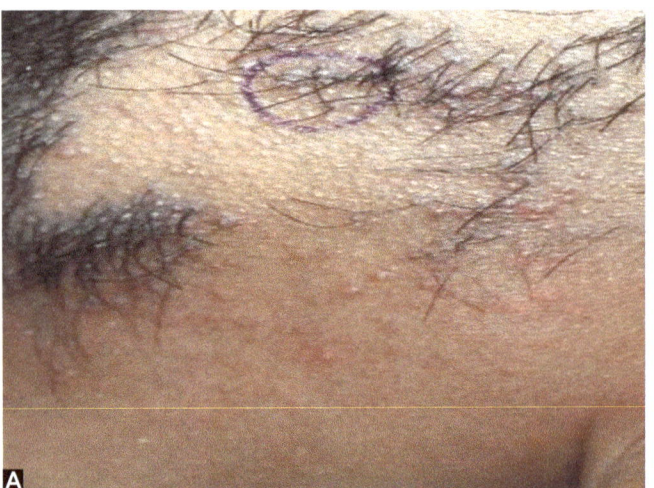
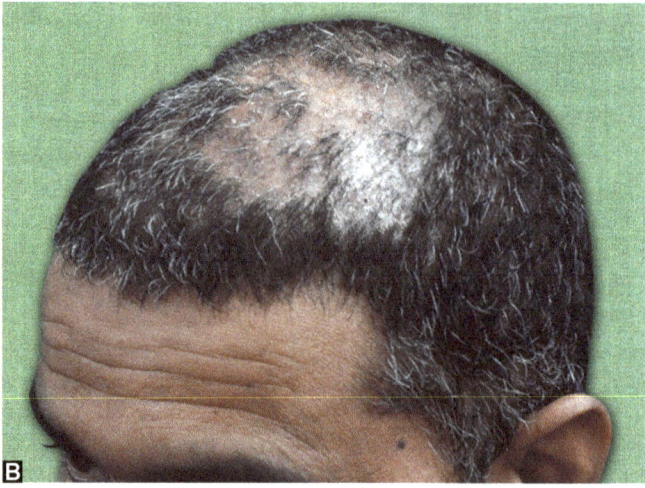

Figs 28A and B: Clinical picture: Lichen planopilaris

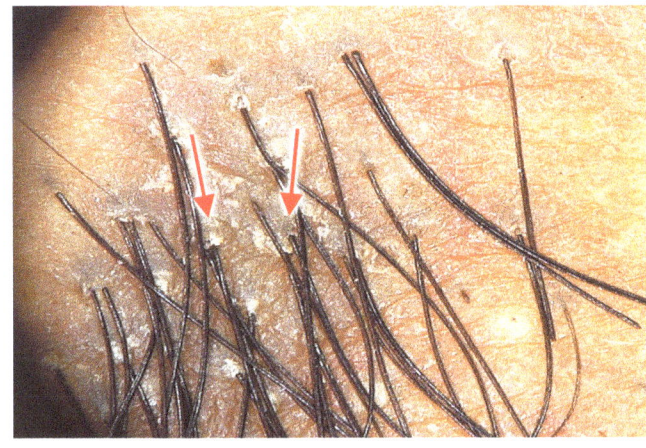

Fig. 29: Peripilar cast: It is one of the most characteristic finding of lichen planopilaris which presents as concentrically arranged layers of scales around the emerging point of the hair shafts. The presence of a group of two to three hair surrounded by a peripilar cast should give rise to a suspicion of lichen planopilaris

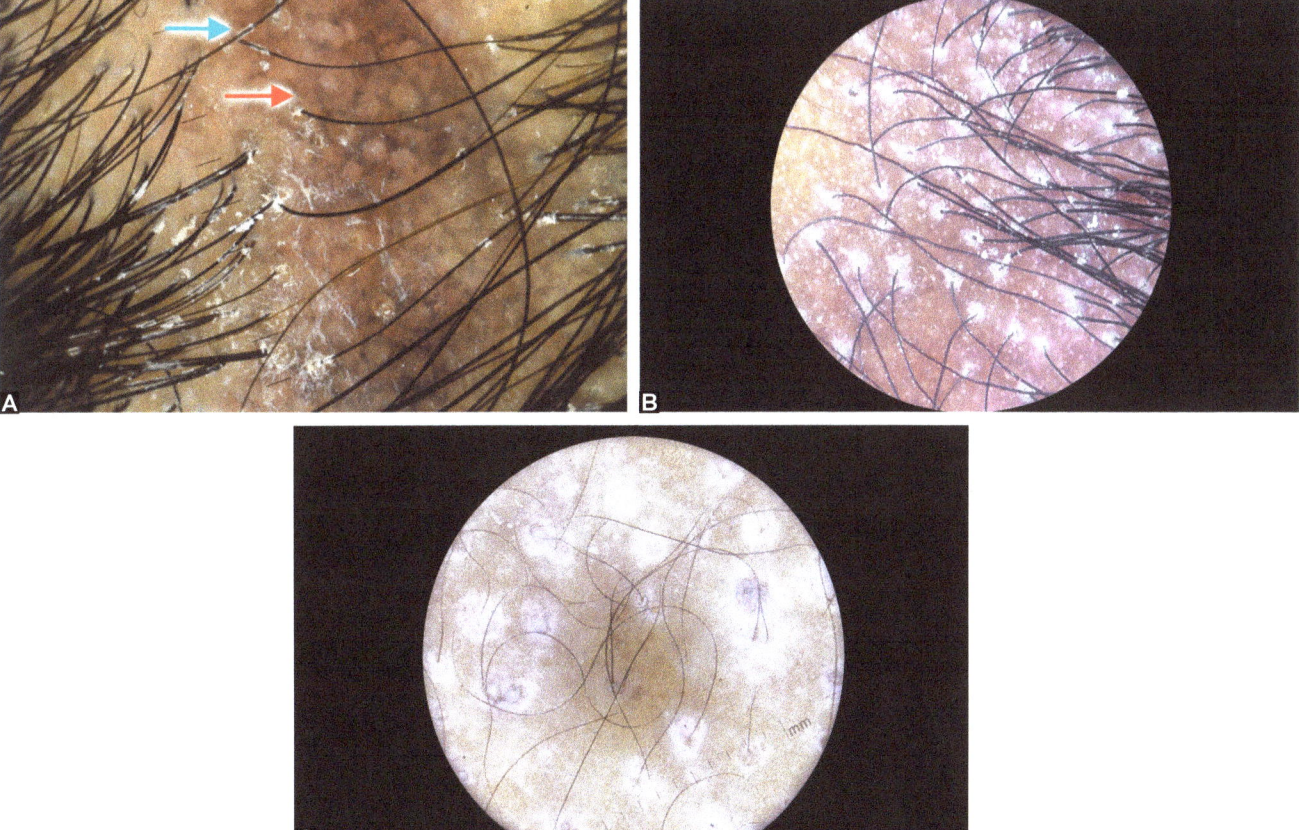

Figs 30A to C: (A) Trichoscopy shows perifollicular scaling, tubular cast (blue arrow) and reticular network of violaceus pigmentation (red arrow). Presence of collar-like or tubular scales which covers approximate 1–3 mm above scalp surface is characteristic of lichen planopilaris (*Courtesy*: Dr Shekhar Neema, Command Hospital, Kolkata); (B) Perifollicular scales, tubular scales and violaceous hue on trichoscopy of lichen planopilaris; (C) Blue-gray dots in trichoscopy seen in lichen planopilaris

features of scarring alopecia like loss of follicular openings. The most common trichoscopic findings include branching capillaries, white patches, follicular plugging, reduced follicular ostia and white dots. Blue-gray dots inside the patch of alopecia referred to as "speckles" pattern may also be seen.[2] Red dots are erythematous polycyclic concentric structures whose presence has been linked to the early active phase of the disease. The blue-gray dots in a speckled pattern corresponds to the melanin incontinence histopathologically which is not just limited to the follicles but also spills over to the interfollicular area. Target pattern blue-gray dots in LPP indicates circular arrangement of melanin around the perifollicular area sparing the interfollicular area unlike DLE wherein blue-gray dots follow a speckled pattern indicating involvement of interfollicular areas with sprinkling of melanin in these areas (Figs 33 and 34).[2]

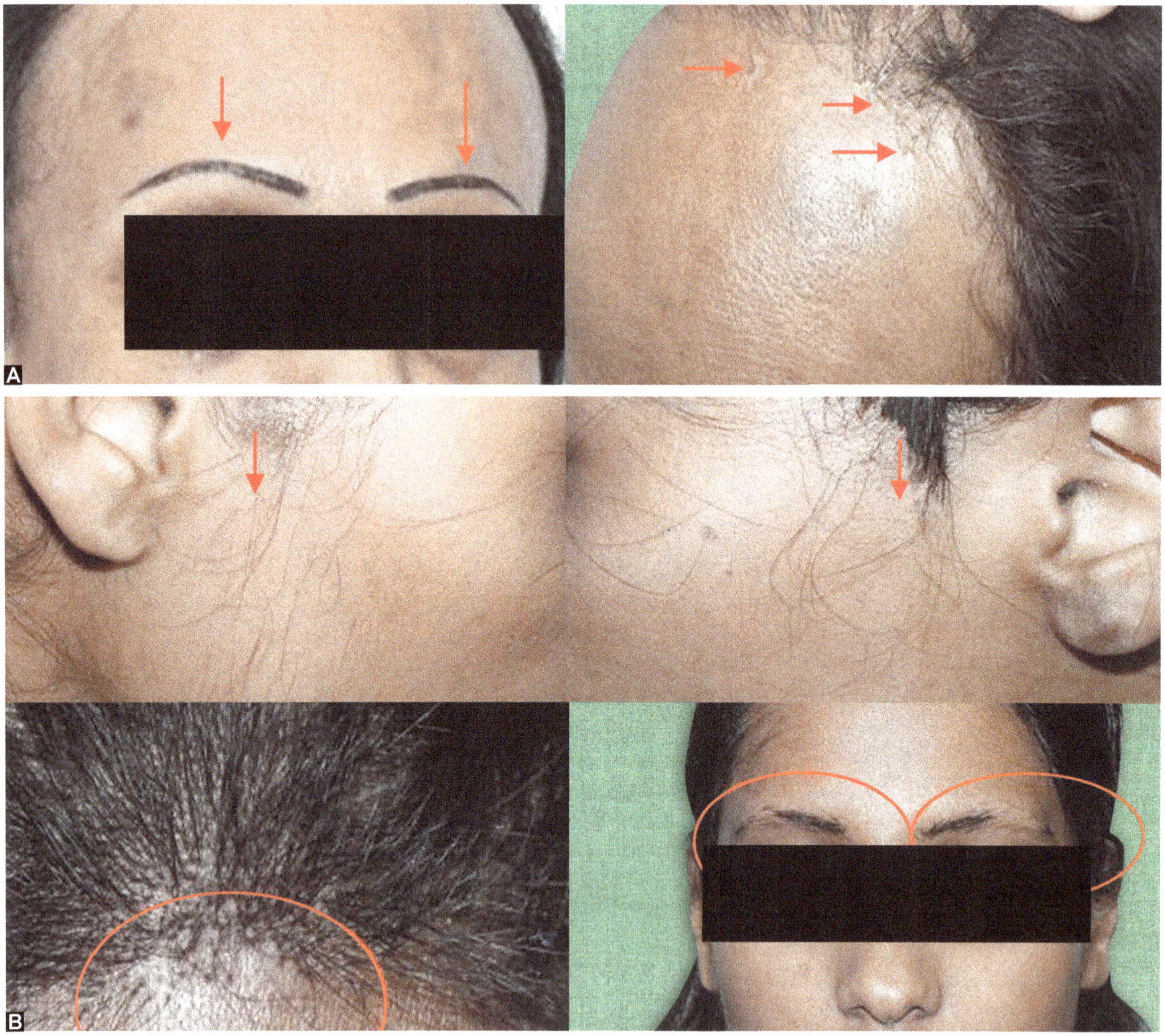

Figs 31A and B: Clinical feature: Frontal fibrosing alopecia shows frontotemporal recession, involvement of sidelocks and eyebrows

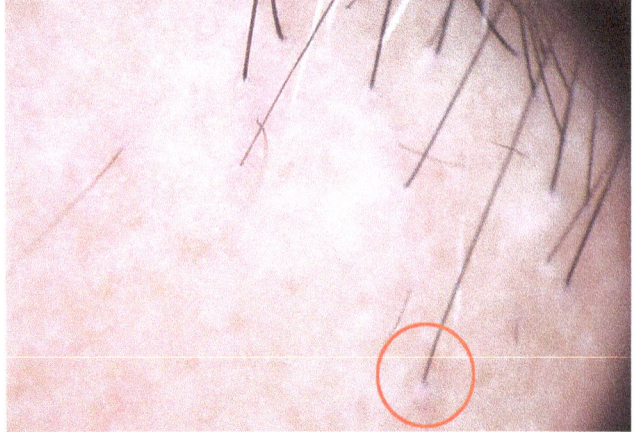

Fig. 32: Trichoscopy shows faint erythema, mild perifollicular scaling, loss of follicular openings and presence of lone hair at hair bearing margin

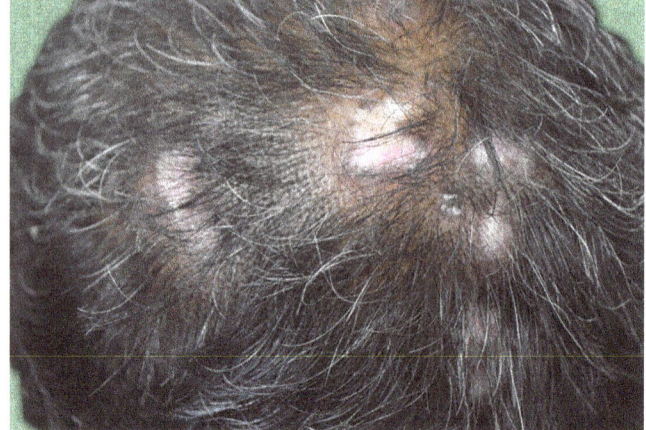

Fig. 33: Clinical picture: Discoid lupus erythematosus
Courtesy: Dr Shekhar Neema, Command Hospital, Kolkata

Chapter 16   Trichoscopy   111

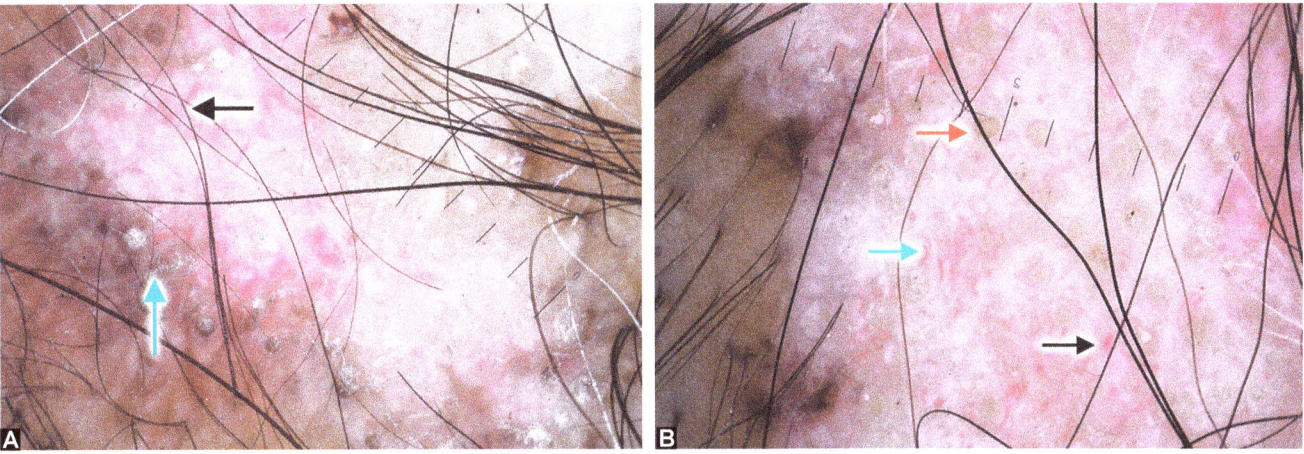

Figs 34A and B: (A) Trichoscopy shows thick arborizing vessels (black arrow), yellow dots (blue arrow). Two types of vessels seen on dermoscopy of DLE are thin arborizing vessels and thick arborizing vessels. Thick arborizing vessels are thicker than hair shaft; (B) Trichoscopy shows thin arborizing vessel (blue arrow), thick arborizing vessel (black arrow) and yellow dots (red arrow)
Courtesy: Dr Shekhar Neema, Command Hospital, Kolkata

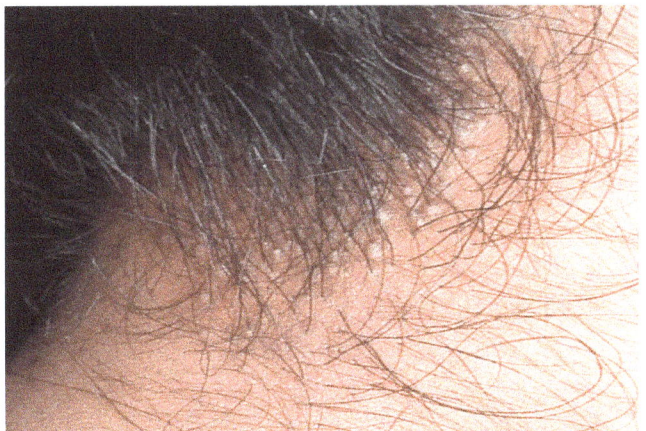

Fig. 35: Clinical picture: Traction alopecia

TRACTIONAL ALOPECIA

This form of alopecia is extremely common amongst women and children, due to hair style and grooming practices. Although most commonly seen in the African descent individuals it can now be seen in different races and ethnicities.

When the frontal and temporal scalps are affected there is preservation of a rim of hair which is also known as Fringe sign. Clinically it presents with recession of hairline or follicular papules (Fig. 35). Dermoscopy shows loss of follicular openings, irregular pinpoint white dots, broken hair and black dots occasionally (Figs 36A and B).

The presence of hair casts around the openings may point towards an ongoing process of traction (Figs 36A and B).

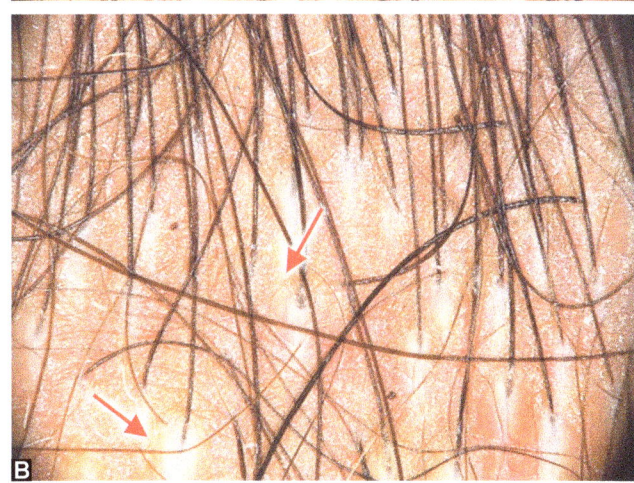

Figs 36A and B: (A) Loss of follicular opening; (B) Irregular pinpoint white dots, broken hair and black dots occasionally

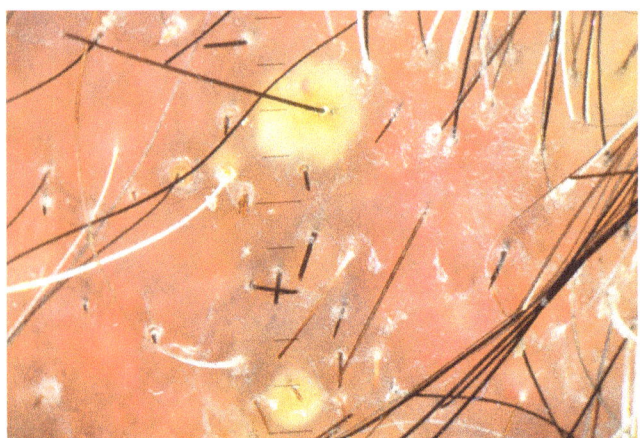

Fig. 37: Folliculitis decalvans: Trichoscopy shows presence of follicular pustules and perifollicular scales. There is background of diffuse erythema
Courtesy: Dr Shekhar Neema, Command Hospital, Kolkata

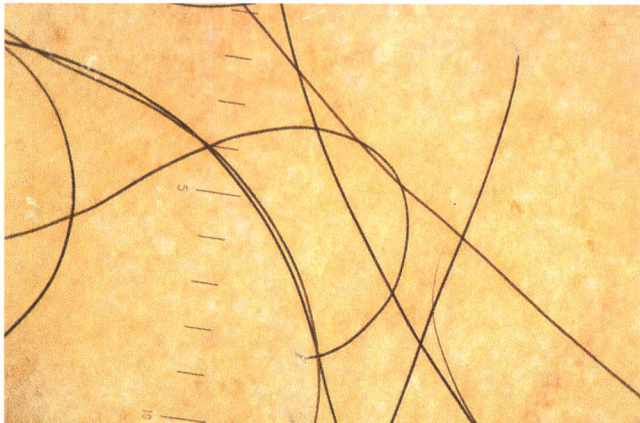

Fig. 38: Pseudopelade of Brocq: Featureless area with no evidence of inflammation and no perifollicular scaling

FOLLICULITIS DECALVANS

It is a type of primary cicatricial alopecia[5] characterized by recurrent follicular pustules, predominantly involving vertex and occipital area of scalp. Trichoscopic features of folliculitis decalvans are presence of tufts of five or more hairs in single follicular unit, presence of follicular pustules, starburst sign and yellowish discharge (Fig. 37). Starburst sign is characteristic feature of folliculitis decalvans and is seen as starburst pattern of epidermal hyperplasia surrounding tuft of hair follicle.

PSEUDOPELADE OF BROCQ

It is primary lymphocytic cicatricial alopecia and is characterized clinically by asymptomatic, irregular patches in central scalp areas. The term has also been used to describe end stage of nonspecific cicatricial alopecia. Trichoscopic features are nonspecific and consists of loss of follicular opening and absence of inflammation (Fig. 38).

CONCLUSION

Trichoscopy of scarring alopecias has multi-faceted advantages. It helps not only in early diagnosis, but helps in determining response to therapy and reactivation of these disorders.

REFERENCES

1. Duque-Estrada B, Tamler C, Sodré CT, Barcaui CB, Pereira FB. Dermoscopy patterns of cicatricial alopecia resulting from discoid lupus erythematosus and lichen planopilaris. An Bras Dermatol. 2010;85:179-83.
2. Ankad BS, Beergouder SL, Moodalgiri VM. Lichen planopilaris versus discoid lupus erythematosus: a trichoscopic perspective. Int J Trichology. 2013;5(4):204-7.
3. Rubegni P, Mandato F, Fimiani M. Frontal fibrosing alopecia: role of dermoscopy in differential diagnosis. Case Rep Dermatol. 2010;2(1):40-5.
4. Vañó-Galván S, Molina-Ruiz AM, Serrano-Falcón C, Arias-Santiago S, Rodrigues-Barata AR, Garnacho-Saucedo G, et al. Frontal fibrosing alopecia: a multicenter review of 355 patients. J Am Acad Dermatol. 2014;70(4):670-8.
5. Rakowska A, Slowinska M, Kowalska-Oledzka E, Warszawik O, Czuwara J, Olszewska M, et al. Trichoscopy of cicatricial alopecia. J Drugs Dermatol. 2012;11:753-8.

Chapter 16 Trichoscopy

TRICHOSCOPY OF SCALY SCALP CONDITIONS

BS Chandrashekhar, Samipa S Mukherjee

INTRODUCTION

Scaly scalp conditions are not uncommon in day-to-day practice. They may range from a simple case of seborrhea capitis to the more extensive scalp psoriasis or seborrheic dermatitis. Although each of these entities have their own characteristic feature, sometimes an overlap between the two may pose a diagnostic dilemma in the mind of the treating physician. It is then that a scaly scalp is approached with an intention to first have a list of differential diagnosis and collecting varied evidences to thus arrive at a conclusive diagnosis.

Scaly scalp includes the following:
- Pityriasis sicca
- Scalp psoriasis
- Seborrheic dermatitis
- Pityriasis amiantacea
- Tinea capitis (infection)
- Mimickers-like nits (infestation)
- Pseudoscales: Color residue or dirt and grit.

While evaluating any scaly condition of the scalp it is worthwhile to bear the following points in mind for the ease of arriving at a diagnosis:
- Evaluation of quality, type and morphology of hair
- Pigment pattern
- Vascular network pattern
- Nature of scales
- Structureless areas
- Evidence of dots.

The nature of scales may vary based on the underlying condition. Different types of scales in permutation and combination with vascular pattern points towards distinct diagnosis. The types of scales encountered on dermoscopy are as follows:
- Silvery micaceous
- Asbestos sheet like
- Greasy yellow
- Adherent or nonadherent
- Perifollicular
- Diffuse sheet like.

SEBORRHEA CAPITIS OR PITYRIASIS SICCA

Seborrhea capitis also known as pityriasis sicca is a common scaly condition of the scalp comprising almost 75% of the scaly scalp conditions (Fig. 39). The etiology is attributed to increased sebum secretion, followed by colonization of the same with *Pityrosporum ovale*. Clinically, it manifests as loose fine white scales on the scalp which may be easily visible to the naked eye and becomes prominent on scratching the area. Seborrhea capitis may mimic other scaly conditions, like scalp psoriasis and seborrheic dermatitis, which require more prolonged treatment with counseling of the patients regarding treatment outcome. Dermoscopy as a noninvasive tool plays an important role in clinically differentiating these mimickers.

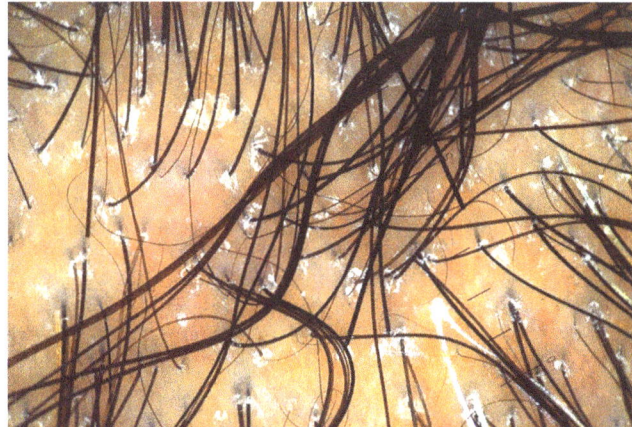

Fig. 39: Pityriasis capitis: Perifollicular scaling seen on dermoscopy
Courtesy: Dr Shekhar Neema, Command Hospital, Kolkata

SCALP PSORIASIS[1,2]

Scalp involvement in psoriasis is often the first and one of the most common site for involvement. This not only causes redness, itching and scaling but may also cause social embarrassment to the patient. Treating scalp psoriasis is often challenging due to the fact that the scalp skin is relatively inaccessible, making topical therapies difficult to apply. The clinical picture may closely resemble that of seborrheic dermatitis posing a diagnostic challenge. Dermoscopy is one of the important tools which helps in differentiating the two conditions. Vascular network pattern is important in addition to the nature of scaling in scalp psoriasis to help in differentiating from other scaly scalp conditions like seborrheic dermatitis or tinea capitis. The pinpoint vessels present as red dots on dermoscopy which corresponds to the thinned out papillary dermis with the squirting papillae. The glomerular vessels appear as red clods and correspond histologically to the dilated tortuous vessels in the dermal papillae, whereas the loops correspond to the tortuous vessel on the dermal papillae. The vascular changes may be apparent on the psoriatic scalp without any intervention or become more accentuated after Auspitz sign. The scales are silvery white, micaceous and are present on the scalp and hair giving rise to the snow on fir-tree appearance (Figs 40A to C). Dermoscopy helps not only in diagnosis but also in follow up of the cases where decrease in the number and size of the red dots and clods point towards response to therapy.

SEBORRHEIC DERMATITIS[2,3]

Seborrheic dermatitis is an inflammatory scaly-scalp condition that produces mild erythema and pruritus on the scalp. Erythema, scaling and small pinpoint follicular pustules may be noted in a few instances. The vascular pattern is of importance as it helps in differentiating from other scaly conditions of the scalp. As the name suggests, it is a dermatitis; most of the pathology happen lower down in the dermis giving rise to a faint vascular pattern. Any pathology presenting below the papillary dermis would reflect as horizontal lines on the skin of the scalp as observed through the dermoscope. The scales are greasy-yellow in color with an adherent nature as described clinically (Figs 41A to C).

PITYRIASIS AMIANTACEA[4]

It is classically defined as a scaly condition of the scalp where the scales are thick and tenaciously adherent to base of groups of the hair shaft (Fig. 42). The scales are so thick that it does not allow visualization of the underlying scalp many a times.

SCALE MIMICKERS: HAIR COLOR RESIDUE AND NITS[5,6]

These are rightly called as mimickers since they resemble scales but are not really scales. They could be a result of the accumulation of exogenous products like hair pomades, hair colorants, dirt and grit or could be the manifestation of any infestation on the scalp. Hair undergoes textural changes due to accumulation of products on the hair shaft leading to an unruly, dry and lusterless appearance. Pigment pattern may be masked by the exogenous pigmentation leading to alteration of the regular reticulate pigmentary pattern (Figs 43A and B, Table 1).

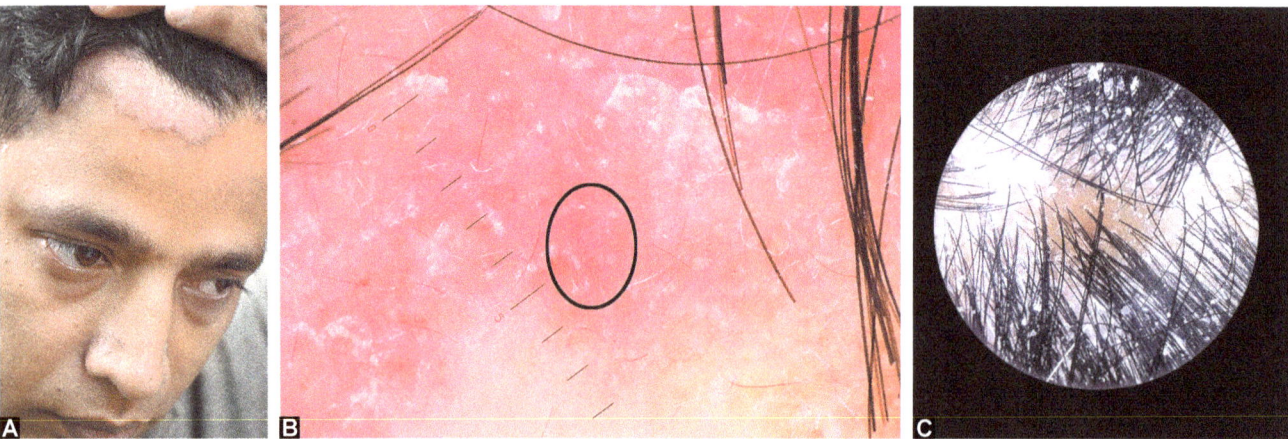

Figs 40A to C: (A) Clinical picture: Scalp psoriasis; (B) Dermoscopy of scalp psoriasis shows presence of white scales and regular arrangement of dilated capillaries, appearing as red dots (*Courtesy*: Dr Shekhar Neema, Command Hospital, Kolkata); (C) Silvery white and micaceous scale giving rise to the snow on fir-tree appearance

Chapter 16 Trichoscopy

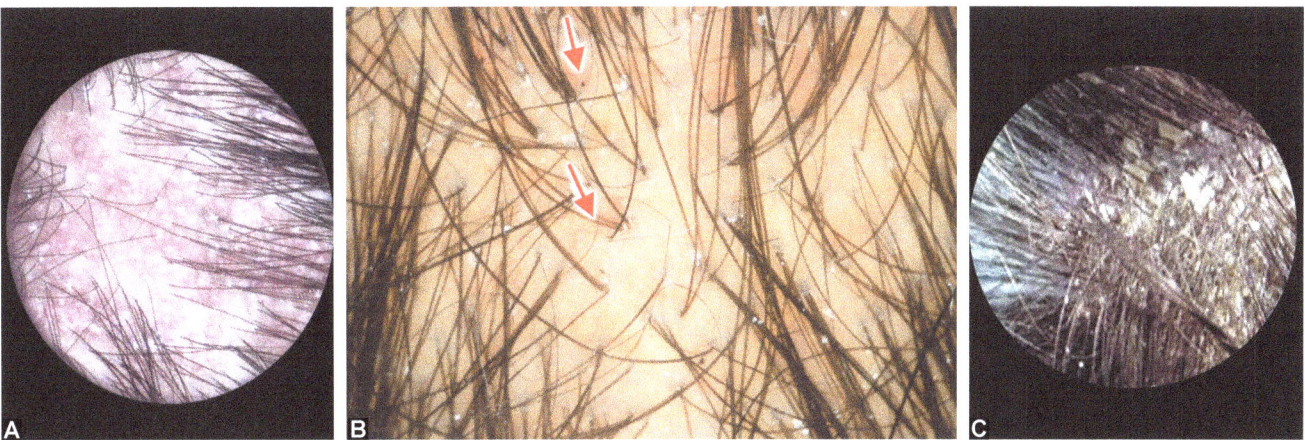

Figs 41A to C: (A) Retained normal reticulate pigmentary pattern; (B) Faint arborizing vasculature is seen in seborrheic dermatitis in contrast to scalp psoriasis which is characterized by presence of red dots (*Courtesy*: Dr Shekhar Neema, Command Hospital, Kolkata); (C) Scales are greasy-yellow in color with an adherent nature

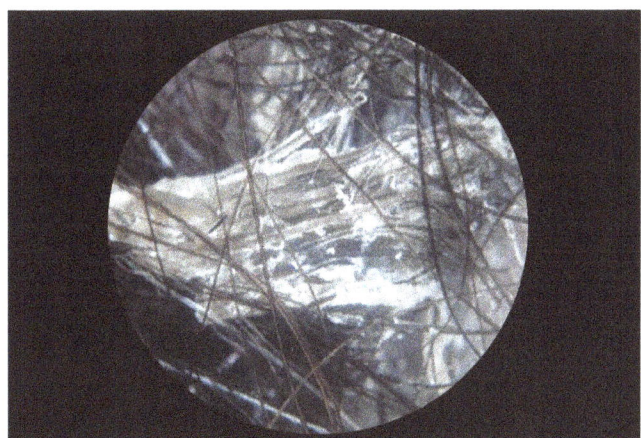

Fig. 42: Pityriasis amiantacea

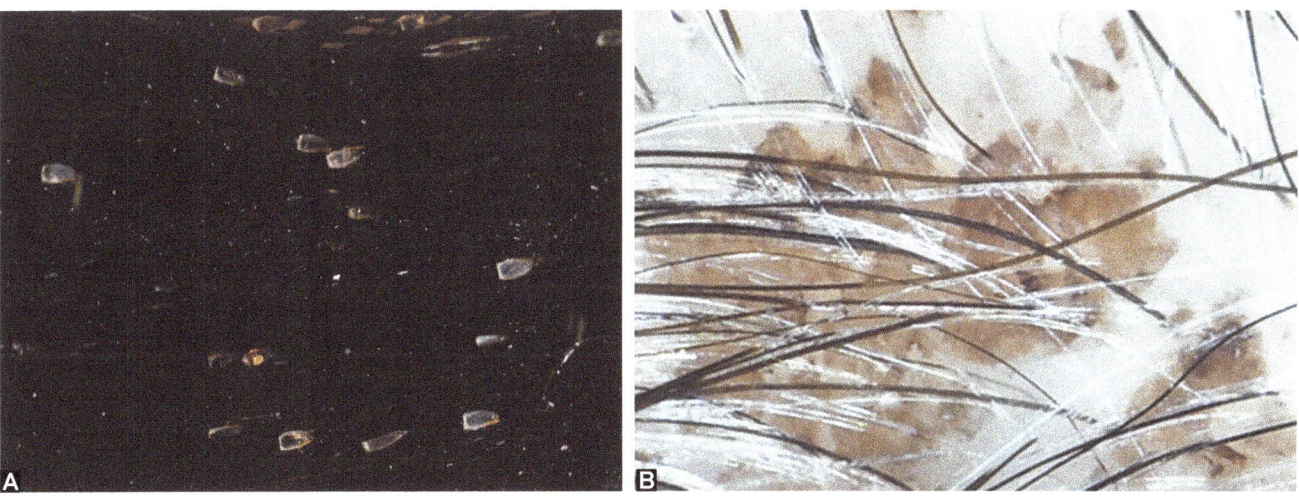

Figs 43A and B: (A) Dermoscopy shows presence of empty and full nits (pseudoscales) (*Courtesy*: Dr Shekhar Neema, Command Hospital, Kolkata); (B) Dermoscopy shows exogenous pigment

Table 1: Difference between scaly-scalp conditions

Parameters	Pityriasis sicca	Scalp psoriasis	Seborrheic dermatitis	Scale mimickers
Evaluation of quality, type and morphology of hair	No change	No change	No change	Unruly, dry, lustureless
Pigment pattern	Reticulate pattern preserved	Reticulate pattern preserved	Reticulate pattern preserved	Masking of reticular pigment pattern
Vascular network pattern	Arborizing faint vasculature	Red dots in regular arrangement	Arborizing faint vasculature	Unaltered
Nature of scales	Fine white scale with perifollicular accentuation	Silvery-white, micaceous	Greasy, yellow scale	Pseudoscales, vary in color and texture
Evidence of dots	Absent	Present	Absent	Absent

CONCLUSION

Scaly conditions of the scalp at times may pose a diagnostic dilemma to the treating physician. An algorithmic step-by-step approach not only helps in arriving at a conclusive diagnosis, but also helps in effectively treating the condition. Dermoscopy is a useful noninvasive diagnostic tool which can be used for the diagnosis of this condition.

REFERENCES

1. Kim GW, Jung HJ, Ko HC, Kim MB, Lee WJ, Lee SJ, et al. Dermoscopy can be useful in differentiating scalp psoriasis from seborrhoeic dermatitis. Br J Dermatol. 2011;164:652-6.
2. Kim KS, Shin MK, Ahn JJ, Haw CR, Park HK. A comparative study of hair shafts in scalp psoriasis and seborrheic dermatitis using atomic force microscopy. Skin Res Technol. 2013;19:e60-4.
3. Zalaudek I, Argenziano G. Dermoscopy subpatterns of inflammatory skin disorders. Arch Dermatol. 2006;142:808.
4. Rudnicka L, Szepietowski JC, Slowinska M, et al. Tinea Capitis. In: Rudnicka L, Olszewska M, Rakowska A (Eds). Atlas of Trichoscopy, 1st edition. London, UK: Springer-Verlag; 2012. pp. 361-9.
5. Lencastre A, Tosti A. Role of trichoscopy in children's scalp and hair disorders. Pediatr Dermatol. 2013;30(6):674-82.
6. Zalaudek I, Argenziano G. Images in clinical medicine. Dermoscopy of nits and pseudonits. N Engl J Med. 2012; 367:1741.

TINEA CAPITIS

BS Chandrashekhar, Samipa S Mukherjee

INTRODUCTION

Hair invasion by dermatophytes in the pediatric age group is not uncommon and most commonly presents with scalp scaling and pruritus. Identification and treatment of the condition is of vital importance to restrict the spread of the disease to family members and peers by close contact. Although potassium hydroxide mount and fungal culture may remain the gold standard for identification and species differentiation of the causative agent, dermoscopy is a noninvasive tool providing definitive diagnostic clues.

CLASSIFICATION

Tinea capitis is clinically classified as inflammatory, noninflammatory or favus. Inflammatory tinea capitis is caused by zoophilic or geophilic fungi and are associated with severe inflammation. Depending on hair shaft involvement by fungal element, it can be classified as ectothrix, endothrix or favus.

Trichoscopic features of tinea capitis are comma hairs, corkscrew hairs, morse code hairs, broken hair, black dots, i-hairs and zigzag hairs (Figs 44 to 48). Comma hairs and corkscrew hairs are most characteristic trichoscopic features of tinea capitis.[1,2] There may be subtle signs of inflammation in the form of increased scalp redness and vasculature which may not be appreciable on a pigmented scalp.

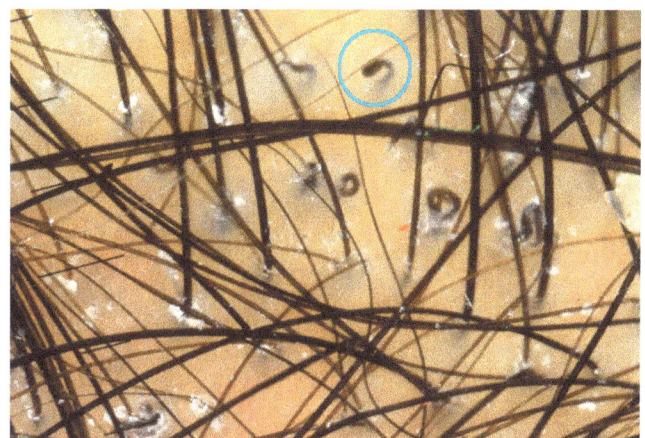

Fig. 45: Digitally magnified image of comma hair (blue circle)
Courtesy: Dr Shekhar Neema, Command Hospital, Kolkata

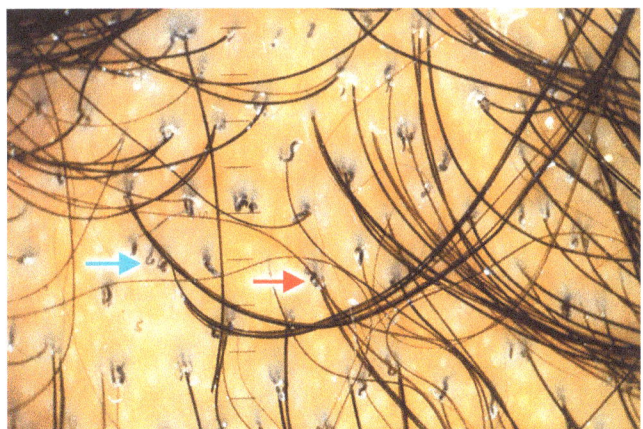

Fig. 44: Trichoscopy shows comma hairs (blue arrow) and corkscrew hair (red arrow). Corkscrew hairs shows presence of multiple twist in comparison to comma hairs
Courtesy: Dr Shekhar Neema, Command Hospital, Kolkata

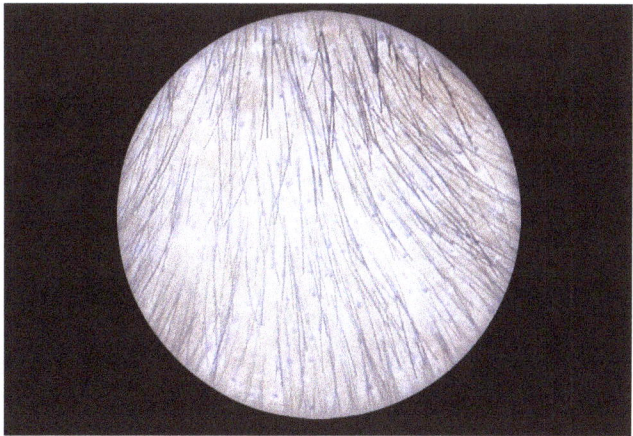

Fig. 46: Multiple comma hairs and corkscrew hairs

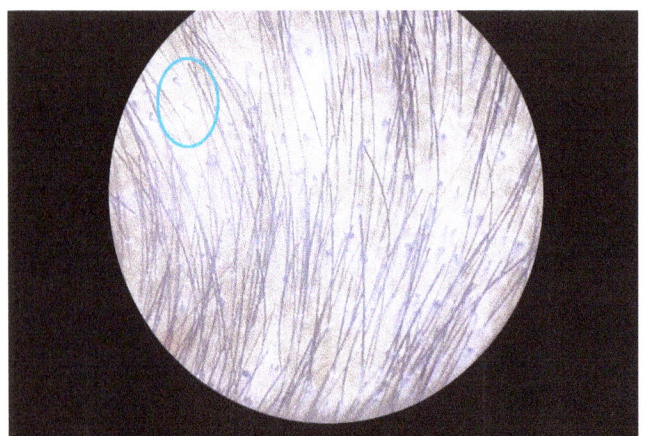

Fig. 47: Comma hairs

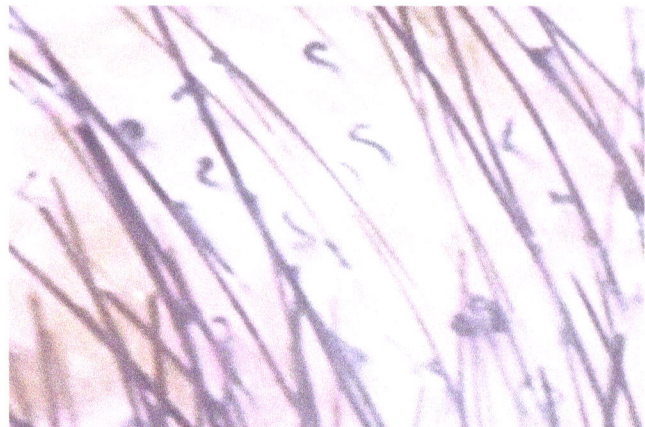

Fig. 48: Multiple comma hairs

CONCLUSION

Tinea capitis needs to be diagnosed correctly and early to prevent spread. Also the treatment is categorically different from the other scaly scalp conditions. Trichoscopy had emerged as a very handy aid in noninvasive diagnosis for this condition.

REFERENCES

1. Slowinska M, Rudnicka L, Schwartz RA, Kowalska-Oledzka E, Rakowska A, Sicinska J, et al. Comma hairs: a dermatoscopic marker for tinea capitis; a rapid diagnostic method. J Am Acad Dermatol. 2008;59(Suppl):S77-9.
2. Hughes R, Chiaverini C, Bahadoran P, Lacour JP. Corkscrew hair: a new dermoscopic sign for diagnosis of tinea capitis in black children. Arch Dermatol. 2011;147:355-6.

SECTION 9

Miscellaneous

Shekhar Neema

Section Outline

- Disorder of Vessels
- Dermoscopy in Nevoid Disorders
- Dermoscopy of Miscellaneous Disorders

CHAPTER 17

Disorder of Vessels

Shekhar Neema

INTRODUCTION

Dermoscopy of vascular structures gives important clues to diagnosis of vascular lesions. Arrangement and characteristics of vessels is also important for diagnosis of inflammatory disorders (inflammoscopy). Vascular arrangement and characteristics of inflammatory disorders have been discussed in their respective chapters; however, in this chapter we will discuss vascular disorders. Dermoscopy has been used for diagnosis of capillary malformation, hemangioma, venous disorders, vasculitis, pyogenic granuloma and other similar diseases. It can give a clue to type and depth of vessels and response to laser therapy can be predicted.

Dermoscopic imaging of vessels require special precautions as excessive pressure can lead to blanching of lesions. Ultrasound gel can be used as interface to prevent excessive blanching of the vascular lesions.[1]

VASCULAR ANOMALIES (MALFORMATIONS AND HEMANGIOMA)

Vascular anomalies are defined as lesions of abnormal vascular development. They are classified as hemangioma and malformation. Hemangiomas are vascular tumors, which grow by cellular hyperplasia in contrast to vascular malformation which results from abnormality in vascular morphogenesis. Malformations can further be classified on the basis of vessel of origin like capillary, lymphatic, venous and arteriovenous malformation.[2]

Vascular Malformation

Two types of vessels have been described in vascular malformation. Type 1 vessels are superficial papillary vessels which appear as red dots, pinpoint or globular structure on dermoscopy. Type 2 vessels are subpapillary vessels and appear as red linear structure on dermoscopy. Type 1 vessels being superficial are more amenable to laser therapy than type 2 vessels; dermoscopy here has prognostic significance (Figs 1 to 3).[3,4]

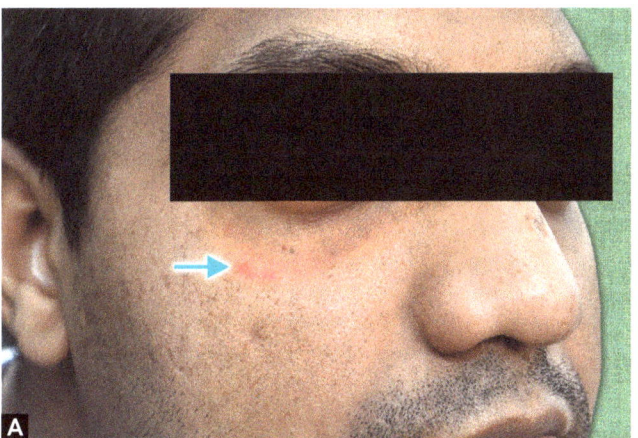 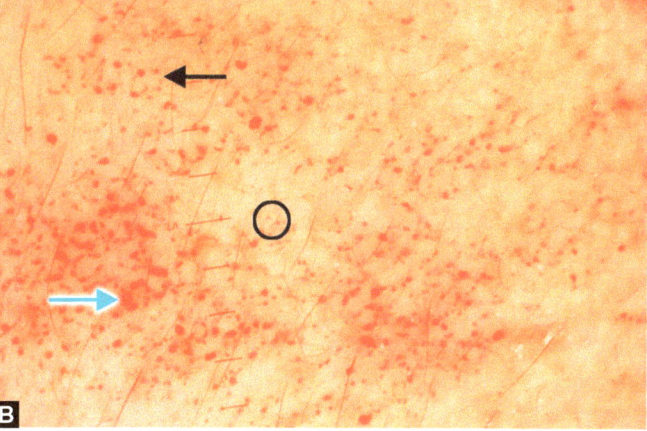

Figs 1A and B: (A) Clinical photograph showing faint capillary malformation (blue arrow); (B) Type 1 vessels appearing as red dots (black arrow), pin point (black circle) or globular structures (Blue arrow)

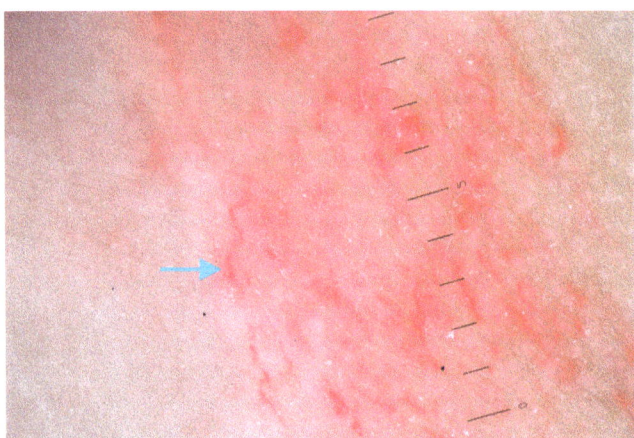

Fig. 2: Type 2 vessels appear as red linear vessels (blue arrow)

Hemangioma

Characteristic dermoscopic features of hemangioma are red lagoons or lacunae. It appears as red colored, varying sized, oval to round structures.[5] It occurs due to proliferation of vessels (Figs 4 and 5).

PYOGENIC GRANULOMA

Pyogenic granuloma, also known as lobular capillary hemangioma, is a common benign vascular lesion of unknown etiology. Trauma, inflammation and infection are considered as possible etiologic factors. It appears as polyp with glistening surface which bleeds easily. Clinical diagnosis of pyogenic granuloma is straight-forward, however, misdiagnosis can occur and it needs to be differentiated from amelanotic melanoma, keratoacanthoma, squamous cell carcinoma, melanocytic nevus, seborrhoeic keratosis and true hemangioma.[6,7]

Dermoscopy can be helpful in diagnosis of pyogenic granuloma. Reddish homogenous areas surrounded by white collarete are most common findings. White rail lines (white lines intersecting the lesion) and ulcers are also quite common dermoscopic findings (Figs 6A to D).[8,9]

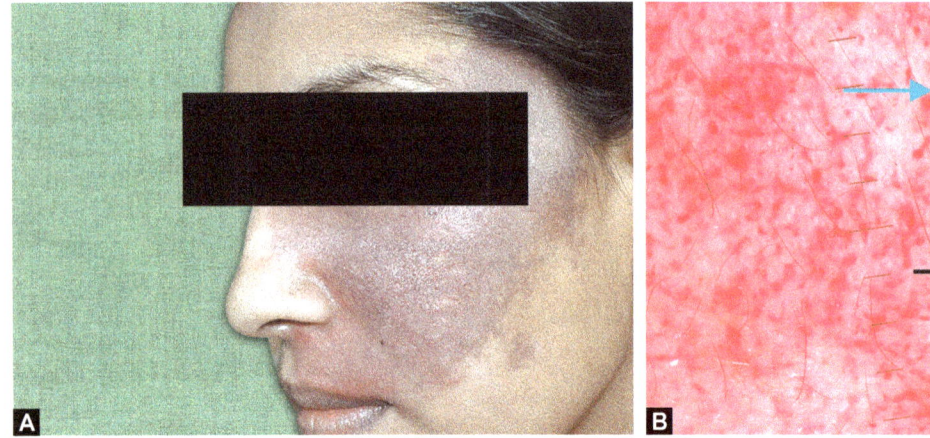
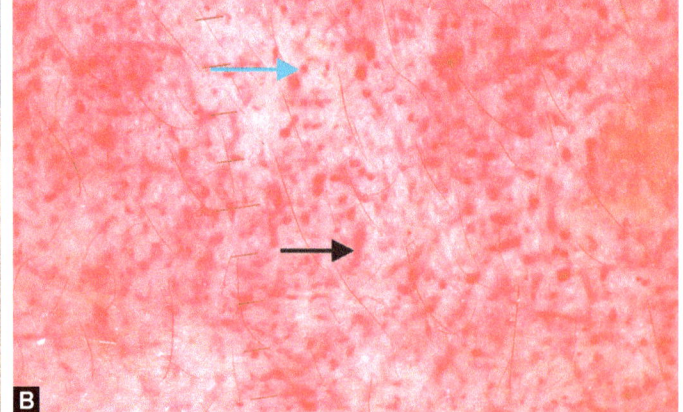

Figs 3A and B: (A) Clinical photograph of capillary malformation; (B) Mixed pattern shows both type 1 (blue arrow) and type 2 vessels (black arrow)

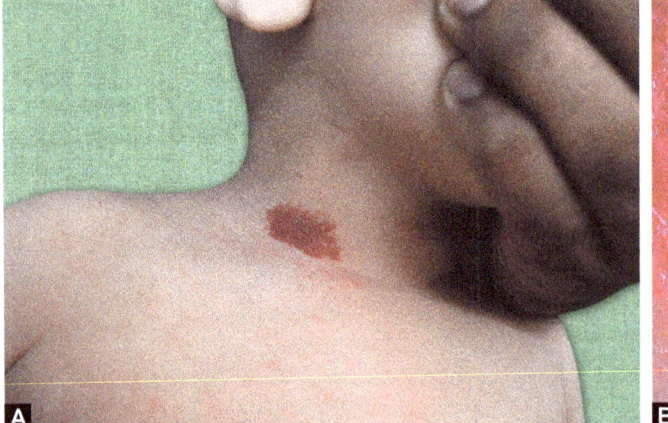
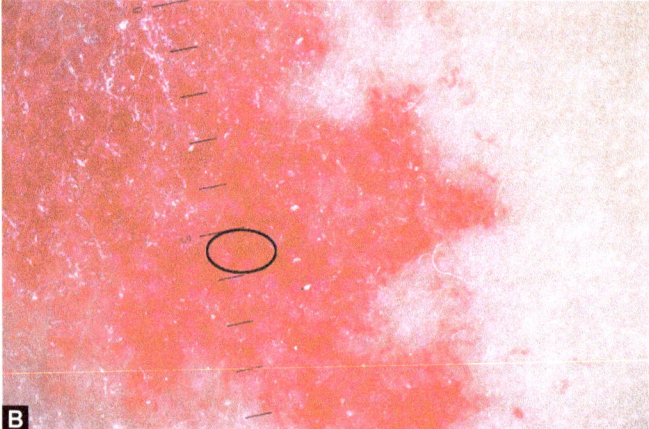

Figs 4A and B: (A) Clinical photograph showing hemangioma in proliferating phase; (B) Proliferating and ectatic vessels appear as red lagoons or lacunae (black circle)

Chapter 17 Disorder of Vessels

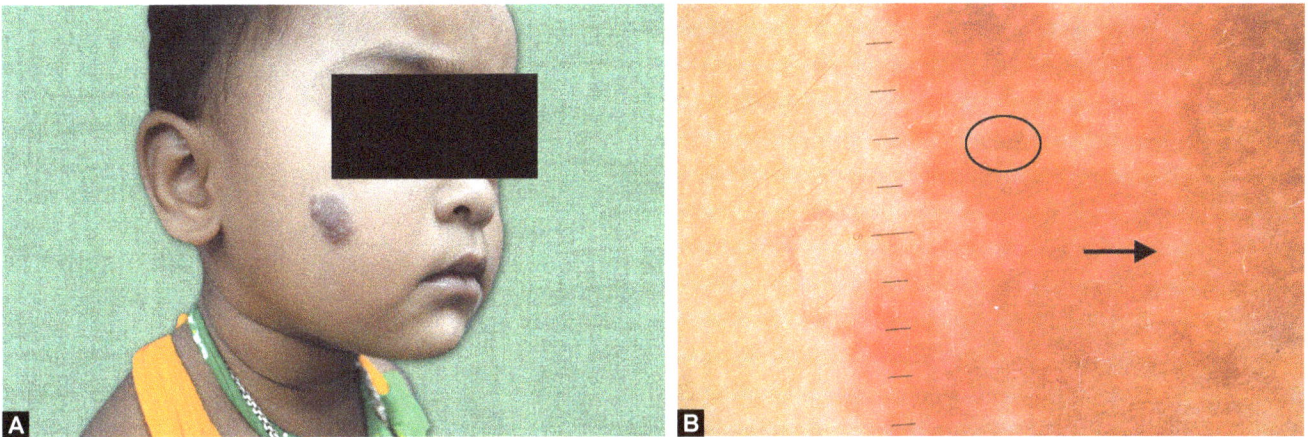

Figs 5A and B: (A) Clinical photograph of infantile hemangioma; (B) Red lagoons are seen (black circle) and areas of regression can be observed (black arrow)

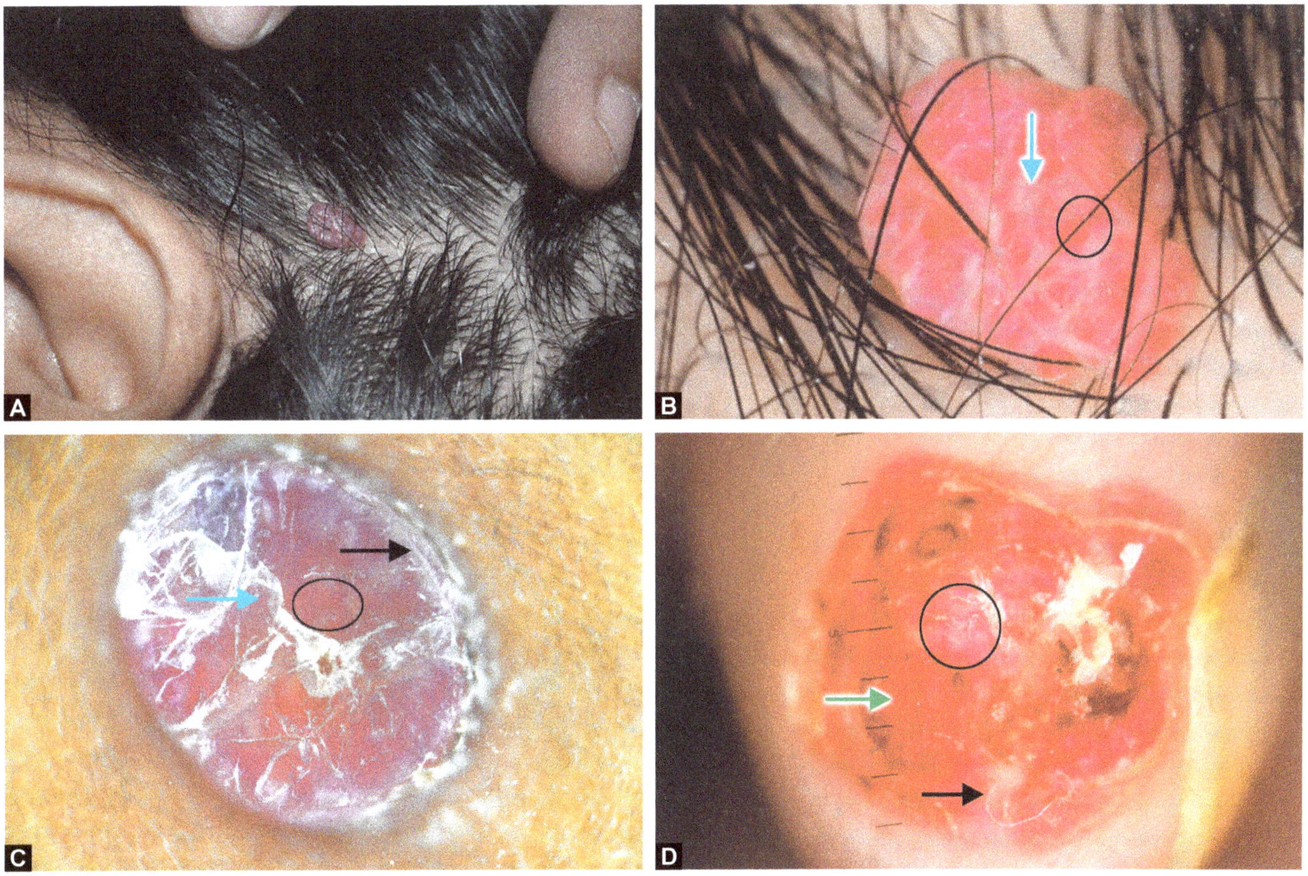

Figs 6A to D: (A) Clinical photograph of pyogenic granuloma; (B) Dermoscopy shows red homogenous areas (black circle) and white rail lines (blue arrow); (C) Dermoscopy shows red homogenous area (black circle), white collarete (black arrow) and white rail lines (blue arrow); (D) Ulcerated pyogenic granuloma shows red homogenous area (black circle), white collarete (black arrow) and area of ulceration (green arrow)

LYMPHANGIOMA CIRCUMSCRIPTUM

It is a superficial lymphatic malformation and accounts for 4% of vascular tumors. It is clinically characterized by translucent vesicles which resemble frogspawn. Differential diagnoses of lymphangioma circumscriptum are angiokeratoma, angiosarcoma, hemangioma, verrucae, molluscum contagiosum and epidermal naevi.[10]

Dermoscopic features of lymphangioma circumscriptum are yellow lacunae surrounded by pale septa and yellow to pink lacunae alternating with red lacunae due to blood (Figs 7A to C).[11,12]

VASCULITIS, VENOUS DISORDERS AND PIGMENTED PURPURIC DERMATOSES

Dermoscopy of vasculitis shows two main dermoscopic features. First is presence of large, homogenous, purpuric areas devoid of definite vascular features. This is seen in noninflammatory purpuric lesions like thrombocytopenia and senile ecchymosis. Second, purpuric dots and globules result from extravasated red blood cells and correlate with inflammatory purpuric lesion (Figs 8A to C).[13]

Stasis dermatitis shows red globules and scales in 10X and glomerular vessels in higher magnification (30X) (Figs 9A and B).

Pigmented purpuric dermatoses (PPD) are a group of chronic disorders characterized by purpura and pigmentation. PPD consists of Schamberg's disease, lichen aureus, eczematoid like purpura of Doucas and Kapetanakis, lichenoid dermatitis of Gougerot and Blum and purpura annularis telangiectoides. Dermoscopic patterns in all subtypes are almost similar and overlap with other inflammatory purpura like leukocytoclastic vasculitis. Dermoscopy shows coppery red background resulting from dermal infiltrates of lymphocytes and histiocytes, red dots and globules resulting from extravasation of erythrocytes and gray dots resulting from hemosiderin laden macrophages (Figs 10A and B).[14]

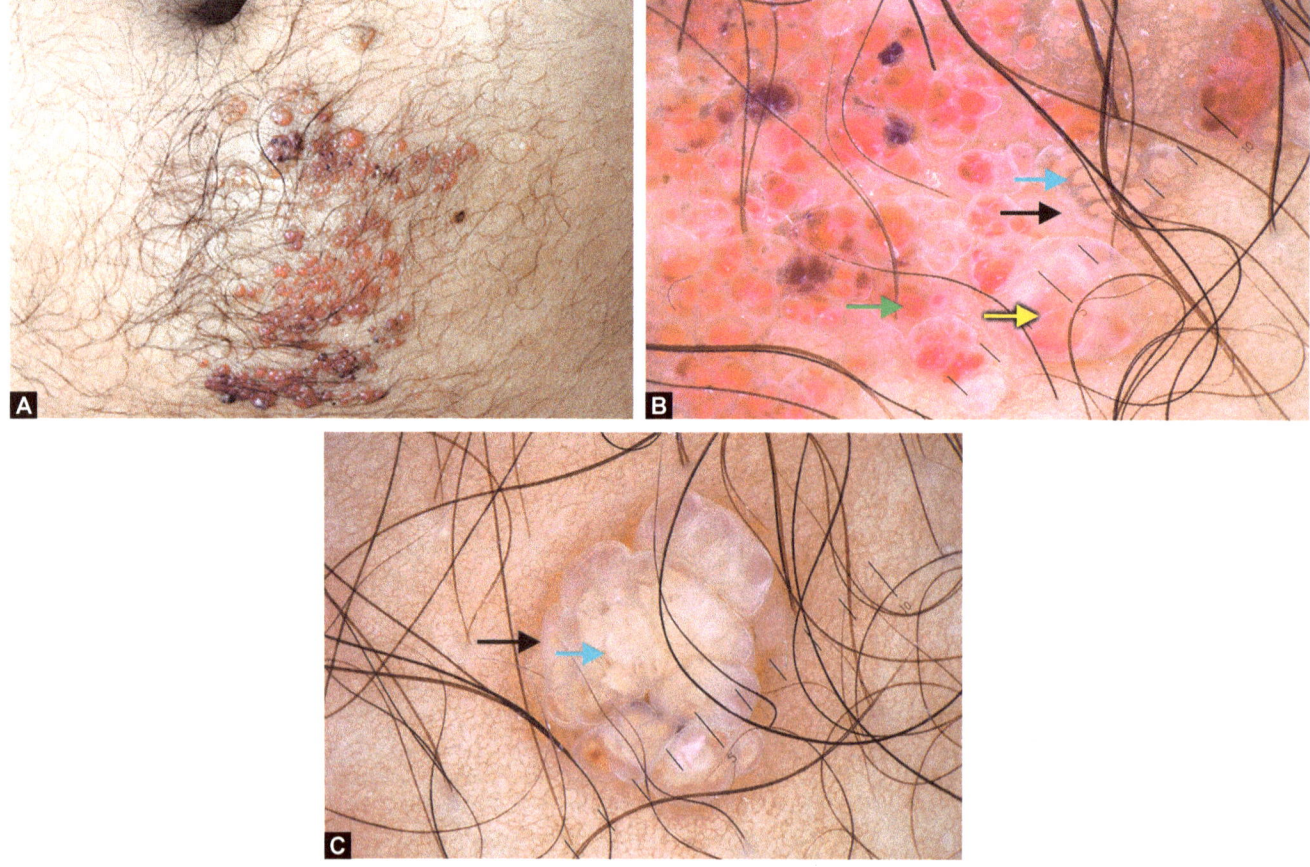

Figs 7A to C: (A) Clinical photograph of lymphangioma circumscriptum; (B) Yellow lacunae (blue arrow) with pale septa (black arrow), yellow to pink lacunae (yellow arrow) and red lacunae (green arrow); (C) Yellow lacunae (blue arrow) with pale septa (black arrow)

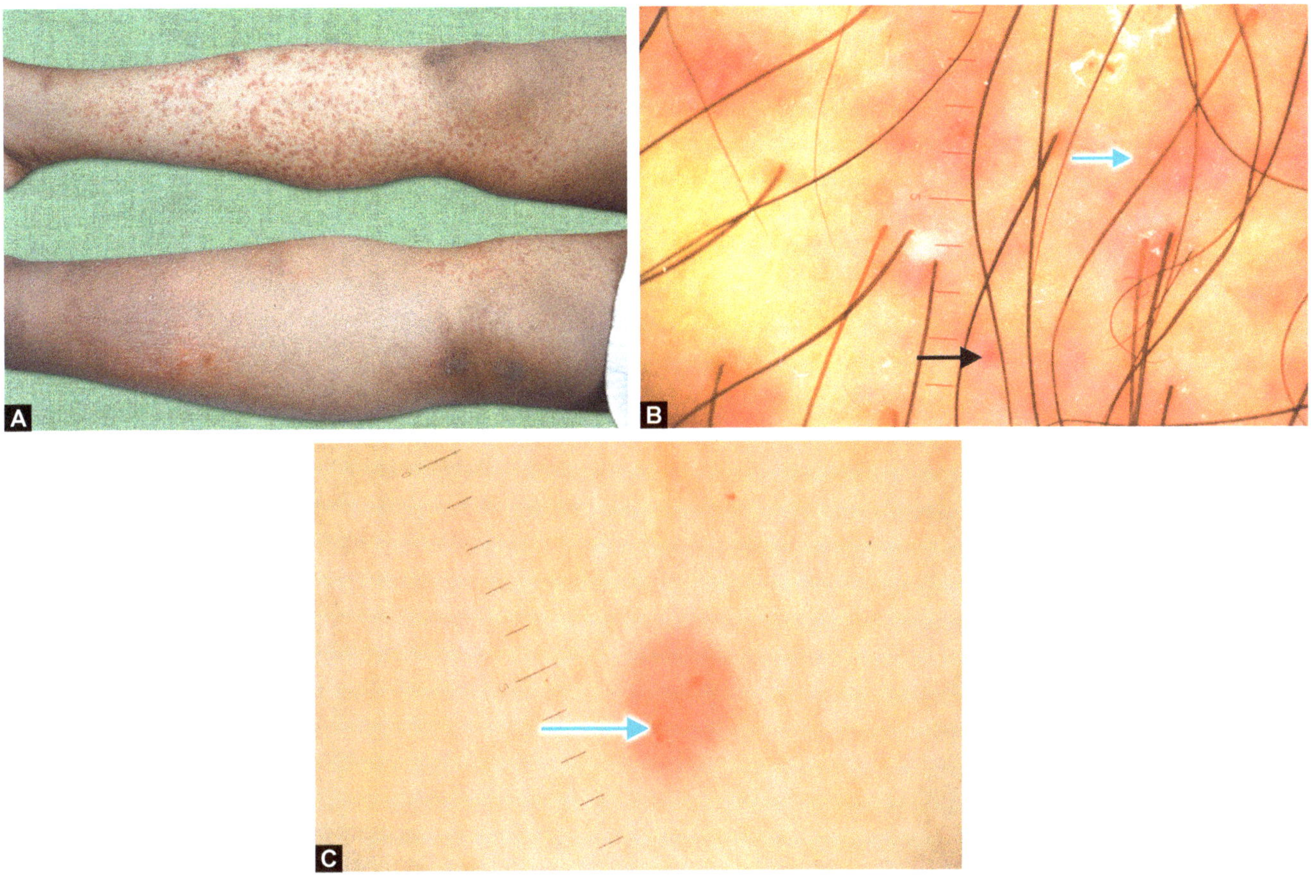

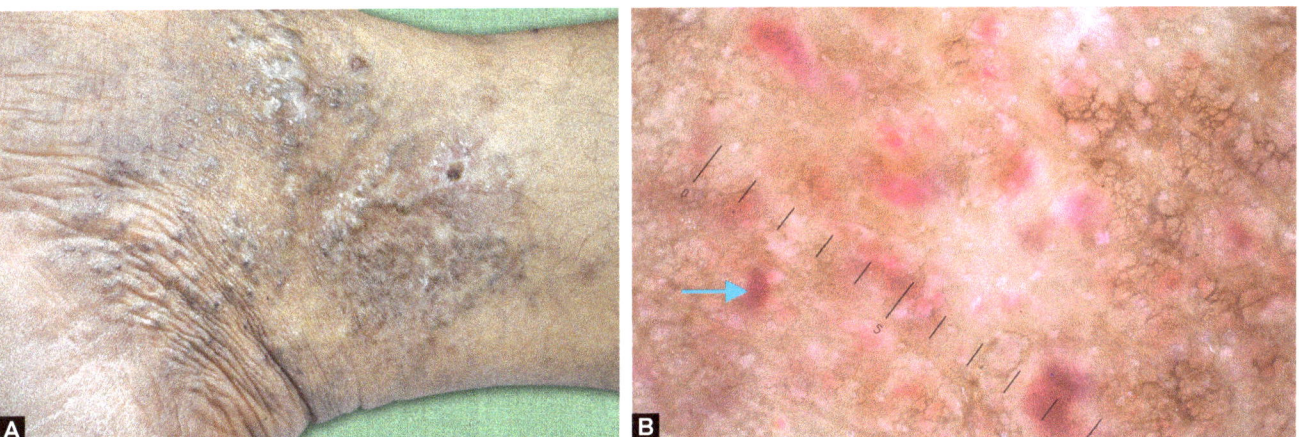

Figs 8A to C: (A) Clinical photograph of cutaneous small vessel vasculitis; (B) Purpuric dots (blue arrow) and globules (black arrow) suggestive of inflammatory purpura; (C) Purpuric globules (blue arrow)

Figs 9A and B: (A) Clinical photograph of stasis dermatitis; (B) Red globules (blue arrow) on dermoscopy

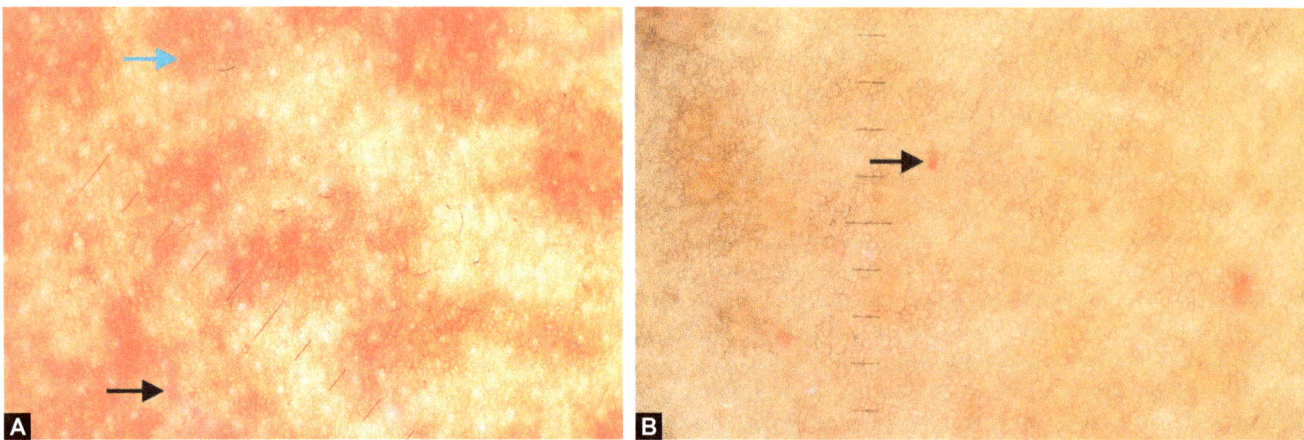

Figs 10A and B: (A) Dermoscopy of pigmented purpuric dermatoses showing coppery red background (blue arrow) and red globules (black arrow). This patient is in active phase as compared to next patient (Fig. 10B), in whom pigmentation has already started clearing; (B) Dermoscopy of pigmented purpuric dermatoses showing diffuse coppery red background and red globules (black arrow)

CONCLUSION

Dermoscopy is a useful tool for diagnosis of lesions of vascular etiology. It can also be used for prognostication in case laser therapy is planned.

REFERENCES

1. Zalaudek I, Kreusch J, Giacomel J, Ferrara G, Catricalà C, Argenziano G. How to diagnose nonpigmented skin tumors: A review of vascular structures seen with dermoscopy. Part I. Melanocytic skin tumors. J Am Acad Dermatol. 2010;63:361-74.
2. Richter GT, Friedman AB. Hemangiomas and Vascular Malformations: Current Theory and Management. Int J Pediatr. 2012;2012:645678.
3. Motley RJ, Lanigan SW, Katugampola GA. Videomicroscopy predicts outcome in treatment of port-wine stains. Arch Dermatol. 1997;133:9021-2.
4. Procaccini EM, Argenziano G, Staibano S, Ferrara G, Monfrecola G. Epilumenescence microscopy for port-wine stains: pretreatment evaluation. Dermatology. 2001;203:329-32.
5. Oiso N, Kawada A. The dermoscopic features in infantile hemangioma. Pediatric Dermatology. 2011;28(5):591-3.
6. Pagliai KA, Cohen BA. Pyogenic granuloma in children. Pediatr Dermatol. 2004;21:10-3.
7. Requena L, Sangueza OP. Cutaneous vascular proliferation. Part II. Hyperplasias and benign neoplasms. J Am Acad Dermatol. 1997;37:887-919.
8. Zaballos P, Llambrich A, Cuellar F, Puig S, Malvehy J. Dermoscopic findings in pyogenic granuloma. Br J Dermatol. 2006;154:1108-11.
9. Zaballos P, Salsench E, Puig S, Malvehy J. Dermoscopy of pyogenic granulomas. Arch Dermatol. 2007;143:824.
10. Patel GA, Schwartz RA. Cutaneous lymphangioma circumscriptum: frog spawn on the skin. Int J Dermatol. 2009;48:1290-5.
11. Arpaia N, Cassano N, Vena GA. Dermoscopic features of cutaneous lymphangioma circumscriptum. Dermatol Surg. 2006;32:852-4.
12. Amini S, Kim NH, Zell DS, Oliviero MC, Rabinovitz HS. Dermoscopic-histopathologic correlation of cutaneous lymphangioma circumscriptum. Arch Dermatol. 2008;144:1671-2.
13. Vázquez-López F, Maldonado-Seral C, Soler-Sánchez T, Perez-Oliva N, Marghoob AA. Surface microscopy for discriminating between common urticaria and urticarial vasculitis. Rheumatology. 2003;42;1079-82.
14. Zaballos P, Puig S, Malvehy J. Dermoscopy of pigmented purpuric dermatoses (lichen aureus): a useful tool for clinical diagnosis. Arch Dermatol. 2003;140:1290-1.

CHAPTER 18

Dermoscopy in Nevoid Disorders

Nilendu Sarma, Balachandran S Ankad

INTRODUCTION

Nevoid disorders are varied group of disorders and consists of conditions like nevus depigmentosus, nevus sebaceous, melanocytic nevi, connective tissue nevi etc. Dermoscopy can be used for diagnosis of these conditions with confidence and differentiate them from other conditions like differentiating nevus depigmentosus and focal vitiligo. It can also be used to detect dysplastic changes and detect early melanoma in congenital melanocytic nevi.

NEVUS DEPIGMENTOSUS

Nevus depigmentosus is a congenital, stable hypopigmented patch. Although single patch is most common, segmental lesion or multiple lesions are found.

A defect in the transfer of melanosomes is proposed as the mechanism of its development. Number of melanocytes in the basal layer remains unchanged, but there is a great reduction in the number of melanosomes in melanocytes. Some membrane-bound aggregated melanosomes were also reported to be present within keratinocytes (Fig. 1).[1]

In dermoscopy, depigmented patches appear to have irregular margin. In the peripheral part, there are numerous depigmented discrete small globular areas within the brown colored background. In more, intensely depigmented central area, white globules coalesce and fill up the area completely. The pigment network is lost and there are no pigmented lines or background at all. Hairs are of normal dark color (Fig. 2).

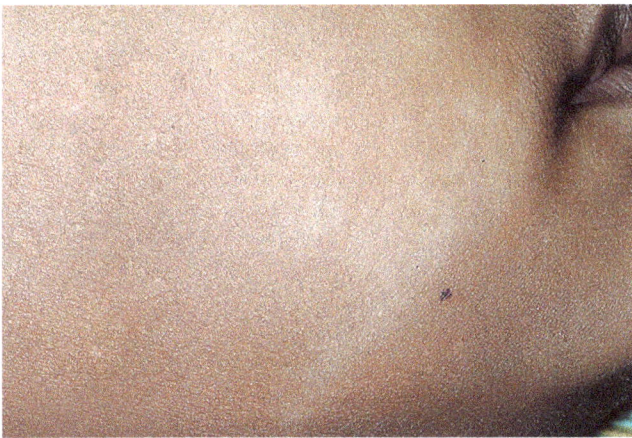

Fig. 1: Linear nevus depigmentosus

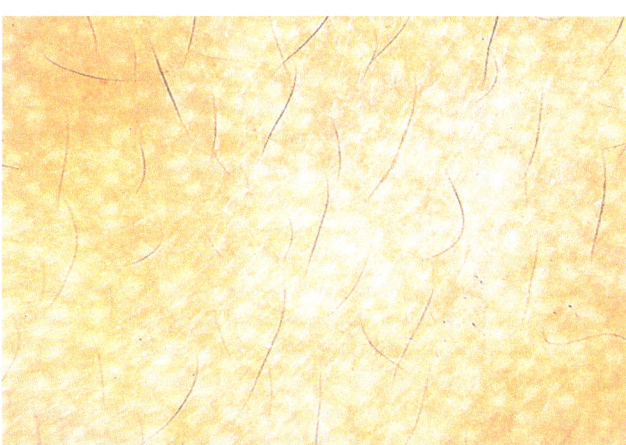

Fig. 2: Depigmented globules, discrete at the periphery and merged at the center obliterating the pigment network completely in nevus depigmentosus

CONGENITAL MELANOCYTIC NEVUS

Melanocytic nevi include a broad spectrum of benign neoplasms derived from melanocytes. They are divided into congenital melanocytic nevi (CMN) and acquired.

Congenital melanocytic nevi are benign proliferations of melanocytes in the form hamartoma presenting as pigmented lesions at birth. Some CMN appear after birth.[2]

Congenital melanocytic nevi are subdivided into junctional, compound and intradermal nevi. Clinically, junctional nevi appear as macular pigmented lesions.

Compound nevi are papular lesion with scanty pigmentation. Intradermal nevi are mammillated tumors with sparse or absent pigmentation.[3]

Recognition of CMN provides diagnostic clue in identifying pigmented lesions and also in differentiating other congenital pigmented disorders.

Studies show that dermoscopy demonstrates specific and characteristic patterns. Not only dermoscopy helps in differentiating CMN from Becker's nevus and other pigmented lesions but also in detecting early malignant changes in CMN.[4]

Junctional Nevus

It appears as macular pigmented lesions at birth. Dermoscopy shows light brown or dark brown pigment network. The thickness of lines is relatively uniform and holes of the network vary in shape and size. Borders usually merge with surrounding skin (Figs 3A and B).[3]

Compound Nevus

Clinically, lesions appear little elevated and less pigmented. Dermoscopy reveals various combinations of network, globules, dots and structureless homogenous areas (Figs 4A and B).[3]

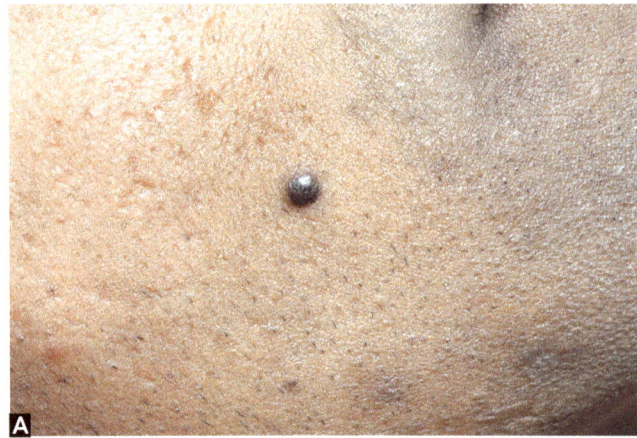
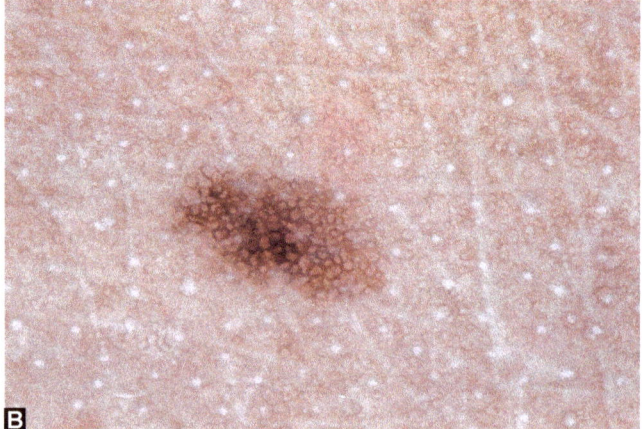

Figs 3A and B: Dermoscopy of junctional nevus showing well-defined pigment network with uniform thickness of lines. Variation in the size and shapes of holes is observed

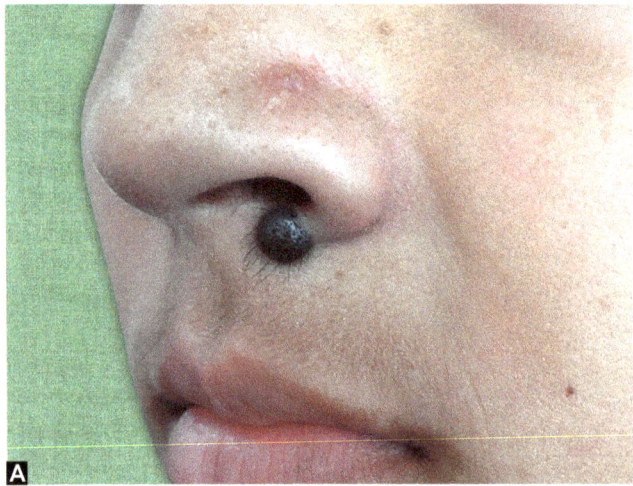
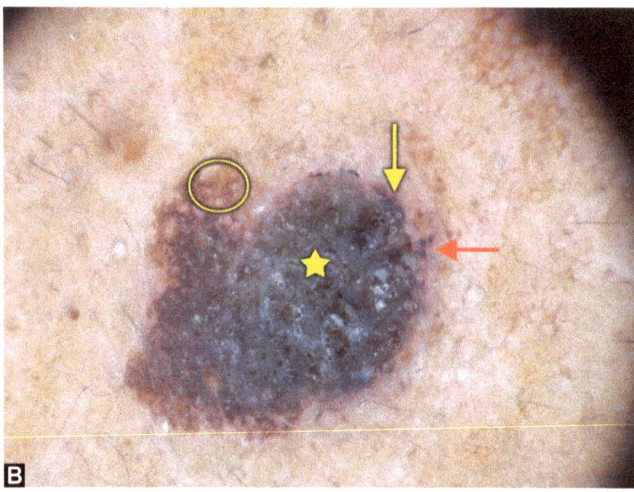

Figs 4A and B: Dermoscopy of compound nevus demonstrates combination of pigment network (yellow circle) with variable thickness of lines. Globules (yellow arrow), dots (red arrow) and bluish structureless areas (yellow star) are seen

Intradermal Nevus

Clinically, it appears as dome-shaped sessile of polypoid lesion with very scanty pigmentation. Dermoscopy reveals sparse or absent pigment network and globules. Cerebriform nevi show sulci and gyri with varying degree of pigment. Occasionally, comma-like vessels, milia-like cysts are seen. Extra hairs can also be seen (Figs 5 and 6).[3]

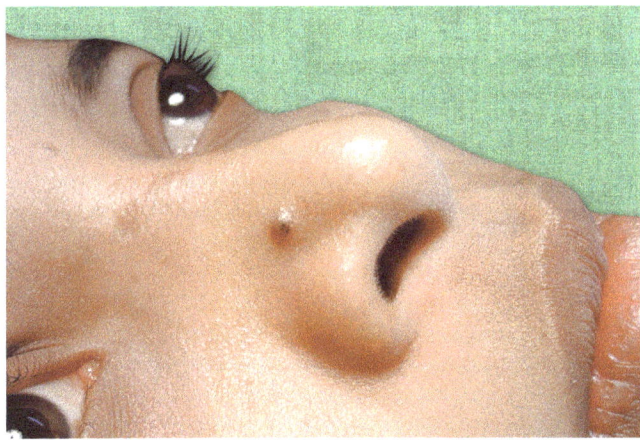

Fig. 5: Intradermal nevus

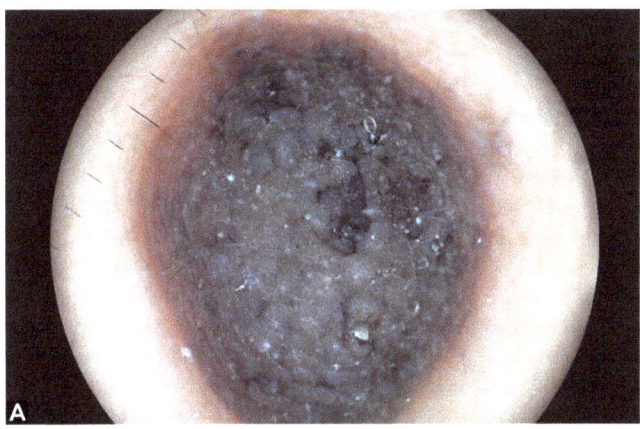

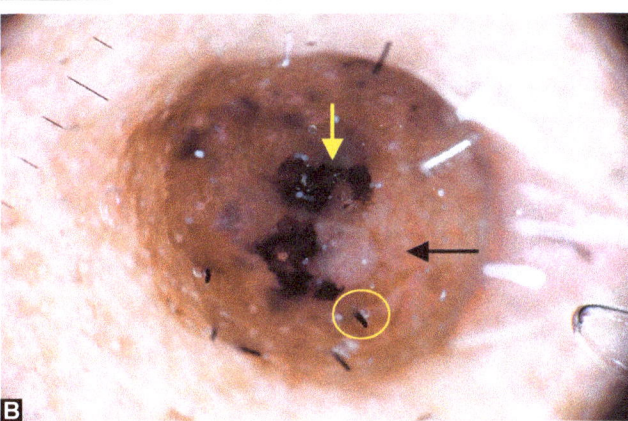

Figs 6A and B: Dermoscopy of intradermal nevus shows: (A) absent pigment network, sulci and gyri with variable, pigmentation; (B) sparse pigmentation (yellow arrow), sulci and gyri (black arrow) and hypertrichosis (yellow circle)

NEVUS SPILUS

Nevus spilus (NS) is characterized by numerous small, darkly pigmented macules or papules on a background pigmentation (Fig. 7). At birth, tan background appears and later on speckles of pigmentation impose on it. Hence, it is referred as "nevus on nevus". Histopathology reveals features of lentigo simplex and speckles show junctional or compound nevus.[5]

Since NS are potential precursors of melanoma, development of melanoma is expected in minority of patients especially when size of NS is very large. Hence, lifelong follow-up is necessary to detect melanoma.6

Dermoscopy is a best method to identify early changes in the lesion. Dermoscopy of speckles demonstrates homogeneous brown pigment network in a branched pattern. Thickness of lines and size and shapes of holes are uniform. Black dots at the center and irregular borders are also observed (Fig. 8).[7]

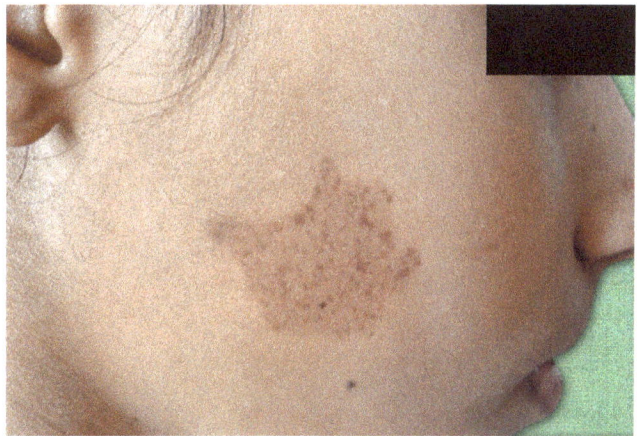

Fig. 7: Clinical photograph of nevus spilus on the right cheek showing irregular tan background and speckled dark macules

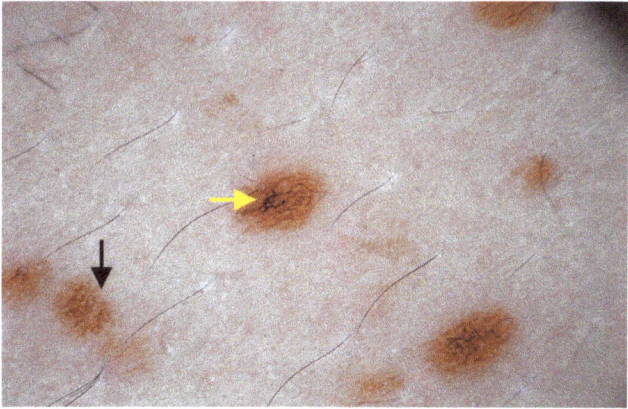

Fig. 8: Dermoscopy of speckles in nevus spilus shows homogeneous branched pigment network with black dots at center (yellow arrow) and irregular borders (black arrow)

Nevus of Ota

Nevus of Ota is a nevus characterized by presence of dermal melanocytes and clinically appears as bluish-gray or bluishbrown patch over the ophthalmic and maxillary branches of trigeminal nerve (Fig. 9).

This is a fairly common nevus among Indians, may involve sclera and rarely oral mucosa and may be sometimes bilateral. This is mostly a congenital condition but may develop during adolescence.

In histology, epidermis appears normal. Dendritic melanocytes may be present in upper as well as deeper dermis and is found to be surrounded by fibrous sheaths.

In dermoscopy, pigment network appears distorted and altered. Pigmented lines are very thick and broad, even much thicker than hypopigmented central area that normally represents dermal papilla. As a result, these hypopigmented areas appear as distinct globular structure surrounded by darker background (Fig. 10).

BECKER'S NEVUS

Becker's nevus, also called Becker's melanosis is a cutaneous hamartoma characterized by circumscribed hyperpigmentation with hypertrichosis (Fig. 11).[8]

Initially, macular brownish pigmentation appears and gradually spreads to become a large irregular blackishbrown patch. Usually, shoulder and upper arms are the common sites; however, any site can be affected.[9]

Dermoscopy demonstrates well-defined pigment network, uniform thickness of lines and also uniform size and shape of holes and perifollicular hypopigmentation (Fig. 12). Occasionally, focal hypopigmentation, skin furrow hypopigmentation and vessels can be observed.[10]

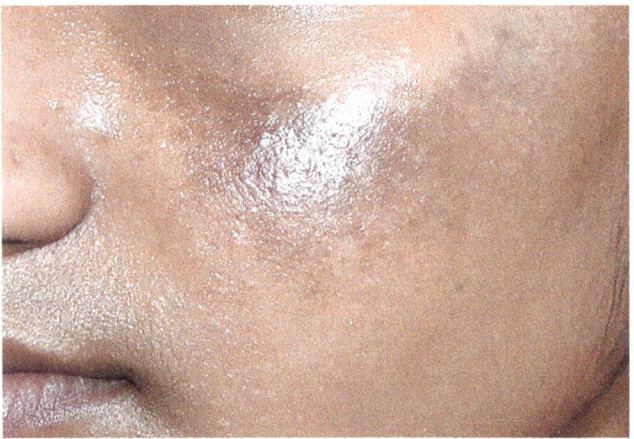

Fig 9: Bluish pigmented patch in nevus of Ota in a young girl

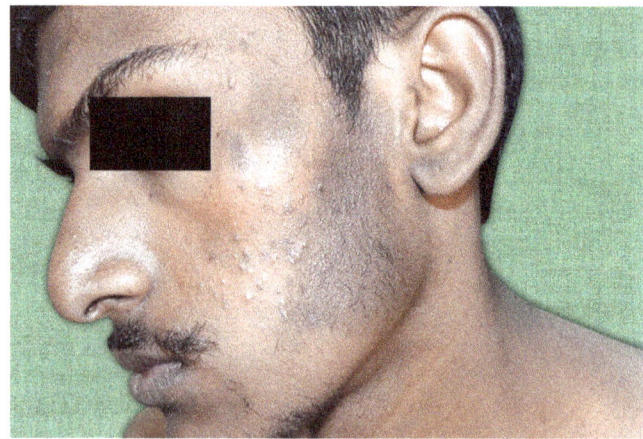

Fig. 11: Clinical photograph of Becker's nevus shows black pigmented patch on the cheek with hypertrichosis and acne

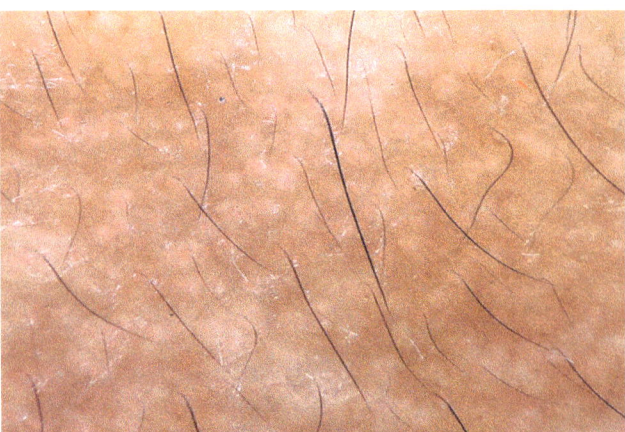

Fig. 10: Hypopigmented globules surrounded by pigmented background in nevus of Ota

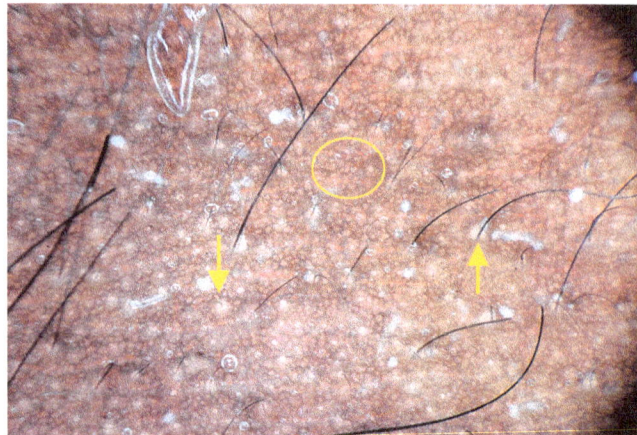

Fig. 12: Dermoscopy of Becker's nevus shows regular reticular pigment network with uniformly thickened lines and with variable size and shape (circle). Perifollicular hypopigmentation (arrows) is observed with hypertrichosis

NEVUS SEBACEOUS

Nevus sebaceous (NS) is a circumscribed hamartomatous lesion composed of sebaceous gland. Three stages of evolution of NS are described such as infantile, childhood and adult stage.[11]

The infantile stage presents as well-defined area of alopecia with smooth surface and yellowish discoloration at birth. Most important differential diagnosis is aplasia cutis, especially membranous type which also appears as alopecia with yellowish discoloration. Dermoscopy is helpful in differentiating both (Fig. 13).[12]

The second stage occurs during childhood and is characterized by a smooth surface with nodularities.

Dermoscopy of this stage show yellow globules in "cobblestone" pattern. Yellowish globules correspond to dermal conglomerations of numerous, hyperplastic sebaceous glands in the histopathology (Fig. 14).[13]

Third stage, i.e. adulthood stage is characterized by verrucous growth of nevus (Fig. 15). Importantly, during this stage, numerous benign and malignant tumors develop in the nevus. Hence, it is very important to follow the nevus for development of such tumors. Dermoscopy plays a very important role in this regard. Dermoscopy of NS in this stage shows "cerebriform" pattern which correlates to epithelial hyperplasia and papillomatosis in the histopathology (Fig. 16).[14]

Syringocystadenoma papilliferum, multiple pigmented trichoblastoma and nodular basal cell carcinoma are reported to develop in NS and in all these cases dermoscopy can be crucial in the early detection of these tumors.[15]

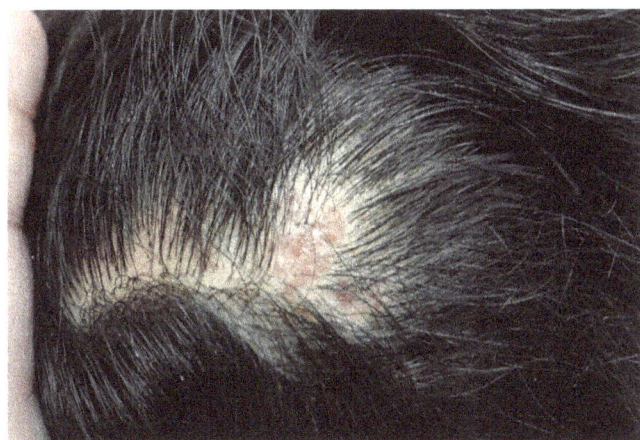

Fig. 13: Clinical photograph of nevus sebaceous in childhood stage showing yellow lobular tumor on the scalp

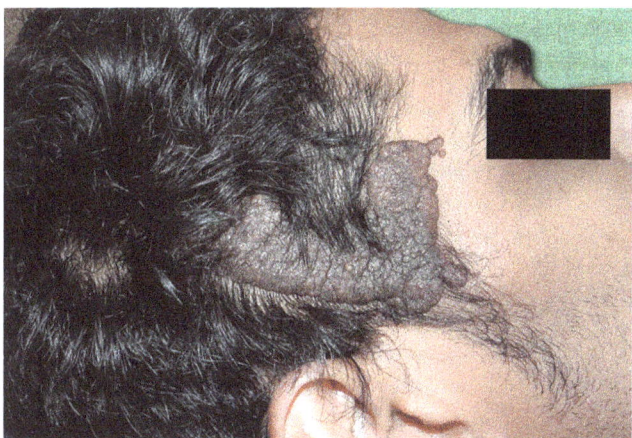

Fig 15: Clinical photograph of adult stage of nevus sebaceous with verrucous tumor on the scalp extending onto the face

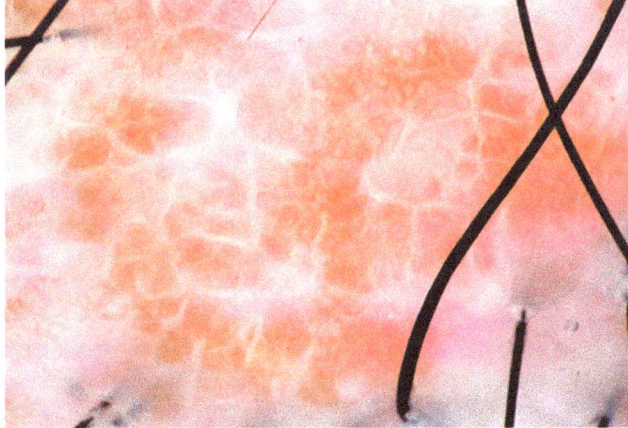

Fig. 14: Dermoscopy of childhood stage of nevus sebaceous showing yellowish globules

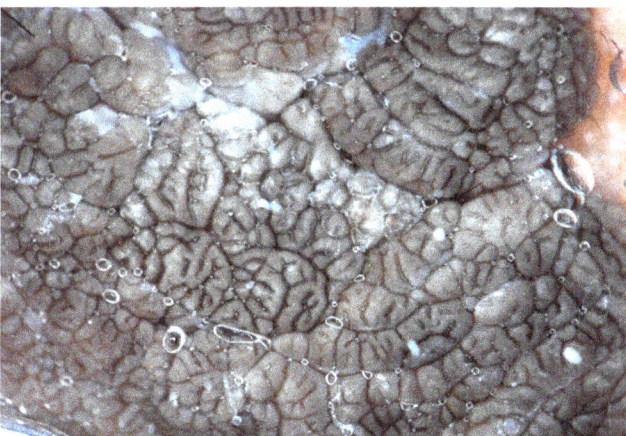

Fig. 16: Dermoscopy showing "cerebriform pattern" of nevus sebaceous in adult stage

EPIDERMAL NEVI

Epidermal nevi are benign hamartoma of skin. Based on the predominant cell types of differentiation, this is divided into keratinocytic nevi (nonorganoid nevi) that contain keratinocytes and organoid nevi that are differentiated into various appendageal tissues like sebaceous glands, hair follicle, apocrine or eccrine glands. Generally, epidermal nevi appear as verrucous. Sometimes, they may show signs of prominent inflammation [e.g. inflammatory linear verrucous epidermal nevus (ILVEN)]. They are generally congenital in origin or may develop early in life.

In histology, there is hyperkeratosis, acanthosis and papillomatosis with focal hypergranulosis. Some of the epidermal nevi show presence of epidermolytic cells in epidermis (epidermolytic epidermal nevi). Other group that do not show these are called nonepidermolytic epidermal nevi.

In dermoscopy, there are islands flower like structures that are composed of many grouped circular structures. These are formed by pigmented lines. Intensity of pigmentation and thickness of these lines are variable. Diameter of the rings they have formed also varies. Frequently, these rings are distributed radially and the outer side show leaf-like extension of pigmented patches. Thus, they appear as a flower (Fig. 17)

The above-mentioned discrete flower-like structures were noted in the nevi that are composed of tiny papular eruptions as shown in the Figure 18.

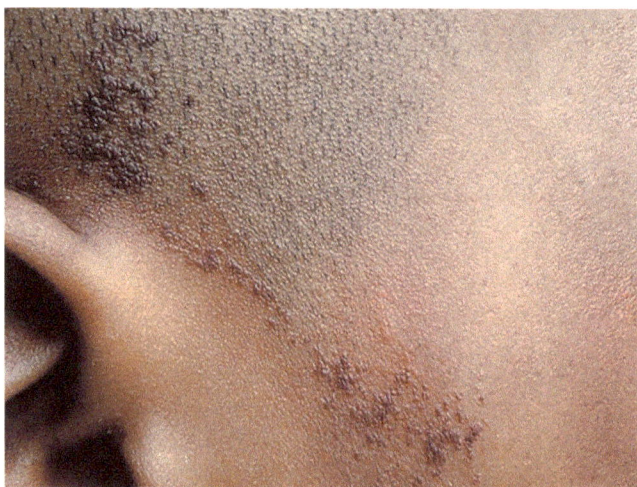

Fig. 18: Epidermal nevus in blaschkoid distribution

SHAGREEN PATCH

A shagreen patch is a firm yellowish-red or pink area of nodules slightly elevated above the surrounding skin and often described as having the texture of an orange peel. It is one of the major criteria of tuberous sclerosis complex.

Usually appears on the lower back, nevertheless, any site can be involved (Fig. 19).16

Since shagreen patch can be confused with smooth muscle hamartoma, correct diagnosis is necessary.

Dermoscopy is a useful diagnostic aid in shagreen patch.

Dermoscopy shows numerous dark brown strands in a "cobblestone pattern". Regular white dots are observed on brown strands. The white dots correspond to eccrine sweat duct openings which are wider than the normal openings and brown strands to papillomatosis and dense collagen bundles (Fig. 20).[17]

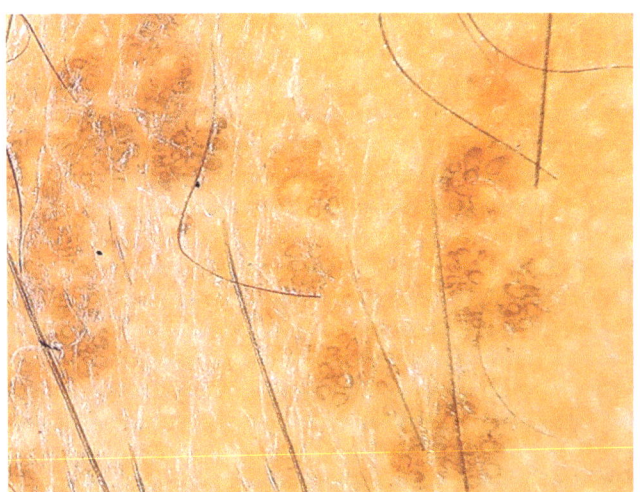

Fig. 17: Flower-like structures in epidermal nevi

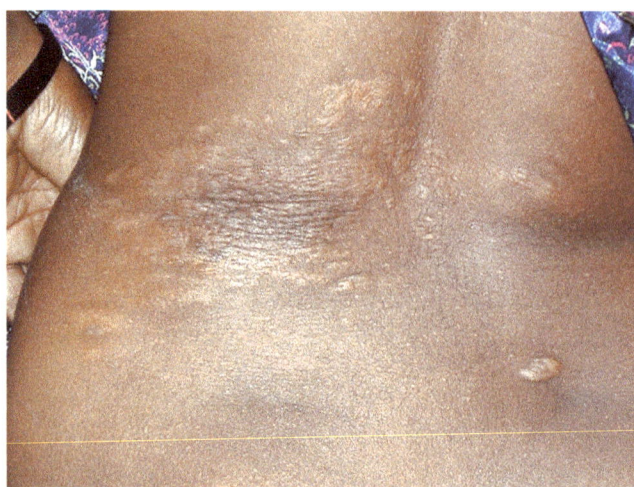

Fig. 19: Clinical photograph of shagreen patch on the back

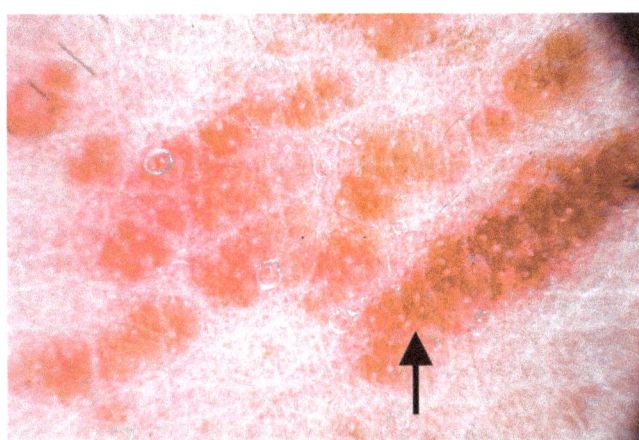

Fig. 20: Dermoscopy of shagreen patch shows dark brown strands with white dots (black arrow)

CONCLUSION

Dermoscopy in nevoid disorders helps not only in diagnosis but also in early detection of malignant transformation. Hence a dermoscopic diagnosis and follow up, along with photographic documentation is recommended for these disorders.

REFERENCES

1. Lee HS, Chun YS, Hann SK. Nevus depigmentosus: clinical features and histopathologic characteristics in 67 patients. J Am Acad Dermatol. 1999;40:21-6.
2. Kittler H, Rosendahl C, Cameron A, Tschandl P. Principal pigmented skin lesions relevant to dermoscopy. In: Kittler H, Rosendahl C, Cameron A, Tschandl P (Eds). Dermatoscopy: An Algorithmic Method Based on Pattern Analysis, 1st edition. Vienna: Facultas. wuv; 2011. pp. 25-49.
3. Malvehy J, Puig S, Braun RP, Marghoob AA, Kopf AW. Melanocytic lesions. In: Malvehy J, Puig S, Braun RP, Marghoob AA, Kopf AW (Eds). Handbook of Dermoscopy, 1st edition. London: Taylor and Francis; 2006. pp. 45-55.
4. Changchien L, Dusza SW, Agero ALC, Korzenko AJ, Braun RP, Sachs D, et al. Age- and site-specific variation in the dermoscopic patterns of congenital melanocytic nevi: An aid to accurate classification and assessment of melanocytic nevi. Arch Dermatol. 2007;143(8):1007-14.
5. Vaidya DC, Schwartz RA, Janniger CK. Nevus spilus. Cutis. 2007;80(6):465-8.
6. Holger A, Haenssle HA, Kaune KM, Thoms KM, Padeken M, Emmert S, et al. Melanoma arising in segmental nevus spilus: detection by sequential digital dermatoscopy. J Am Acad Dermatol. 2009;61(2):337-41.
7. Prodinger C, Tatarski R, Laimer M, Ahlgrimm-Siess V. Large congenital nevus spilus—improved follow-up through the use of in vivo reflectance confocal microscopy. Dermatol Pract Concept. 2013;3(2):55-8.
8. Lambert JR, Willems P, Abs R, Van Roy B. Becker's nevus associated with chromosomal mosaicism and congenital adrenal hyperplasia. J Am Acad Dermatol. 1994;30:655-7.
9. Patrizi A, Medri M, Raone B, Bianchi F, Aprile S, Neri I. Clinical characteristics of Becker's nevus in children: report of 118 cases from Italy. Pediatr Dermatol. 2012;29(5):571-4.
10. Ingordo V, Iannazzone SS, Cusano F, Naldi L. Dermoscopic features of congenital melanocytic nevus and becker nevus in an adult male population: An analysis with a 10-fold magnification. Dermatology. 2006;212:354-60.
11. Morioka S. The natural history of nevus sebaceous. J Cutan Pathol. 1985;12:200-13.
12. Neri I, Savoia F, Giacomini F, Raone B, Aprile S, Patrizi A. Usefulness of dermatoscopy for the early diagnosis of sebaceous naevus and differentiation from aplasia cutis congenita. Clin Exp Dermatol. 2009;34:e50-2.
13. Kim NH, Zell DS, Kolm I, Oliviero M, Rabinovitz HS. The dermoscopic differential diagnosis of yellow lobular like structures. Arch Dermatol. 2008;144:962.
14. Ankad BS, Beergouder SL, Domble V. Trichoscopy: The best auxiliary tool in the evaluation of nevus sebaceous. Int J Trichol. 2016;8:5-10.
15. De Giorgi V, Massi D, Trez E, Alfaioli B, Carli P. Multiple pigmented trichoblastomas and syringocystadenoma papilliferum in naevus sebaceous mimicking a malignant melanoma: A clinical dermoscopicpathological case study. Br J Dermatol. 2003;149:1067-70.
16. Darling TN, Moss J, Mausner M. Dermatologic manifestations of tuberous sclerosis complex (TSC). In: Kwiatkowski DJ, Whittemore VH, Thiele E (Eds). Tuberous Sclerosis Complex: Genes, Clinical Features and Therapeutics. Wenham: Wiley-Blackwell; 2010. pp. 285-309.
17. Gundalli S, Ankad BS, Ashwin PK, Kolekar R. Dermoscopy of shagreen patch: A first report. Our Dermatol Online. 2015;6(3):331-3.

19
CHAPTER

Dermoscopy of Miscellaneous Disorders

Sukesh MS

INTRODUCTION

In this chapter, dermoscopic features of few common conditions and some rare conditions with characteristic features are discussed.

PHRYNODERMA

Phrynoderma is a type of follicular hyperkeratosis presenting with discrete, keratotic, follicular, brown or skin colored, acuminate papules with central keratinous plug localized to elbows, knees, buttocks and extensor extremities mostly bilaterally symmetrical, with various nutritional deficiency disorders implicated in the etiology (Figs 1 and 2). Phrynoderma predominantly occurs in children and adolescents aged between 5 years and 15 years and is also noticed in lactating mothers. In generalized disease, the lesions also appear on the trunk and face (Figs 3A to C).

Dermoscopy reveals hyperpigmented follicular papules, big brown-black keratin plugs with perifollicular pigmentation and collarete of scales. The surrounding skin appears dry, scaly and pigmented (Figs 4 and 5).[1] Sometimes, the characteristic "horn sign" can be seen (Figs 6A to C). These distinct clinical features help in differentiating phrynoderma from other common follicular keratotic disorders such as keratosis pilaris (KP), lichen spinulosis and follicular lichen planus (LP) (described below).

KERATOSIS PILARIS

Keratosis pilaris is a common autosomal dominant disorder of follicular hyperkeratosis characterized by multiple

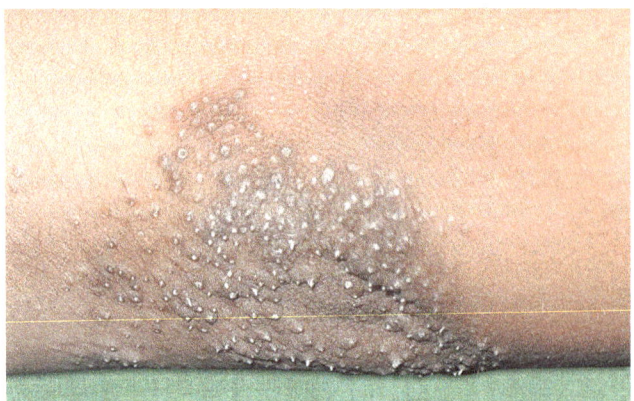

Fig. 1: Numerous hyperpigmented, clustered follicular papules with prominent horny plugs on elbow

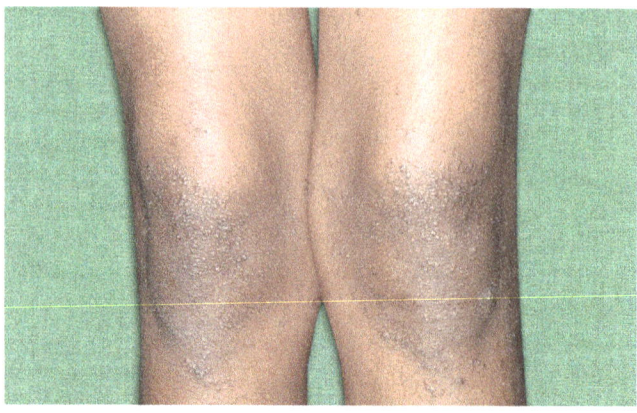

Fig. 2: Multiple hyperpigmented follicular papules with marked variability in size present on and around the knee

Chapter 19 Dermoscopy of Miscellaneous Disorders

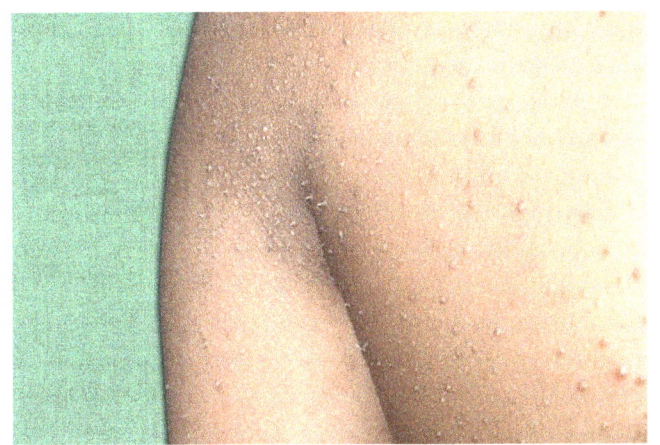
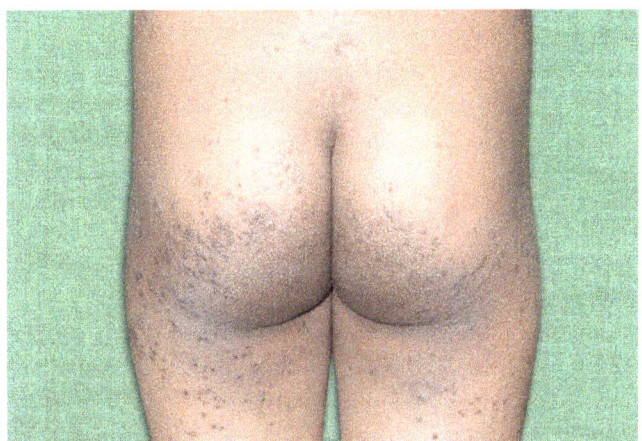
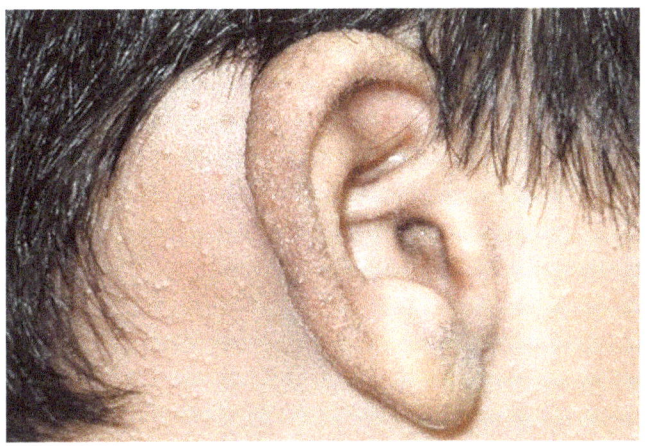

Figs 3A to C: Extensive involvement of: (A) trunk, (B) buttocks, and (C) earlobes in phrynoderma

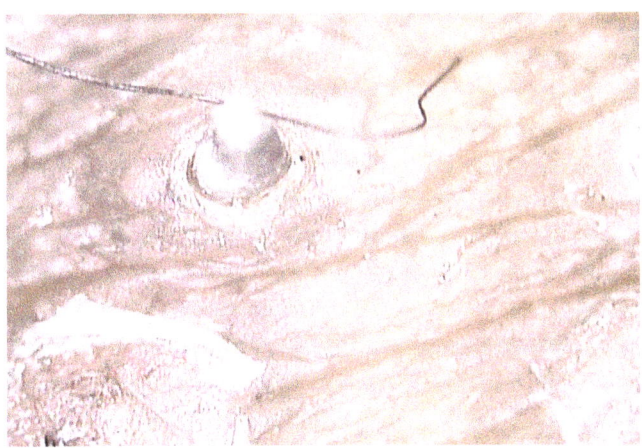
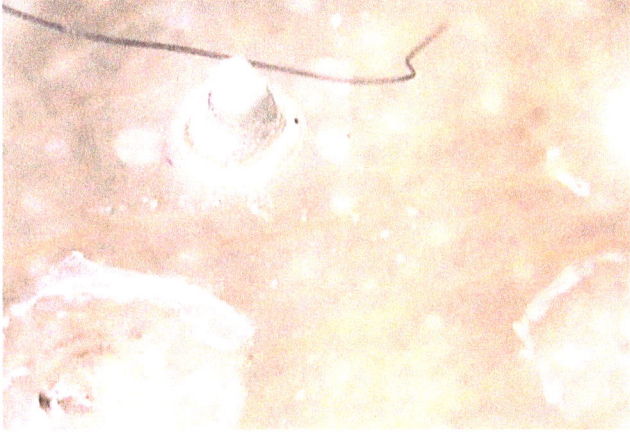

Figs 4A and B: Dermoscopy of phrynoderma shows hyperpigmented follicular papules, big brown-black keratin plugs with perifollicular pigmentation and collarets of scales in nonpolarized and polarized mode, respectively

small gray-white, keratinous plugs in the follicular orifices, approximately 1 mm in size, resembling gooseflesh with varying degrees of perifollicular erythema or inflammation. KP lesions often contain a fine-coiled, brittle hair.[2] The common affected body sites are the extensor surfaces of the upper aspect of arms, thighs, face, buttocks and eyebrows (Figs 7 and 8).

Dermoscopy, in mild cases, shows vellus hair, frequently twisted or coiled, surrounded by peripilar casts or scaling. Around 1–3 vellus hair may emerge together. In more severe

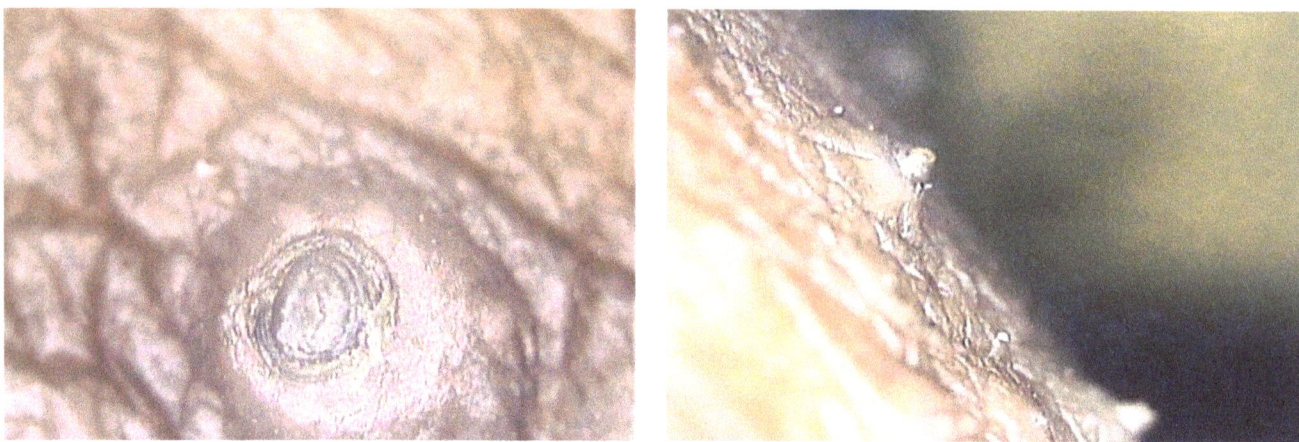

Figs 5A and B: Follicular papules with follicular plugs, better seen on tangential view on dermoscopic examination

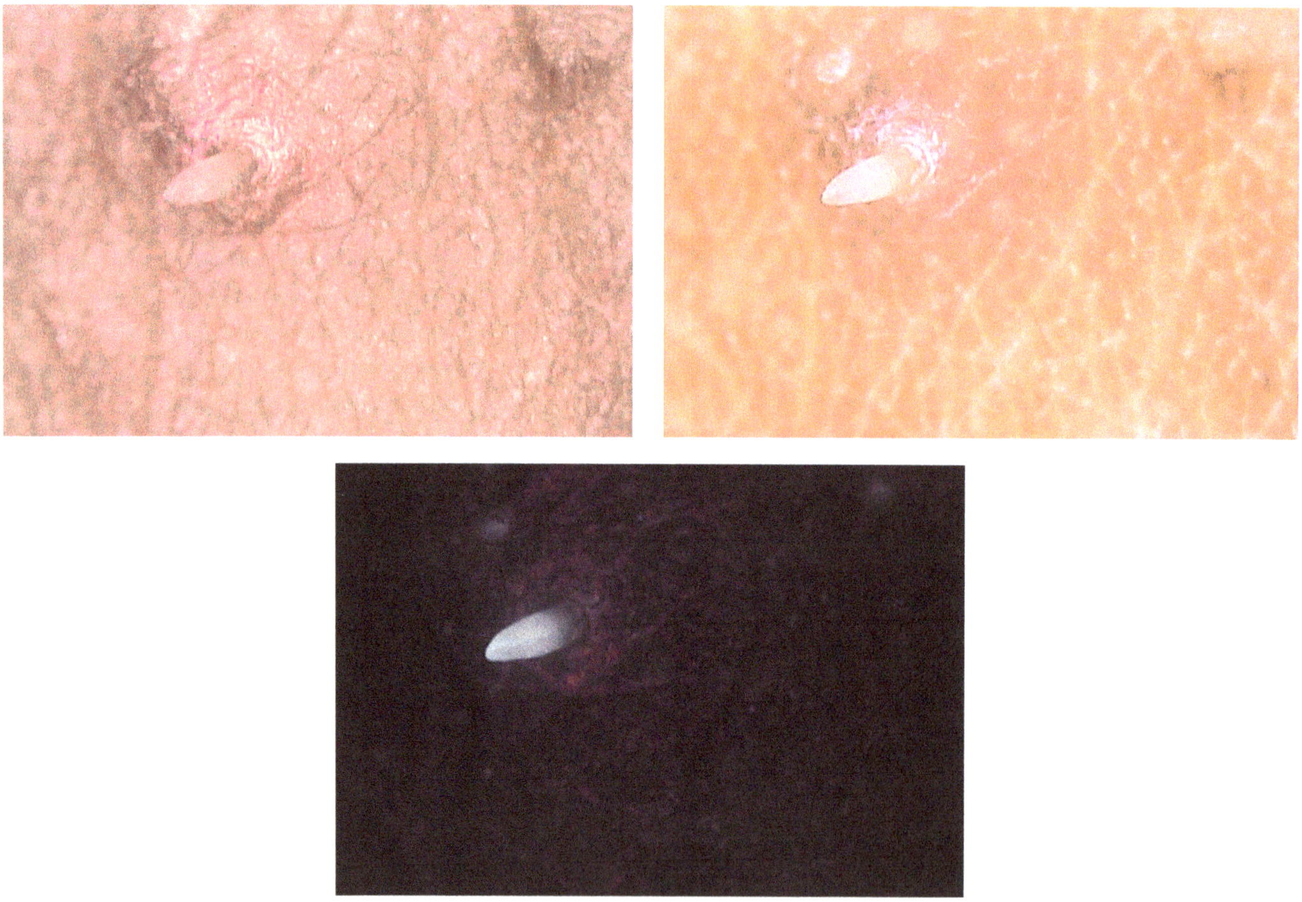

Figs 6A to C: "Horn sign"—follicular plug which is also fluorescent under UV light

cases, vellus hair are coiled and embedded in the horny layer. Perifollicular erythema and hyperpigmentation (pigmented KP) can also be sometimes seen, especially in the fairer skin (Figs 9 and 10). These dermoscopic findings are correlated with classic histopathologic findings described as distention of the follicular orifice by a keratinous plug that may contain one or more twisted hair.[3] Even after the coiled hair shaft, embedded in the uppermost epidermis is dislodged from it with the help of a needle, it continues to maintain its coiled nature.

Chapter 19　Dermoscopy of Miscellaneous Disorders　137

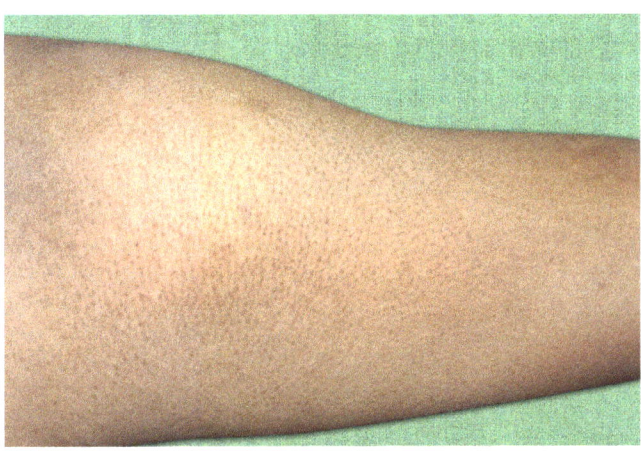 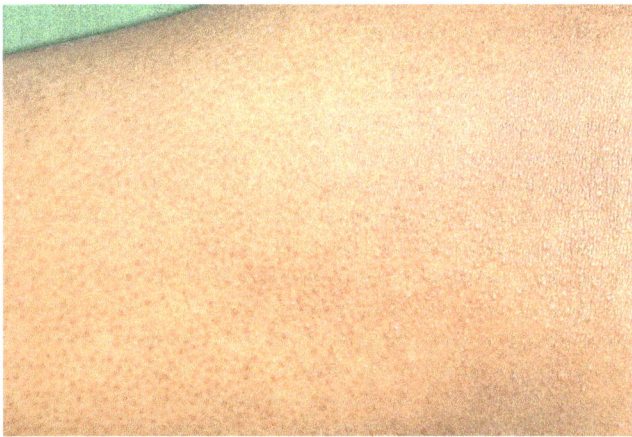

Figs 7A and B: Numerous tiny erythematous follicular papules with mild variability in size noted on extensor aspect of elbows

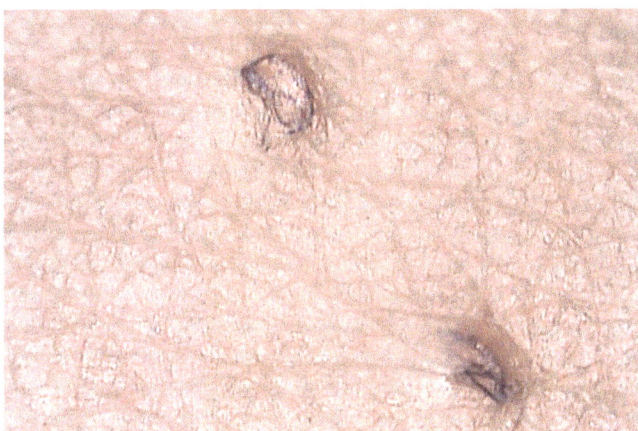 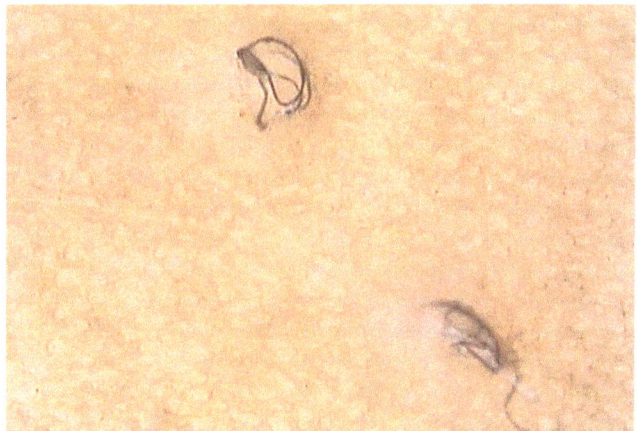

Figs 8A and B: Dermoscopy of keratosis pilaris reveals coiled hair better seen on polarized light

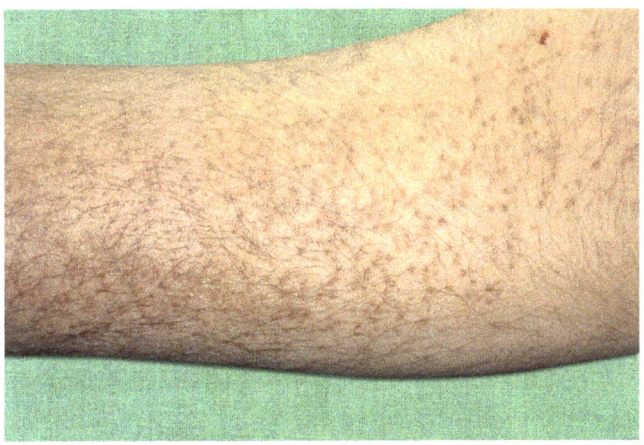 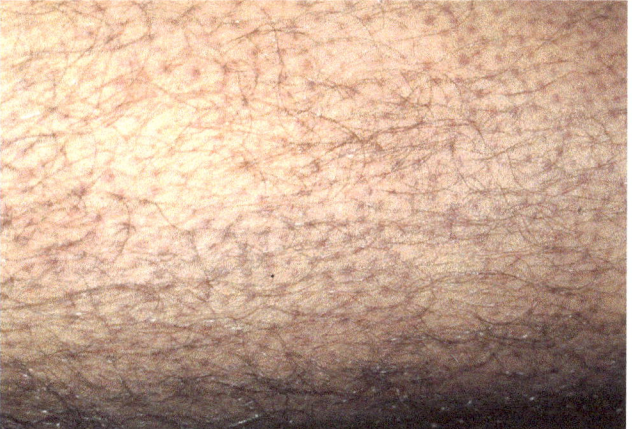

Figs 9A and B: "Pigmented KP"—marked hyperpigmentation around the follicular papules

Dermoscopy is also helpful in differentiating KP rubra from follicular LP that shows similar clinical features of follicular spinous papules on the body. In follicular LP, dermoscopy shows follicular keratotic plugs without broken or twisted hairs.[4]

TRICHOSTASIS SPINULOSA

Trichostasis spinulosa (TS) is a relatively underdiagnosed disorder of hair follicles that retain successive telogen hair. TS may appear as an isolated finding (primary TS)

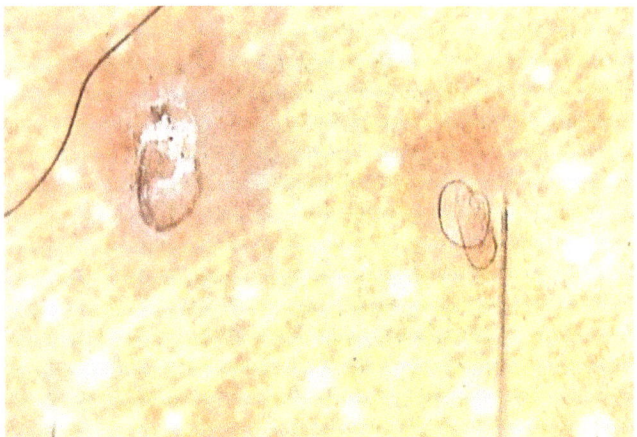 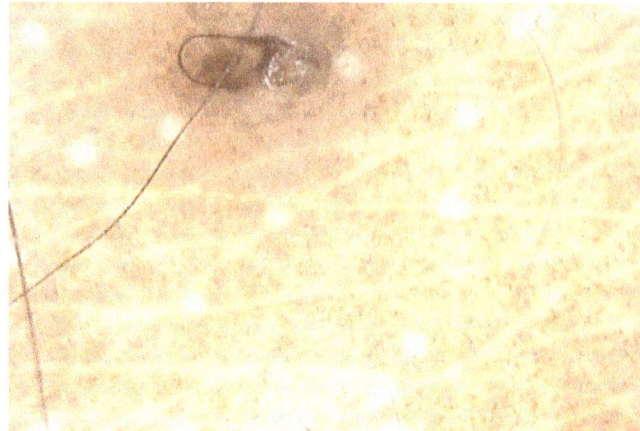

Figs 10A and B: Dermoscopy of pigmented keratosis pilaris (KP) showing marked perifollicular hyperpigmentation with coiled hair

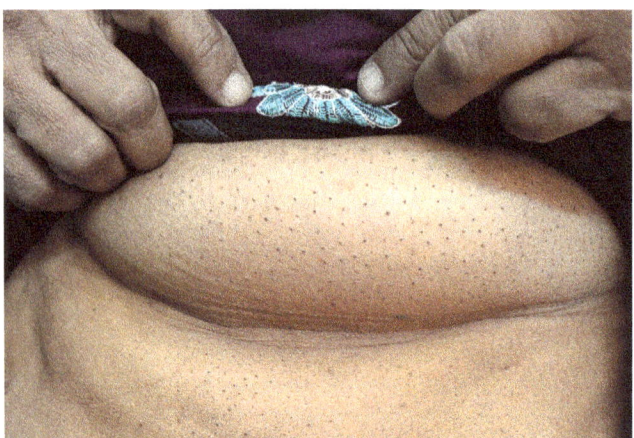 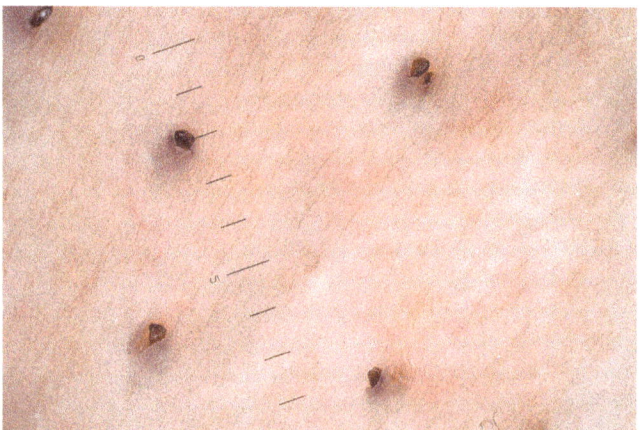

Fig. 11: Multiple tiny hyperpigmented follicular lesions noticed on the trunk

Fig. 12: Dermoscopy reveals multiple vellus hair bundled in a funnel-like structure (hair tuft) clinching the diagnosis of trichostasis spinulosa

or in association with expansile nondestructive lesions that narrow hair infundibulum, such as melanocytic nevi, seborrheic keratoses, syringomas, or nodular basal cell carcinomas (secondary TS) (Fig. 11).[5]

Dermoscopy helps to identify the characteristic hair tuft and clearly shows multiple vellus hair erupting through the follicles,[5] which is not clearly visible to naked eye. Under dermoscope, plucked hair show multiple vellus hair bundled in a funnel-like structure (Fig. 12).[6]

Dermoscopy is helpful in diagnosing TS from trichofolliculoma and intradermal nevus. Dermoscopy of trichofolliculomas show multiple units of hair tufts which are the result of folliculosebaceous hamartomas around a central pore.[6] Dermoscopy of intradermal nevi shows a sparse pigment network, multiple comma-like blood vessels that are typical of intradermal melanocytic nevi, a few peripheral vellus hair and a small hair tuft emerging from the central punctum.6 However, in TS-retained hair shafts within follicles with infundibular keratosis are noticed.

FOLLICULAR LICHEN PLANUS

Localization of LP to follicles is described clinically as lichen planopilaris. Three clinicopathological variants have been described. The first is characterized clinically by individual keratotic follicular papules and histologically by a lichenoid inflammatory cell infiltrate confined to the follicular epithelium. The second consists of erythematous to violaceous plaques, studded with follicular papules; the histological appearance is that of a lichenoid inflammatory cell infiltrate that affects both follicular and interfollicular areas. The third occurs as follicular papules of the scalp with concomitant or subsequent cicatricial alopecia. In this variant, the histological hallmark is a lichenoid, follicular and interfollicular inflammation, associated with or followed by scarring.[7]

The first variant mentioned above presents with violaceous or hyperpigmented, follicular, hyperkeratotic papules distributed on the trunk and medial aspects of proximal extremities (Figs 13A and B).[7]

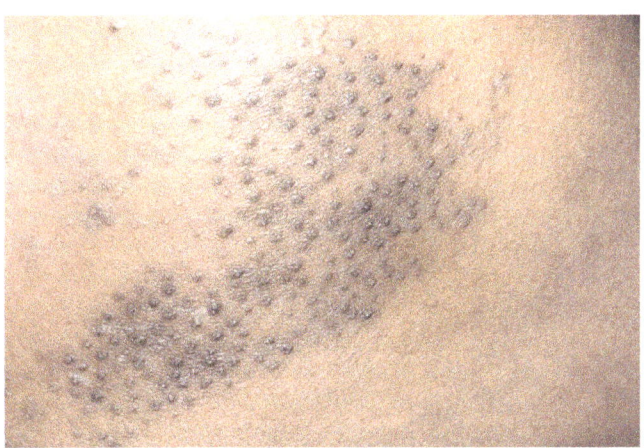 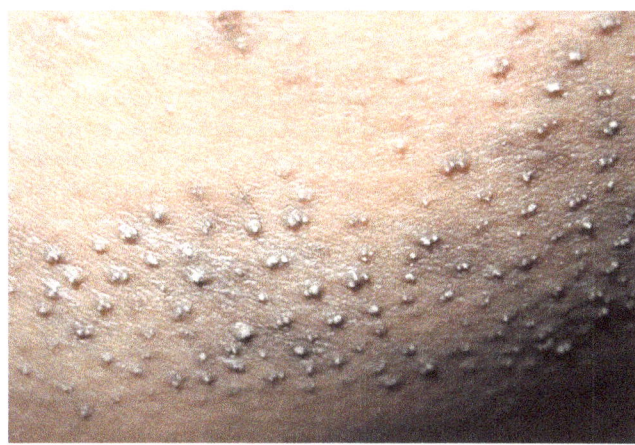

Figs 13A and B: Multiple grouped violaceous to hyperpigmented follicular papules with moderate variability in size seen in follicular lichen planus

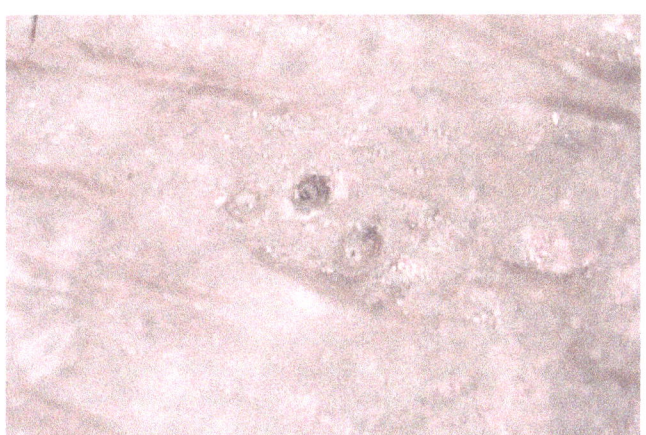 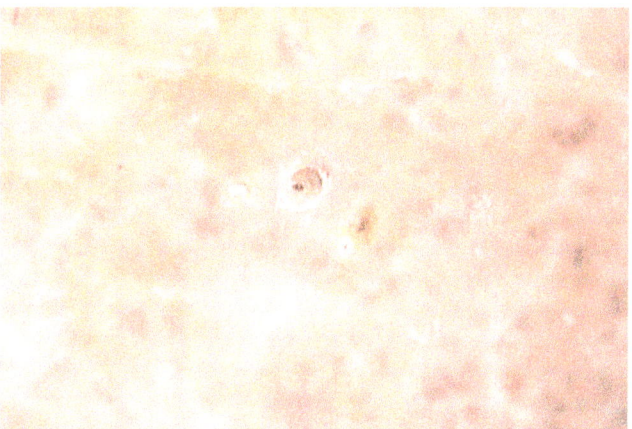

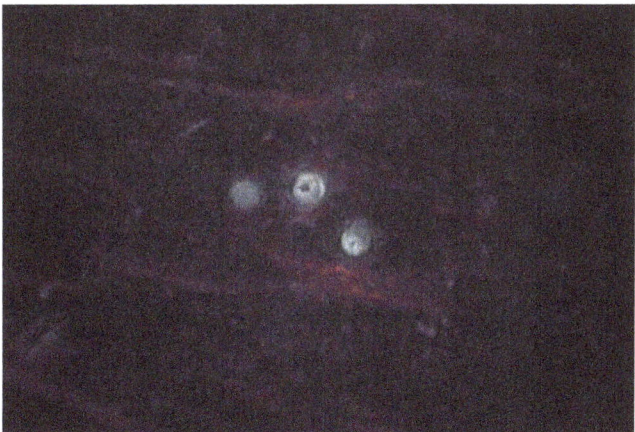

Figs 14A to C: Dermoscopy of follicular lichen planus reveals follicular papules with plugs fluorescent under UV light, perfollicular pigment globules better appreciated on polarized mode

Dermoscopy reveals follicular papules with keratinous plugs and violaceous globules in surrounding skin (Figs 14 and 15). These features help to differentiate from phrynoderma, KP and follicular eczema.

FOLLICULAR ECZEMA

Follicular eczema presents with grouped follicular papules which are either skin colored or hypopigmented forming discoid patches, predominantly over the extensor aspect

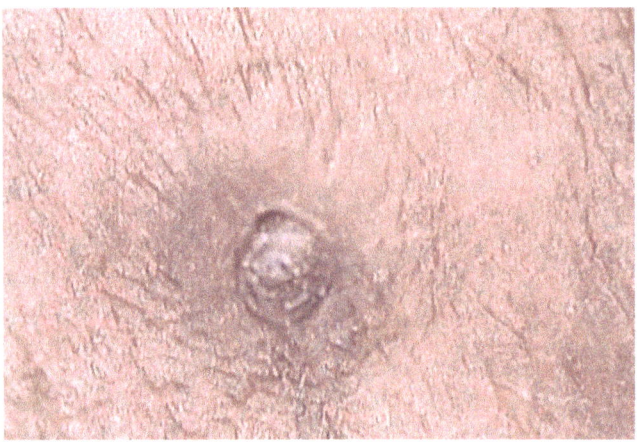 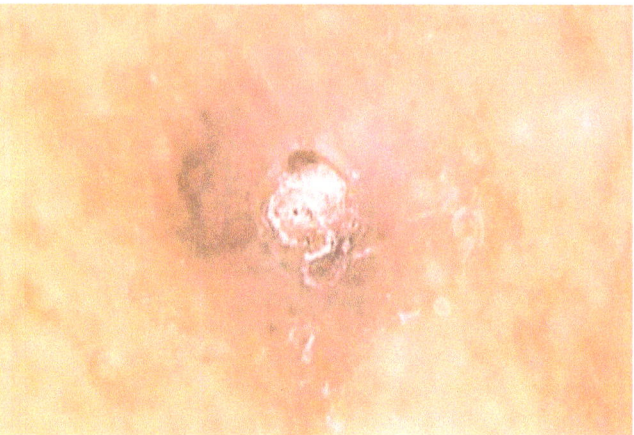

Figs 15A and B: Hyperpigmented papule with plug, accentuation of pigment on polarized light noted in follicular lichen planus

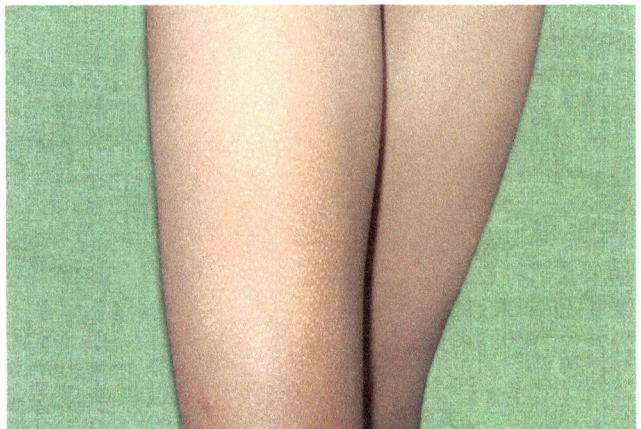 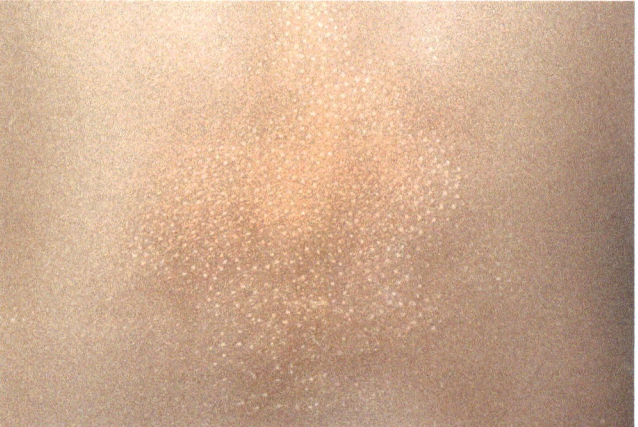

Figs 16A and B: Follicular eczema presenting with multiple hypopigmented follicular papules with mild variability in size and moderate clustering forming a patch on the anterior aspect of thigh

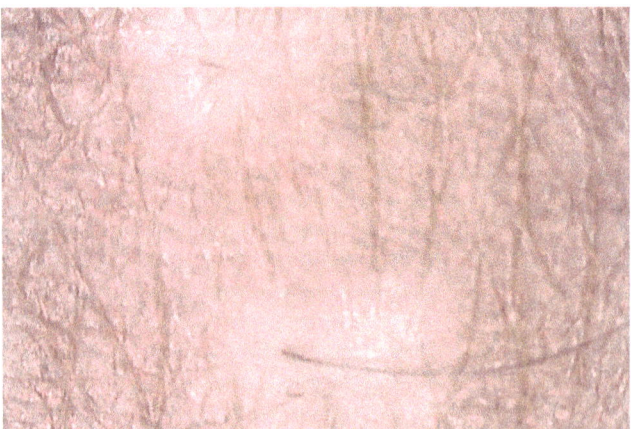 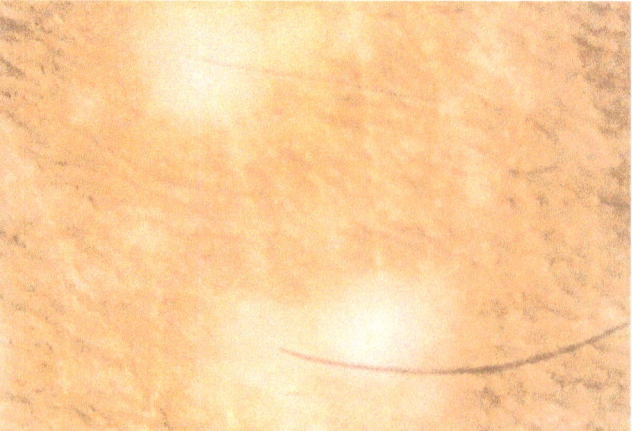

Figs 17A and B: Dermoscopy of follicular eczema reveals hypopigmented follicular papules with scaling, hypopigmentation better seen in polarized light

of forearms and legs with biopsy showing spongiotic dermatitis localized to the upper portion of hair follicle. They are usually associated with generalized xerosis (Figs 16A and B).[8]

Dermoscopic features include tiny hypopigmented follicular papules with tiny whitish yellow plugs, perifollicular collarette of scales and hypopigmentation and erythema and presence of hair present without twisting (Figs 17 and 18).

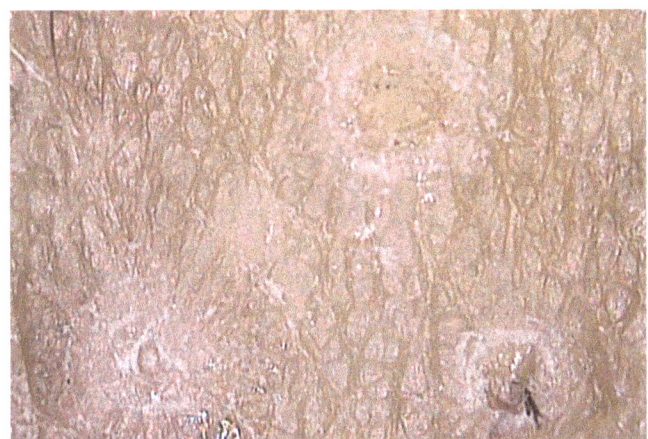 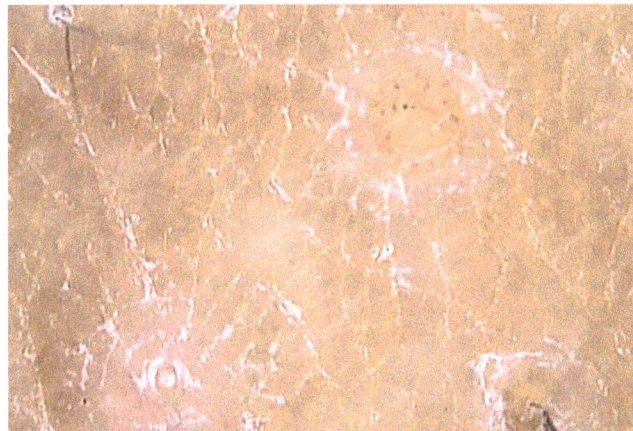

Figs 18A and B: Dermoscopy shows perifollicular collarette of scales with xerosis of surrounding skin

SEBACEOUS HYPERPLASIA

Sebaceous gland hyperplasia may present as a solitary or multiple flesh-colored facial papules. The clinical dermoscopic features are very subtle.

Dermoscopy shows multiple sebaceous gland aggregates in the form of pale yellow lobules. Sometimes, the ostium of the gland is visible as a central follicular opening (comedolike openings). The yellowish nodules are surrounded by groups of orderly winding, scarcely branching vessels. The vessels may extend toward the center, but they never cross it (Fig. 19). They are not arborizing as noticed in basal cell carcinoma. Their pattern can be described clearly by the term "crown vessels" and this vascular pattern is specific for hyperplastic sebaceous glands.[9]

ROSACEA

Dermoscopy highlights the vascular alterations of erythematotelangiectatic rosacea (ER), by revealing large polygonal vessels. Intense vasodilatation, which represents a major pathophysiologic alteration of the disease, results in a characteristic morphologic pattern of dermoscopic vascular polygons. Telangiectasias may also be detected on chronically sun-damaged, atrophic facial skin, but they usually lack the characteristic polygonal arrangement. Because this polygonal pattern has not been reported in any other skin disease, it stands as a useful criterion for the diagnosis of ER.[10]

Additional dermoscopic findings of ER include follicular plugs, white scales and, rarely, features related to the presence of Demodex mites, namely "demodex tails" and whitish amorphic follicular material.

In papulopustular rosacea, dermoscopy highlights clinically invisible pustules, follicular plugs and polygonal vessels (Fig. 20).[11]

Fig. 19: Dermoscopy of sebaceous hyperplasia shows multiple sebaceous gland aggregates with multiple comedo-like openings (arrow head) and curvilinear crown vessels

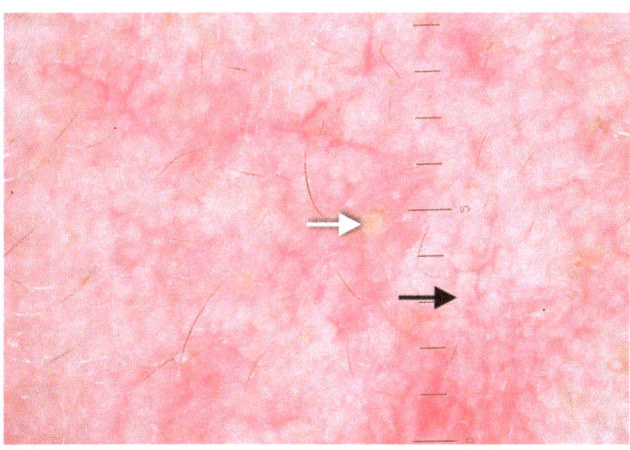

Fig. 20: Dermoscopy of papulopustular rosacea highlights tiny pustules (white arrow) and characteristic polygonal vessels (black arrow)

Dermoscopy facilitates in differentiating it from seborrheic dermatitis. In seborrheic dermatitis, dermoscopy reveals dotted vessels combined with yellow scales whereas pathognomonic polygonal vessels are characteristic of rosacea.

HUMAN PAPILLOMAVIRUS INFECTIONS

Dermoscopy has been shown to be valuable in the diagnosis and treatment monitoring of human papillomavirus (HPV) infections.

Common warts (verruca vulgaris) dermoscopically display multiple densely packed papillae, each containing a central red dot or loop, which is surrounded by a whitish halo. Hemorrhages represent a possible additional feature, appearing as irregularly distributed, small, red to black, tiny dots or streaks (Fig. 21). Dermoscopy of plantar warts typically reveals multiple prominent hemorrhages within a well-defined, yellowish papilliform surface in which skin lines are interrupted. Dermoscopy of plane warts typically reveals regularly distributed, tiny red dots on a light brown to yellow background.[12,13]

In contrast to the warts, dermoscopy of corn reveals a translucent central core known as a nucleus with presence of skin lines (dermatoglyphics) and absence of dotted vessels. Dermoscopy of callus reveals a homogeneous opacity and absence of dotted vessels.[12]

POROKERATOSIS

Porokeratosis is a clonal disorder of keratinization clinically characterized by sharply demarcated, atrophic, annular lesions with a distinct keratotic edge corresponding histologically to the presence of the cornoid lamella, a column of parakeratotic cells extending through the stratum corneum (Fig. 22).[14]

Dermoscopy reveals a characteristic raised, hyperkeratotic border (usually a double line–inner hypopigmented and outer hyperpigmented) surrounded by ectatic and dotted vessels.[14] Also, the papillary dermis beneath the cornoid lamella contains a moderately dense, lymphocytic infiltrate and dilated capillaries. Therefore, brownish pigmentation on the inner side of the raised track and a peripheral vascularization can be seen.[15] Liquefactive degeneration of the basal layer of the epithelium is sometimes present and occasionally provokes melanophagia and, in these cases, some blue-gray coarse granules can also be observed.[16]

The classical raised hyperkeratotic border (inner hypopigmented and outer hyperpigmented) at the circumference of the lesion is made clearly noticeable by dermoscopy, thus clinching the diagnosis (Figs 23 to 25).

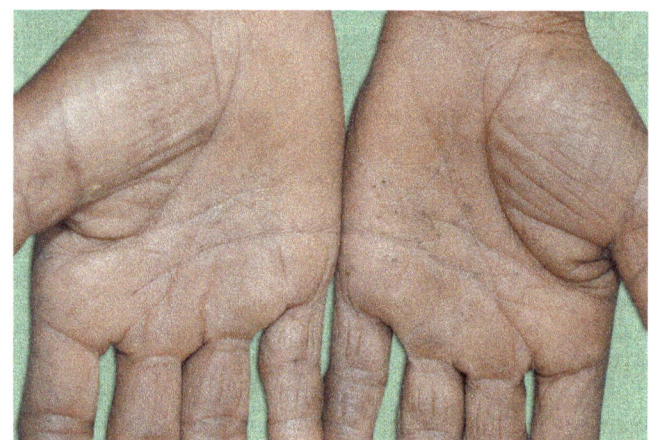

Fig. 22: Multiple discrete irregularly scattered tiny hyperpigmented macules noted over bilateral palms

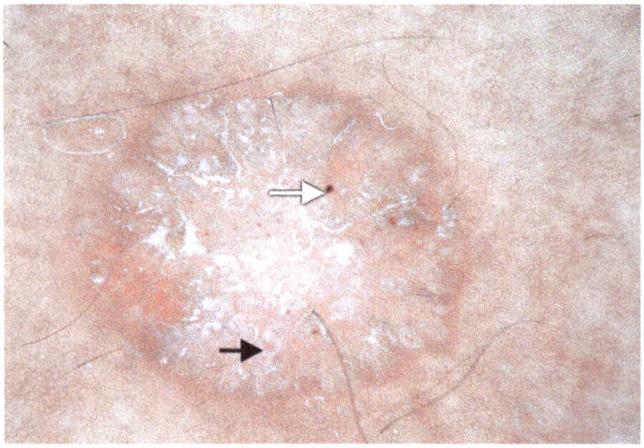

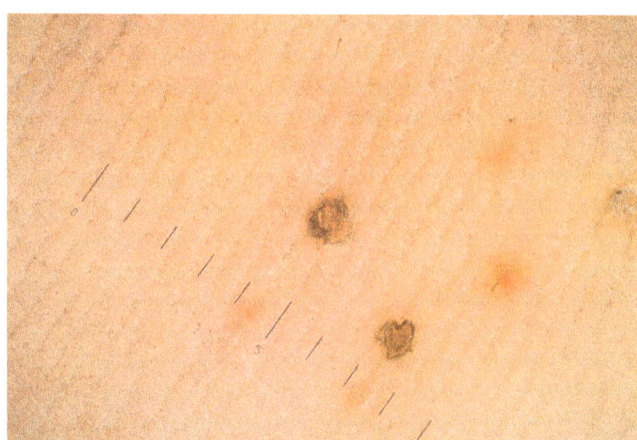

Fig. 21: Dermoscopy shows multiple densely packed papillae, each containing a central red dot or loop (black arrow), which is surrounded by a whitish halo. Hemorrhages seen as irregularly distributed, small, red to black, tiny dots or streaks (white arrow)

Fig. 23: Dermoscopy clearly highlighting the classical raised hyperkeratotic border (inner hypopigmented and outer hyperpigmented) at the circumference of the lesion

ARSENIC KERATOSIS

The earliest and most common manifestations of chronic arsenicism are dermatological and therefore recognition of hallmark lesions is often key to making the initial diagnosis. The most common cutaneous effects of arsenic involve pigmentary changes concentrated on the trunk and hyperkeratotic papules and/or plaques on the palms and soles (Fig. 26).[17]

Dermoscopy examination in the initial stages reveal keratosis present as barely visible papules, less than 2 mm in size, which usually occur on the background of indurated skin and have a grit-like texture. Over time, these lesions may progress to form raised and punctate papules, which may resemble corns. Papules may grow up to 10 mm in length and may coalesce to form larger verrucous plaques. Usually, the lesions are yellow, although they can appear slightly brown or dark (Fig. 27).[18]

TERRA FIRMA-FORME DERMATOSIS

Terra firma-forme dermatosis (TFFD) is characterized by dirt-like skin lesions that disappear after rubbing with alcohol (Fig. 28). The histology of TFFD shows epidermal acanthosis with papillomatosis; the prominent lamellar hyperkeratosis is characteristic showing a tendency to form compact orthokeratotic whorls.

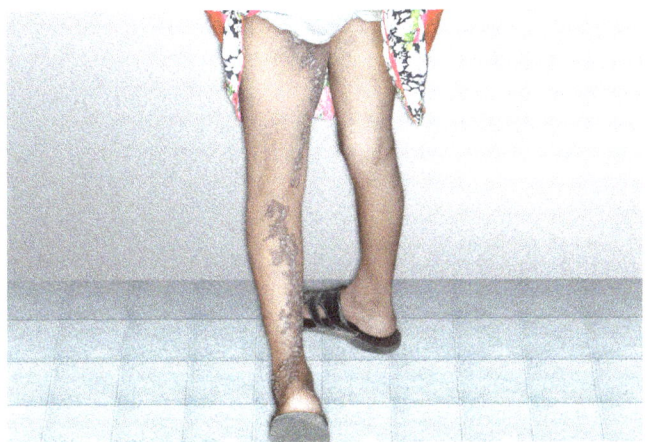

Fig. 24: Clinical photograph shows linear hyperkeratotic lesion involving entire lower leg. Differential diagnosis of tuberculosis verrucosa cutis, linear verrucous epidermal nevus were considered

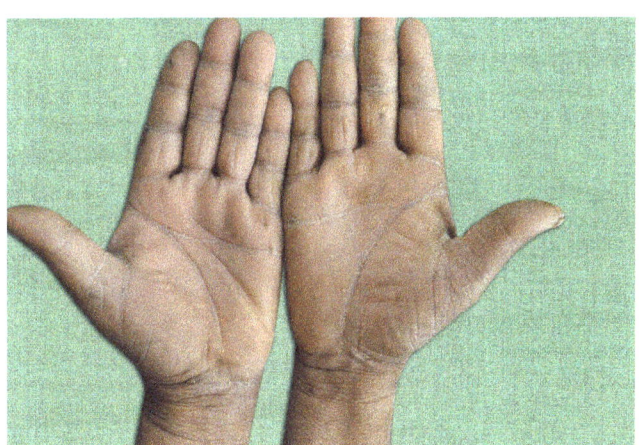

Fig. 26: Arsenic keratosis presenting with hyperkeratotic papules and plaques on bilateral palms

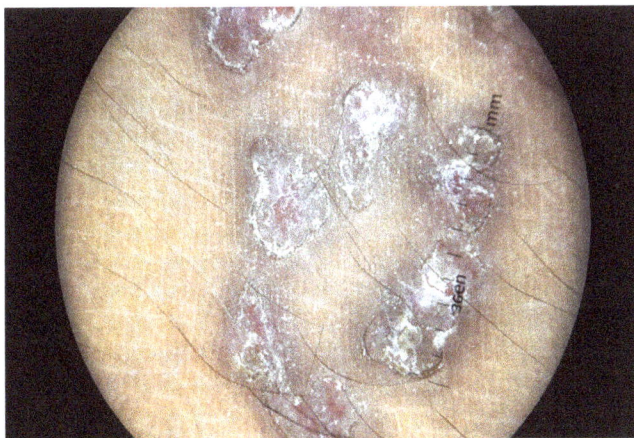

Fig. 25: Dermoscopy clearly highlighting the classical raised hyperkeratotic border (inner hypopigmented and outer hyperpigmented), diagnosis of linear porokeratosis was made, which was confirmed on histopathology

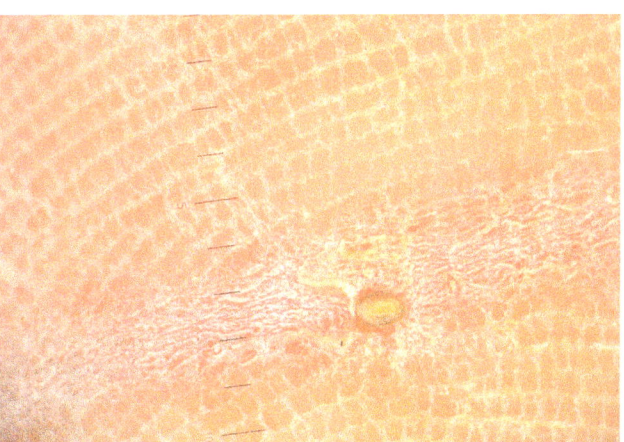

Fig. 27: Dermoscopy of arsenic keratosis reveals raised punctate papule which resemble a corn on the background of indurated dry skin with rough texture

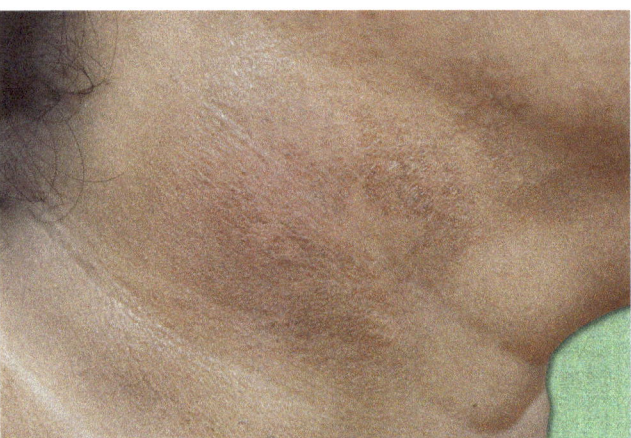

Fig. 28: Terra firma-forme dermatosis (TFFD) presenting with dirt-like lesions over the neck

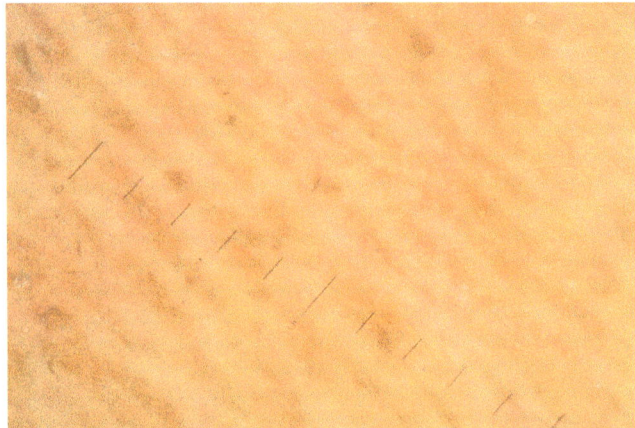

Fig. 29: Dermoscopic features of terra firma-forme dermatosis (TFFD) show polygonal plate-like brown scales arranged together giving a mosaic pattern or tile-like pattern, interrupted by furrows. These features completely clear after rubbing with isopropyl alcohol

Dermoscopic features of TFFD show large polygonal plate-like brown scales arranged together giving a mosaic pattern or tile-like pattern that is interrupted in furrows (Fig. 29). These features disappear completely after isopropyl alcohol swabbing of the lesions. It is distinguished from dermatosis neglecta by a history of good hygienic measures, absence of cornflake-like brownish scales and successful disappearance of pigmentation with isopropyl alcohol in the former and adequate clearance of lesions with soap and water in the latter.[19]

ACKNOWLEDGEMENTS

The author wish to thank:
1. Dr Pradnya Joshi, Lecturer, Department of Dermatology, Rajiv Gandhi Medical College and Chatrapati Shivaji Maharaj Hospital, Kalwa, for contributing clinical and dermoscopic pictures of phrynoderma, keratosis pliaris, follicular lichen planus and follicular eczema.
2. Dr Manas Chatterjee, Professor and Head, Department of Dermatology, INHS Asvini, Mumbai, for contributing clinical and dermoscopic pictures of trichostasis spinulosa, porokeratosis and arsenic keratosis.
3. Dr Balachandra Ankad, Professor and Head, Department of Dermatology, SN Medical College, Bagalkot, for contributing dermoscopic picture of common wart.
4. Dr Shekhar Neema, Assistant Professor, Department of Dermatology, Command Hospital, Kolkata, for contributing dermoscopic pictures of sebaceous hyperplasia, papulopustular rosacea and terra firmaforme dermatosis.
5. Dr Subrata Malakar, Director, Rita Skin Foundation, Kolkata, for contributing pictures of linear porokeratosis.

CONCLUSION

The motley conditions discussed in this chapter all pose a diagnostic challenge with a multitude of differential diagnosis for each. Dermoscopy helps in rapid OPD diagnosis and obviates the need of biopsy.

REFERENCES

1. Ragunatha S, Jagannath KV, Murugesh SB. A clinical study of 125 patients with phrynoderma. Indian J Dermatol. 2011;56:389-92.
2. Hwang S, Schwartz RA. Keratosis pilaris: a common follicular hyperkeratosis. Cutis. 2008;82:177-80.
3. Thomas M, Khopkar US. Keratosis pilaris revisited: is it more than just a follicular keratosis? Int J Trichology. 2012;4(4):255-8.
4. Panchaprateep R, Tanus A, Tosti A. Clinical, dermoscopic, and histopathologic features of body hair disorders. J Am Acad Dermatol. 2015;72(5):890-900.
5. Pozo L, Bowling J, Perrett CM, Bull R, Diaz-Cano SJ. Dermoscopy of trichostasis spinulosa. Arch Dermatol. 2008;144:1088.
6. Naveen KN, Shetty SR. Trichostasis spinulosa: An overlooked entity. Indian Dermatol Online J. 2014;201;5(Suppl S2):132-3.
7. Matta M, Kibbi AG, Khattar J, Salman SM, Zaynoun ST. Lichen planopilaris: a clinicopathologic study. J Am Acad Dermatol. 1990;22:594-8.
8. Sardana K, Arora P, Mishra D. Follicular eczema: a commonly misdiagnosed dermatosis. Indian Pediatr. 2012;49(7):599.
9. Zaballos P1, Ara M, Puig S, Malvehy J. Dermoscopy of sebaceous hyperplasia. Arch Dermatol. 2005;141(6):808.
10. Lallas A, Argenziano G, Longo C, Moscarella E, Apalla Z, Koteli C, et al. Polygonal vessels of rosacea are highlighted by dermoscopy. Int J Dermatol. 2014;53(5):e325-7.
11. Lallas A, Argenziano G, Apalla Z, Gourhant JY, Zaballos P, Di Lernia V, et al. Dermoscopic patterns of common facial inflammatory skin diseases. J Eur Acad Dermatol Venereol. 2013;28(5):609-14.

12. Bae JM, Kang H, Kim HO, Park YM. Differential diagnosis of plantar wart from corn, callus and healed wart with the aid of dermoscopy. Br J Dermatol. 2009;160(1):220-1.
13. Lee DY, Park JH, Lee JH, Yang JM, Lee ES. The use of dermoscopy for the diagnosis of plantar wart. J Eur Acad Dermatol Venereol. 2009;23:726-7.
14. Delfino M, Argenziano G, Nino M. Dermoscopy for the diagnosis of porokeratosis. J Eur Acad Dermatol Venereol. 2004;18:194-5.
15. Vargas-Laguna E, Nagore E, Alfaro A, Botella-Estrada R, Sanmartín O, Requena C, et al. Monitoring the evolution of a localized type of porokeratosis using dermatoscopy (Article in Spanish). Actas Dermosifiliogr. 2006;97:77-8.
16. D'Amico D, Vaccaro M, Guarneri C, Borgia F, Cannavó SP, Guarneri F. Videodermatoscopic approach to porokeratosis of Mibelli: a useful tool for the diagnosis. Acta Derm Venerol. 2001;81:431-2.
17. Sengupta SR, Das NK, Datta PK. Pathogenesis, clinical features and pathology of chronic arsenicosis. Indian J Dermatol Venereol Leprol. 2008;74:559-70.
18. Pratt M, Wadden P, Gulliver W. Arsenic Keratosis in a Patient from Newfoundland and Labrador, Canada: Case Report and Review. J Cutan Med Surg. 2016;20:67-71.
19. Abdel-Razek MM, Fathy H. Terra firma-forme dermatosis: Case Series and dermoscopic features. Dermatol Online J. 2015;21(10).

Index

Page numbers followed by *f* refer to figure

A

Acanthosis nigricans 30, 32, 32*f*
Acne 130*f*
Acral lentiginous melanoma 83*f*
Actinic keratosis, dermoscopy of 84, 143*f*
Alopecia areata 64*f*, 100, 101*f*, 102*f*, 103*f*
Amyloidosis, macular 108*f*
Androgenetic alopecia 25*f*, 101*f*, 103*f*
Angiokeratoma 16*f*, 76, 77*f*
Arsenic keratosis 107*f*, 143
Ash leaf macule 39, 40, 40*f*
Auspitz sign 46*f*

B

Basal cell carcinoma 9, 15*f*, 17*f*, 83
    dermoscopy of 81
Becker's melanosis 130
Becker's nevus 130, 130*f*
    dermoscopy of 130*f*
Blaschkoid distribution 132*f*
Borderline lepromatous Hansen's disease 68, 70*f*
Bowen's disease 16*f*, 18*f*, 77, 77*f*, 84, 84*f*
    dermoscopy of 84
Broken hair 102, 104, 105*f*
Bull's eye sign 103, 103*f*

C

Capillary loops
    enlargement of 92
    loss of 92
Comet-tail appearance 36, 37*f*
Comma
    hairs 117*f*, 118*f*
    vessels 13, 14, 14*f*
Congenital atrichia 106, 107*f*
Contact dermatitis 28*f*
Corkscrew
    hair 117*f*
    vessels 13, 16
Crista cutis 32*f*
Cutaneous amyloidosis, primary 31
Cutaneous small vessel vasculitis 125*f*

D

Deep vessels 13*f*
Depigmented areas, dermoscopy of 65*f*
Dermatitis 47*f*
Dermatofibroma 75, 75*f*, 76*f*
Dermatomyositis 92, 92*f*
Dermatophytosis 56
Dermlite dermoscopes 7, 9*f*
Dermoscopy 3, 4, 12, 127, 142*f*
    basics of 1
    principles of 4
Discoid lupus erythematosus 63, 63*f*, 64*f*, 108, 110*f*
Dowling-Degos disease 32
Dry trichoscopy 100*f*
Dyschromia, maturational 29

E

Eczema, follicular 139, 140*f*
Epidermal nevus 132, 132*f*
Erosive lichen planus 50*f*
Erythema
    dyschromicum perstans 29, 29*f*
    perifollicular 98*f*
Erythematous plaque 70*f*

F

Fitzpatrick's dimple sign 75
Fixed drug eruption 33, 34*f*
Flame hairs 105*f*
Follicular lichen planus, dermoscopy of 139*f*
Follicular papules
    hyperpigmented 135*f*, 139*f*
    hypopigmented 140*f*
Frontal fibrosing alopecia 100*f*, 108
Fungal infections 56

G

Gland, sebaceous 101*f*
Glomerular vessels 13, 15*f*, 16, 77*f*
Granulomatous disorders 61
    dermoscopy of 67

H

Hair 97
    diameter diversity 100
    dust 104, 105
    morphology of 113
Hairpin vessels 12-14, 14*f*, 15*f*, 78*f*, 79, 83*f*
Hansen's disease 68, 70
Heine delta 20 dermoscope 10*f*
Hemangioma 121, 122, 122*f*
    infantile 123*f*
Hematoma, subungual 89, 90, 90*f*
Hemorrhage 81*f*, 92*f*, 142
    capillary 92
    perifollicular 104
    splinter 91*f*
Honeycomb pattern 98*f*
Horn sign 136*f*
Human papillomavirus 142
    infection 56, 142
Hybrid dermoscopes 4
Hyperpigmented
    follicular papules, multiple 134*f*
    macule, dermoscopy of 33*f*
Hyperplasia, sebaceous 14*f*, 79, 79*f*, 141
Hypertrichosis 129*f*, 130*f*
Hyponychium 89
Hypopigmentation 35
Hypopigmented
    follicular papules, multiple 140*f*
    macule, dermoscopy of 33*f*

I

Idiopathic guttate hypomelanoses 36, 37*f*
Indian Association of Dermatologists, Venereologists and Leprologists 35
Intradermal nevus 129, 129*f*
    dermoscopy of 129*f*

J

Junctional nevus 128
    dermoscopy of 128*f*

K

Keratoacanthoma 77, 78*f*, 82
Keratosis
    actinic 84*f*, 85
    pilaris 134
        dermoscopy of 137*f*
Kitamura and Dowling-Degos disease 31
Kitamura, acropigmentation of 33
Koebner's phenomenon 35, 37*f*

L

Lacunae 13, 16, 16*f*
Leukotrichia 35
Lichen
    planopilaris 108, 108*f*, 109*f*
    planus 47, 49, 49*f*, 90
        follicular 134, 138, 139*f*, 140*f*
        hypertrophicus 50*f*
        pigmentosus 27, 27*f*-29*f*
        sclerosus et atrophicus 64, 64*f*, 65*f*
    spinulosis 134
    striatus 50, 50*f*
Light-emitting diode 3
Lupus vulgaris 67, 68*f*

Lymphangioma circumscriptum 124, 124f

M

Macular amyloidosis, dermoscopy of 31f
Macule
    hyperpigmented 33f
    hypopigmented 33f
Malignant cutaneous tumors, dermoscopy of 81
Malignant melanoma, dermoscopy of 82
Melanocytic nevus, congenital 128
Melasma 25, 26f
Milia-like cyst 78, 78f
Molluscum contagiosum 56, 58f
Morphea 65
Moth-eaten appearance 78f
Multiple vellus hairs, multiple 101f, 107f

N

Nail
    bed 89
    fold
        capillaries, dilatation of 65f
        dermoscopy of 65f
    melanonychia 90
    plate 89, 90f
    psoriasis 48, 48f, 91f
    unit 89
Nevus
    anemicus 39, 40f
    depigmentosus 39, 40, 40f, 41f, 127, 127f
    of Ota 130, 130f
    sebaceous 131, 131f
        cerebriform pattern of 131f
    spilus 129, 129f
Nonpigmented actinic keratosis 84
Nonscarring alopecias, trichoscopy of 100

O

Onycholysis 48f
    linear 91f
    traumatic 89
Onychomycosis 89, 90, 91, 91f
    dermoscopy of 59f
Onychoscopy 87, 89
Oral
    hydroxychloroquine sulfate 91f
    lichen planus 50, 50f

P

Palmoplantar psoriasis 48, 49f
Papular eruption 106, 107f
Papule
    follicular 136f, 137f, 139f
    hyperkeratotic 143f
    hyperpigmented 140f
    punctate 143f
Papulopustular rosacea, dermoscopy of 141f
Papulosquamous disorders 43, 45
Pediculus humanus capitis 55
Perfollicular pigment globules 139f
Peripheral white scales 51f
Peripilar
    cast 109f
    sign 100, 101f
Phrynoderma 134, 135f
    dermoscopy of 135f
Pigtail hair 102, 102f
Pityriasis
    amiantacea 113, 114, 115f
    capitis 113f
    rosea 47, 51, 51f
    rubra pilaris 51
    sicca 113, 116
    versicolor 56, 58f
Pityrosporum ovale 113
Plaque psoriasis, chronic 45f, 46f
Polymorphous vessels 13, 16
Porokeratosis 142
    linear 143f
Post-kala-azar dermal leishmaniasis 68, 69f
Pseudomonas superinfection 89, 90, 90f
Pseudomonilethrix hair 102
Pseudopelade of Brocq 112, 112f
Pseudopodia 37f
Pseudoscales 98f, 113, 115f
Psoriasis 9, 45, 46f, 47, 90
Pyogenic granuloma 90, 122, 123f

Q

Quadrichrome 35

R

Riehl-like melanosis 28
Rosacea 141

S

Scabies 55
Scales 59f, 99, 99f
    mimickers 114, 116
    nature of 113
    perifollicular 58f
        collarette of 141f
Scalp
    pigmentation 100
    psoriasis 47, 47f, 48f, 113, 114, 114f, 115f, 116
    dermoscopy of 114f
Scarring alopecias, trichoscopy of 108
Scleroderma 92
Sclerosis, systemic 65, 65f, 92f
Sebaceous hyperplasia, dermoscopy of 141f
Seborrhea capitis 113
Seborrheic dermatitis 48, 113, 114, 115f, 116
Seborrheic keratoses 78, 78f
Shagreen patch 132, 132f
    dermoscopy of 133f

Skin
    benign tumors of 75
    premalignant tumors of 75
    surface microscopy 4
    tumors 73
Sparse pigmentation 129f
Squamous cell carcinoma 77, 82, 83f
    dermoscopy of 82, 83f
Starry sky appearance 58f
Sulcus cutis 32f
Superficial fine telangiectasia 56, 81, 83
Systemic lupus erythematosus 92, 92f

T

Target sign 103, 103f
Telangiectatic vessels 13, 15, 15f
Telogen effluvium 104
    acute 104
    chronic 104, 104f
Terra firma-forme dermatosis 143, 144f
Tinea capitis 113, 117
Tinea faciei 59f
Toe nails, transverse leukonychia of 89
Traction alopecia 111, 111f
Triangular alopecia, congenital 106, 107f
Trichoptilosis 106f
Trichoscopy 64f, 95, 97, 105f, 109f, 111f
Trichostasis spinulosa 137, 138f
Trichotillomania 104, 105f
Trichrome 35
    appearance 36
Tuberculosis verrucosa cutis 67
    plaque of 69f
Tubular cast 109f
Tulip hair 106f

U

Ulceration 81

V

Vasculitis 124
Verrucae vulgaris 56f
Verrucous epidermal nevus, linear 143
Vessels
    disorder of 121
    morphology of 13
    structural arrangement of 13, 16
Videodermoscopy 107f
Viral infections 56
Vitiligo 35, 36, 36f, 40, 40f
    inflammatory 35
    nonsegmental 35
    segmental 35
    stable 37f

W

Warts 89
    hyperkeratotic 57f
    plantar 57f
Wickham's striae 45, 49, 50, 49f, 50f

www.ingramcontent.com/pod-product-compliance
Lightning Source LLC
Chambersburg PA
CBHW040541220526
45473CB00016B/2990